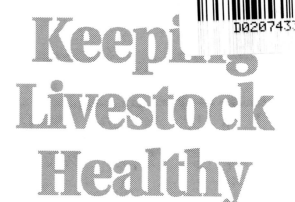

Keeping Livestock Healthy

*A Veterinary Guide
to Horses, Cattle, Pigs,
Goats & Sheep*

N. Bruce Haynes, D.V.M.

A Garden Way Publishing Book

STOREY

Storey Communications, Inc.
Schoolhouse Road
Pownal Vermont 05261

Edited by Deborah Balmuth
Cover design by Meredith Maker
Cover illustration by Brigita Fuhrmann
Text design by Cynthia McFarland
Text production by Therese G. Lenz
Indexed by Northwind Editorial Services

Copyright ©1994, 1985 by Storey Communications, Inc.

Originally published 1978 copyright © by Garden Way, Inc.

All rights reserved. No part of this book may be reproduced without written permission from the publisher, except by a reviewer who may quote brief passages or reproduce illustrations in a review with appropriate credits; nor may any part of this book be reproduced, stored in a retrieval system, or transmitted in any form or by any means — electronic, mechanical, photocopying, recording, or other — without written permission from the publisher.

The information in this book is true and complete to the best of our knowledge. All recommendations are made without guarantee on the part of the author or Storey Communications, Inc. The author and publisher disclaim any liability in connection with the use of this information. For additional information please contact Storey Communications, Inc., Schoolhouse Road, Pownal, Vermont 05261.

Garden Way Publishing was founded in 1973 as part of the Garden Way Incorporated Group of Companies, dedicated to bringing gardening information and equipment to as many people as possible. Today the name "Garden Way Publishing" is licensed to Storey Communications, Inc., in Pownal, Vermont. For a complete list of Garden Way Publishing titles call 1-800-827-8673. Garden Way Incorporated manufactures products in Troy, New York, under the Troy-Bilt® brand including garden tillers, chipper/shredders, mulching mowers, sicklebar mowers, and tractors. For information on any Garden Way Incorporated product, please call 1-800-345-4454.

*Printed in the United States by **Capital City Press***

First printing, October 1994

Library of Congress Cataloging-in-Publication Data

Haynes, N. Bruce, 1926–
    Keeping livestock healthy : a veterinary guide to horses, cattle, pigs, goats & sheep / N. Bruce Haynes . — 3rd ed.
            p.   cm.
        "A Garden Way Publishing book."
        Includes bibliographical references (p.   ) and index.
        ISBN 0-88266-884-6
        1. Livestock—Diseases.   2. Livestock—Diseases—Prevention.   I. Title.
    SF751.H39   1994
    636.089'6—dc20   94-26886
                        CIP

Contents

Author's Note to the Third Edition

AS I REFLECT ON OVER A HALF CENTURY OF ASSOCIATION with the livestock industry and the veterinary profession, I am amazed at the changes and the progress which have occurred. Thanks to improvements in nutrition, housing, breeding, and disease prevention, an ever-dwindling number of livestock producers provides high-quality food for an increasing domestic population with enough left over to share with the world.

My colleagues in the veterinary profession can be justly proud of their contributions which in this short span of time have brought about the advent of antibiotics, eradication of hog cholera, almost total eradication of bovine tuberculosis and brucellosis, and development of vaccines for protection of livestock from a variety of potentially devastating diseases. We should also note the success of veterinarians in protecting our livestock from serious foreign animal diseases such as rinderpest, foot and mouth disease, African horse sickness, and African swine fever. No less important are the advances made in anesthesia and surgical techniques for the comfort and health of individual animals.

Clearly great strides have been made in veterinary medicine, but changes in the profession unrelated to medical education per se are occurring now which have important implications for the livestock owner. Historically, veterinary medicine has been a combination of art and science. Because our patients cannot communicate with us, we must have a thorough knowledge of their normal behavior and attitude to recognize the departure from normal induced by disease. We must also be aware of their nutritional and housing needs since these have a major effect on health. This knowledge is part of the art of veterinary medicine and the most successful veterinarians are those skilled in both art and science.

It wasn't many years ago that experience with farm animals was a prerequisite for graduation from veterinary college. This is no longer the case and it is now possible, indeed probable, that some veterinarians graduate without ever having laid a hand on one of the so-called minor species — sheep and goats — not to mention exotic species such as llamas. For many reasons the "art" of veterinary medicine is giving way to the science.

The second major change in the veterinary profession of interest to livestock owners is in the composition of the student body of the veterinary colleges. In the not too distant past, women as veterinarians were a rarity. Now, almost seventy-five percent of new graduates are women.

The foregoing discussion of changes in the veterinary profession is not to imply that new veterinarians are incompetent. Indeed, their technical training is superb and they are familiar with techniques and equipment that students of my generation could only dream about. They have the ability to step into a laboratory or clinic setting anywhere and do a commendable job. And, although some may lack the animal experience required of their predecessors they certainly have been taught the pathogenesis of animal diseases and methods of prevention or control.

It is this training and the employment opportunities it provides that contributes in part to what I perceive to be a coming problem for the small livestock enterprise. For many reasons — among them working conditions, physical ability, technical challenge, and personal preference — the percentage of new veterinary graduates who enter livestock practice is steadily declining. If this trend continues I foresee the day when, except in geographic areas where livestock concentrations are adequate to support practitioners specializing in large animal practice, it will be difficult to find veterinarians equipped to handle livestock problems.

With this eventuality in mind, it behooves the livestock owner to learn as much as possible about animal health from books such as this. Working cooperatively, a knowledgeable owner and a veterinarian can apply both the "art" and the "science" of veterinary medicine for the benefit of animals everywhere.

N. Bruce Haynes, D.V.M.
June 1994

Preface

THIS BOOK IS BASED ON THE AUTHOR'S CONVICTION after forty years experience in private practice, as extension veterinarian at Cornell University, and as a veterinary consultant, that the great majority of farm animal disease problems are preventable. On economic grounds alone any sick animal, no matter how effective the treatment or how speedy the recovery, represents a loss. A less tangible but certainly very real argument for disease prevention is the pain and suffering disease causes.

Farm animals provide us with food, fiber, financial income, and pleasure. In return we owe them comfortable quarters, adequate feed, compassion — and good health. Since the objective is to keep animals healthy, the reader will find that this is not a book on how to treat sick animals. Instead it attempts to explain the nature of the disease process and outlines methods of preventing illnesses of the major farm animal species. If, by applying the information it contains, the reader is enabled to keep his animals healthier, it will have served its intended purpose.

Last, this book is dedicated to my colleagues in the veterinary profession, past and present, whose collective talent and skill made it possible.

N. Bruce Haynes, D.V.M.

I

PREVENTING DISEASE

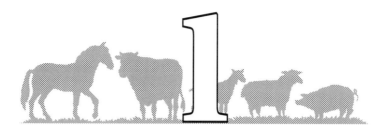

The Nature of Disease

ALTHOUGH MOST PEOPLE TEND to think of disease as the result of infection, this accounts for only part of the ills that come to man and animals. Looked at in the broadest sense, disease is any condition that results in a departure from normal function. Certainly the infectious agents such as viruses and bacteria produce the most dramatic and contagious diseases resulting in epidemics in man and epizootics in animals. But, there are other important factors as well. Among these are heredity, nutrition, parasitism, accident and injury, and environmental stress. To this list, man must be added as an indirect and occasionally direct cause of animal disease problems. Let's take a detailed look at some of these causes of disease.

Microorganisms

The term microorganisms is applied to those living organisms that are microscopic in size. These may be unicellular such as bacteria, yeasts, and protozoa, multicellular such as molds, or without cellular structure such as viruses. All have the capacity to reproduce at astonishing rates under favorable conditions and some have a remarkable capacity for surviving adverse conditions. For example, the virus causing foot and mouth disease will survive boiling and, in the frozen state, most viruses will last for years. Some bacteria, such as those causing anthrax, under adverse conditions enter a dormant phase called sporulation. Spores will exist in the soil for years reverting to virulence when the opportunity arises. It has been reported that viable anthrax spores have been found in the tombs of the Egyptian pharaohs! Knowledge of the characteristics of potentially harmful microorganisms is important to the control of infectious diseases and will be discussed in later chapters with the specific animal disease they cause.

There are thousands of species of microorganisms in the world and they are arbitrarily divided into two broad groups, the good guys called saprophytes and the bad guys called pathogens. A few, depending on circumstances, will fit either category. We could do without the pathogens but our survival depends on the saprophytes. All of the higher forms of life depend on the action of saprophytic organisms in the digestive tract for the utilization of conventional diets. Herbivorous animals, such as cows, are especially dependent on microorganisms for the conversion of cellulose in plants to usable forms of energy. Other organisms help to reduce complex protein molecules to their component parts, and themselves, as they die off, provide some nutritional value to the animals. The ability of ruminants such as the cow to utilize economical non-protein nitrogen sources such as urea and biuret to meet part of their dietary protein need is dependent entirely on the action of microorganisms in the rumen.

Because saprophytic organisms in the digestive tract are so important to digestion, it's important in terms of animal health to maintain an environment conducive of their well-being. Radical changes in the cow's diet such as an abrupt shift to large amounts of grain will increase rumen acidity, unfavorable to some bacteria, resulting in indigestion. Oral administration of large amounts of antibiotics or smaller doses over a longer period will destroy many of the useful organisms in the digestive tract, causing diarrhea and other digestive upsets.

Clearly the saprophytes are important to our health but they are important in other ways too. For example, while we rarely think of it, without these beneficial organisms we wouldn't have sauerkraut, cheese, vinegar — or beer. Even worse, without them biodegradable waste would not disappear and our planet would be buried under a layer of refuse, sewage, and even leaves. So the next time someone mentions bacteria don't throw up your hands in horror! Remember that in every society, even the one-celled variety, there are both good guys and bad guys and we can't get along without the good ones. But we do have to contend with the bad guys, so let's look now at how the animal body copes with pathogens.

Disease Resistance

Most pathogens are parasitic in that they survive at the expense of their host. Many tend to have an affinity for certain tissues. For example, the viruses of rabies and equine encephalomyelitis prefer to attack the cells of the nervous system as does the bacterium *Listeria monocytogenes,* which causes circling disease. *Streptococcus agalactiae* is rarely found outside the udder of the cow while some species of staphylococci will invade tissues anywhere when circumstances are favorable. Some members of the mold family such as *Trichophyton spp.* prefer the skin, where they cause ringworm. Others such as *Aspergillus spp.* prefer the internal body surfaces such as the lungs and reproductive tract. The list goes on and on.

Aside from tissue preference, pathogens also vary in their mode of action. Some will invade and destroy body cells. Others such as *Clostridium tetani* produce metabolic poisons called toxins which are harmful. Some molds never invade the body at all but produce toxins in feedstuffs called mycotoxins that are equally harmful when consumed by the animal. Last, pathogens vary in their affinity for some animal species. While this host specificity is not absolute, it is sometimes helpful in arriving at a diagnosis. For example, rabies can affect any animal while Eastern encephalomyelitis virus will be found only in horses, man, and some birds. Therefore, that disease can be ruled out in a cow with evidence of central nervous system disease.

The first line of body defense against the invasion of pathogens is the skin and mucous membranes. Mucous membrane is the highly specialized epithelial tissue that lines the body cavities that are exposed to the environment, such as the digestive tract. This tissue acts partly as a mechanical barrier to the invasion of bacteria, yeasts, and molds. But, in addition, the mucous membranes contain cells that produce fluids that tend to wash away invaders. The respiratory tract epithelium lining the trachea and bronchi also is lined with cells that have hair-like projections called cilia. These move with rhythmic undulating regularity to help wash out bacteria and particulate matter. Because of the extremely small size of virus particles, this protective screen is much less effective in preventing viral infections. In fact, some viruses readily invade between the cells of the mucous membranes to produce disease.

If the integrity of this first line of defense is breached by cuts, abrasions, burns, etc., infection may result. **Note that infection and disease are not synonymous.** Infection means only that the organism is in the body. Depending on a number of factors, it may or may not produce disease and, in fact, each of us and our animals carry a number of potential pathogens at any given time without any evidence of disease. This accounts for the epizootics that frequently occur when animals from a variety of sources are brought together such as at fairs and shows. Unaffected carriers of a contagious infection will transmit the infection to all the others and disease may result if they are susceptible. **Thus, bringing your animals into contact with others carries an element of risk that must be weighed against the potential benefits.**

Let's use a cut in the skin as an example of how the primary bacterial defense mechanism works. At the moment skin integrity is destroyed, a chain of events is set in motion which determines whether disease will result or not. First there is bleeding which tends to wash out any bacteria which may have been carried into the wound. Concurrently, large numbers of specialized white blood cells called phagocytes appear at the site which have the capacity to engulf and destroy bacteria. If the invading force of bacteria is small, that's the end of it and healing occurs. If, however, the invading force is large, inflammation occurs with heat and swelling produced and some discharge of pus. Pus is an accumulation of dead bacteria and tissue cells. When pus accumulates in a closed wound it is called an abscess. As a part of the defense mechanism, abscesses become walled off with connective tissue to prevent extension of the infection and in some cases may persist for weeks or months after active infection has subsided. These are sometimes referred to as sterile abscesses.

In response to the need at the wound site, the healthy body rapidly will produce additional white blood cells, called leucocytes, and if the invaders get beyond the point of introduction, leucocytes will attack wherever needed. Thus, with active bacterial infection, there is almost always an increase in the white blood cell count called leucocytosis. The opposite is called leucopenia and it is commonly seen with viral diseases. A white cell count is useful therefore in determining the presence of a bacterial infection and in distinguishing between a bacterial and a viral infection.

Under normal circumstances this first line of defense is adequate to cope with most common infections. If it weren't, every cut and scratch would be the beginning of disaster. But failures do occasionally occur with serious results. The capacity of the body to produce leucocytes in response to need is reduced in the presence of malnutrition, during long-term disease, as a result of stress, when cortico-steroid drugs, have been recently used, in patients undergoing cancer chemotherapy, and as a result of a few specific diseases such as acquired immune deficiency syndrome (AIDS) in people. Under these circumstances invading bacteria are carried via the blood stream to all parts of the body, a condition called bacteremia or septicemia. These migrating bacteria multiply rapidly creating microabscesses wherever they may lodge. The kidney, liver, and brain are frequent sites of secondary infection, the serious implications of which are obvious. While, in this era of antibiotics, septicemic infection is not the catastrophe it once was, it is still serious and requires prompt and correct specific and supportive therapy.

Viral Infections

While the foregoing is true of infection with bacteria, yeasts, and molds, it does not hold true for viral infections. Viruses are so small they can slip through tissues with minimal disruption and tissue response. Viruses generally don't result in pus formation and phagocytosis is not an important factor in defense against viral infections. In fact, an engulfed virus will often continue replicating in the phagocyte and actually be carried therein via the blood stream to its preferred tissue site. Once at that site it will begin destroying tissue cells or causing cell alteration in the case of tumor-inducing viruses. When viruses are circulating in the blood stream, the condition is called viremia and it is during this phase, early in the disease, that an infected animal poses the greatest risk to others. The first evidence that viral infection has taken place may be fever, which in itself has some protective effect as far as defense is concerned. A body temperature rise of only a few degrees will make the body a less desirable place from the virus's point of view. A prolonged fever, however, has detrimental effects on the body such as dehydration, so it becomes a fine line in therapeutic judgment how long to let a fever continue and when to reduce it with the aid of drugs such as aspirin.

Immunity

Defense against viral infections relies heavily on a complex mechanism called immunity. While immunity may be considered a secondary, although important, defense against the larger pathogens such as bacteria, it is the primary defense against viral infections. It is highly selective in that immunity against one organism will not protect against another. There are a few minor exceptions to this rule which will be mentioned under specific diseases.

The science of immunology is developing rapidly and new frontiers are being explored daily. It's not surprising then that new concepts are coming to light that help to explain the successes and failures of the immune system. In its simplest terms, immunity results when the body produces a protein (antibody) in response to stimulation by a foreign protein (antigen). **Pathogens are foreign proteins.** Antibody found in the globulin fraction of the blood (humoral antibody) combines physically or chemically with the antigen to inactivate it. In the normal animal, some immunity begins to develop whenever infection occurs. If the invading organism is low in virulence or present in small numbers, immunity develops fast enough so that clinical disease either doesn't occur or if it does, recovery results. If all the defense mechanisms including immunity are overwhelmed, death usually results. Drugs, in part, are used to buy time for the animal to develop immunity by holding the infection in check and preventing secondary infections. **Unfortunately, with few exceptions, drugs have virtually no effect against viruses.** The exceptions include a drug, acyclovir, moderately effective against the Herpes simplex virus responsible for cold sores and genital herpes in man.

The primary sites of humoral antibody development are the liver, bone marrow, and in the young animal, the thymus gland. Lymphoid tissue such as tonsils and lymph nodes plays a role that is less clear. Certain cells in other tissues respond to antigens by producing another type of antibody called interferon, which appears to block the entry of viruses into target cells. Interferon production is more rapid than humoral antibody and it exerts its effect locally at the site of infection. Vaccines such as the intranasal vaccine for infectious bovine rhinotracheitis take advantage of this phenomenon. In general, however, it takes about two weeks for a protective level of antibody to be produced either in response to infection or vaccination. **For this reason, vaccination after a disease appears in a herd is usually of little value.**

Types of Immunity

With this brief background of immunology we can take a look at immunization and immunizing agents. Basically there are two types of immunity: active and passive.

Passive Immunity
Passive immunity occurs without the active participation of the antibody production system of the immunized animal. For example, blood serum from an immune animal contains antibody which when injected into another compatible animal will make the latter immune. This is mechanical transfer of immunity in which the recipient plays no part; therefore it is passive immunity. However, because only antibody, not antigen, is transferred, the recipient's immune system is not stimulated and he will be immune only as long as the transferred antibody

lasts, which may be as short as two weeks or as long as six months. Passive immunity, although of short duration, has the advantage of being immediate. Unfortunately, antiserum or its antibody containing fraction, gamma globulin, is not without risk and is expensive precluding routine use in veterinary medicine.

In nature, passive immunity results from transfer of maternal antibody to the offspring via colostrum. Colostrum, or first milk, contains about twice the total solids of normal milk. Much of this excess is globulin containing the same antibodies as found in the dam's blood. The developing fetus has a very limited capacity for antibody production and therefore most animals are born with little or no immunity. If we stop to think how vulnerable the newborn is to infection and about the stress to which it is subjected at birth, it's not hard to visualize how important it is that newborns acquire some immunity as rapidly as possible. Nature has provided for this by equipping colostrum with high concentrations of antibody and at the same time providing a mechanism for the newborn to absorb antibody molecules intact.

Antibody is a complex protein that, when ingested by an adult, is broken down into its amino acid components prior to absorption. This digestive process destroys its usefulness as an immunizing agent. The newborn, however, has an undeveloped intestinal epithelium which permits absorption of intact antibody. But this capacity diminishes rapidly, being almost gone twenty-four hours after birth. **It is vitally important therefore that the newborn animal receive colostrum as soon as possible after birth — even by hand feeding if necessary.** Once this specialized absorptive capacity disappears, colostrum has value primarily as a nutrient, although it continues to provide some local protection against diseases affecting the digestive tract. Surplus colostrum is valuable and should not be discarded. It can be stored in clean covered containers at room temperature for 7–10 days or frozen and stored for months while still retaining antibody content sufficient to protect other newborns if the need arises.

Active Immunity

Active immunity occurs when the animal itself produces antibody in response to antigen. It may be the result of infection and recovery or may result from deliberate exposure to antigen as through vaccination. The duration of active immunity may range from several months to a lifetime depending on the stimulative effect (antigenicity) of the organism involved. Some organisms, notably those having limited local effect on the animal, are not strong antigens and attempts to produce vaccines to protect against them have not been very successful. Examples of these are the several species of bacteria causing mastitis in cattle. Conversely, some, such as the virus causing virus diarrhea in cattle, produce a strong lifetime immunity.

We have talked about passive and active immunity. There is a situation in which both mechanisms come into play, complementing each other. When the dam develops active immunity in response to infection, she will pass that immunity on to her offspring via colostral antibody to produce a temporary passive immunity in the newborn. However, since her infection resulted from natural exposure, in many cases the pathogen will still be on the premises and will infect the newborn. While this infection usually will not result in disease due to the passive immunity the newborn animal has acquired, the constant exposure to the infectious agent will stimulate active antibody production to reinforce the colostral antibody providing protection long after the passive immunity has disappeared.

From this one might conclude that the best time to vaccinate an animal for maximum protection would be during the period of passive immunity. Such is not the case and frequency of exposure makes the difference. Vaccines (antigens) given once or even twice would be rapidly inactivated by the maternal antibody. On the other hand, natural exposure in our hypothetical illustration takes place daily. Thus while the maternal antibody is gradually dissipating, repeated exposure to infection is stimulating active antibody production. It is possible in the laboratory to measure circulating antibody, the measurement being called antibody titer. Ideally one should determine maternal antibody titer periodically in the young animal and vaccinate when it declines. Unfortunately this is not an economical practice. **Therefore, in most cases, attempts to immunize permanently by vaccination should be postponed until most of the maternal antibody is gone. This is usually at about six months of age.** An exception to this rule of thumb is the situation where the disease does not exist. For example, calves are vaccinated against brucellosis even though the herd may be free of infection solely because many states require it as a prerequisite to interstate shipment. In this case, they should be vaccinated at the minimum legal age.

Immunization

Medical research has been able to capitalize on this immunity phenomenon by producing a variety of immunizing agents for protection against infectious diseases, and we are now able to protect man and animals against the great majority of serious illnesses. Although all immunizing agents are commonly called vaccines, there are three basic types, each with important differences.

The first and simplest is antiserum. This is the serum component of whole blood which contains antibody. It is produced by hyperimmunizing animals either through vaccination or actual infection, so that they produce a high level of antibody. Blood is then taken from them and refined, so that the finished product contains a high percentage of globulin, the protein fraction containing antibody. The resulting product has the advantage of producing immediate immunity when injected, but its duration is very short. It does not stimulate immunity in the animal to which it is given, but merely passively transfers antibody to that animal. Antiserum is quite perishable, relatively expensive, and must be kept under refrigeration until used. It must also be used in the specific species from which it was prepared. For example, bovine antiserum should not be given to a horse because it may produce a very severe allergic type response. There are times, however, when immediate protection is necessary and antiserum is the best way to provide it.

Bacterins by definition are killed bacterial cultures. These are produced by growing bacteria in artificial media in the laboratory and then killing the bacteria with chemicals, ultraviolet light, irradiation, or gene modification. They represent a method of getting a specific bacterial protein (antigen) into the animal without risk of clinical disease. After the bacteria are destroyed the culture is refined and then packaged for marketing as a single organism antigen such as **Leptospira pomona** bacterin or mixed bacterins prepared from cultures of more than one organism. The effectiveness of bacterins as immunizing agents is determined by the antigenicity of the organism, the number of killed organisms present in the product, the quality of its manufacture, and the addition of special adjuvants to delay absorption following injection. Bacterins are widely used to protect against leptospirosis, blackleg, malignant edema, swine erysipelas, and a variety of other diseases. **Bacterin-induced immunity is usually of medium duration and rarely lasts over one year. Two or more doses may have to be given to yield satisfactory protection.**

Vaccines

Immunizing agents are commonly lumped together as "vaccines," but the term technically is reserved for those products containing living antigen, although new technological advances have made this definition less accurate. One of the earliest and still widely used vaccines in veterinary medicine is the *Brucella abortus* strain 19 vaccine designed to protect cows against brucellosis. This vaccine is a living culture of a variant of *Brucella abortus*. The variant retains the antigenic identity of the naturally occurring organism, but generally doesn't cause clinical disease although there have been exceptions where it caused both systemic and local infection. These exceptions are always a risk where living immunizing agents are used.

The most common vaccines used today are for protection against virus diseases in animals and humans. Viruses generally will not survive long except in living tissue. Therefore, the production procedures for viral vaccines differ significantly from those used for bacterins or bacterial vaccines. The virus must first be adapted to an unusual host cell and propagated through serial passage until it ultimately loses its virulence and capacity to produce disease, a process called attenuation.

The early viral vaccine work utilized living chick embryos as the unusual host. Since then, however, virologists have developed techniques of culturing living tissue cells in the laboratory and this has greatly simplified the production of viral vaccines. Tissues commonly used, for example, are kidney cells taken from swine or sometimes laboratory animals such as hamsters. The end result is safer products, better standardization, and greater antigenicity.

Spectacular advances in molecular biology in recent years have made it possible to incorporate only the immunogenic portion of some organisms in a vaccine. More effective *E. Coli* vaccines have been produced this way. In a few cases, where sufficient antigenic material cannot be produced by separating it from the pathogen, antigenic genetic material can be placed in other harmless organisms, a process called gene cloning. These organisms are then propagated in quantity to produce vaccine. Undoubtedly, even more exotic techniques will be devised to produce vaccines as time goes on.

Sometimes, because of the nature of the disease or for convenience, it is desirable to use a mixed vaccine. Shipping fever in cattle, for example, is caused by the interaction of viruses and bacteria and a vaccine is available containing antigenic fractions of several viruses as well as the *Pasteurella spp.* responsible for the disease. Leptospira bacterin may contain fractions of one or all of the several species of leptospira known to cause disease.

Although commercial mixed vaccines are available, remember that these have been tested and proven effective. Do not mix vaccines on the farm because, mixed together, they may be incompatible and rendered totally ineffective. If it is desirable to use two or more vaccines concurrently keep them separate and use different injection sites.

The modified live virus (MLV) vaccines have an important disadvantage; although they generally produce a long-lasting immunity, they occasionally will cause the illness because most are a compromise between antigenicity and attenuation. The most effective in producing immunity are those with the least attenuation. Thus, when given to an animal weakened by malnutrition, stress, or those without a responsive immune mechanism, clinical disease may result. **Their use should be restricted to healthy animals not under stress** and they should be given at a stage in life when economic effects will be minimized if the animal does get sick. Largely because of the risk associated with MLV vaccines, new vaccines utilizing inactivated virus have been developed. They produce immunity of shorter duration but are not as hazardous to use.

Generally the killed virus vaccines need to be given annually to maintain a protective antibody titer whereas the MLV vaccines such as bovine virus diarrhea vaccine will produce immunity lasting several years.

Planned Infection

There is another technique of producing immunity which is really planned infection with the actual or closely related disease organism. A disease such as infectious bronchitis in chickens, for example, exerts its principal effect economically by lowering egg production. This loss is averted by deliberately exposing young birds to the virus before they begin laying. This technique is almost universally applied by commercial poultry growers. It has also been demonstrated that hog cholera can be prevented by infecting swine with the virus causing bovine virus diarrhea. This virus does not produce apparent disease in swine but does exert a blocking effect against hog cholera virus. This method was never widely used and with total eradication of hog cholera in the United States, the need for immunization has disappeared.

There is one obvious and important disadvantage in the planned infection approach to disease control that is best exemplified by the use of rhinopneumonitis virus in horses. This virus causes a mild upper respiratory infection but it also causes abortion, a matter of serious concern on breeding farms. To minimize abortions from this disease, all horses on the farm are deliberately infected at a time when risk of abortion is minimal so that mares have a good antibody titer during pregnancy. This practice results in wide dissemination of virus and precludes any possibility of eradicating the disease. Fortunately, this method of immunization against equine rhinopneumonitis has fallen out of favor.

Summary

We will talk more about immunization against specific diseases but there are several important points to remember. The need to vaccinate depends on the prevalence of a disease, the risk of disease transmission and the degree of risk one is willing to assume. A single animal kept in the backyard and never in contact with others of its species does not share the same risk as an animal in a large commercial herd to which new animals are frequently added. For the former, vaccination is less important but for the latter would be essential.

Once a decision to vaccinate has been made, then you need to keep in mind that as a general rule killed products do not produce as long an immunity as modified live vaccines although killed products are safer to use. **In any case, bear in mind that vaccination and immunity are not synonymous**. Vaccination is not a simple mechanical procedure that automatically produces immunity. Under the best of circumstances no vaccine is 100 percent effective. They must be properly handled from point of manufacture to point of injection. Generally this means refrigeration, protection from sunlight, and use prior to expiration date. Lastly, for maximum immune response, vaccines must be given at the proper time to healthy animals. Once a disease appears in a herd, vaccination is of very limited value and, in some cases, may actually be harmful.

There are a great variety of vaccines available and often several types to protect against the same disease. In a matter as important as immunization, the prudent livestock owner would be well advised to seek the advice of a veterinarian on the necessity of vaccination and the best to use. Don't forget that this should be done before the disease appears.

Other Causes of Disease

If animal diseases were limited to those caused by infectious organisms the diagnostic problem would be greatly simplified. Unfortunately this is not the case and other factors must always be considered.

Nutrition

Nutrition is a factor often overlooked. When animals roamed wild, nutritional deficiencies were less of a factor because the animal would eat a variety of grasses and leaves when these were available. Although this diet was inadequate and precluded maximum growth rate and productivity, the variety generally prevented some of the mineral and vitamin deficiencies we see today. The chief nutritional problem of animals in the wild was outright starvation. While that is a rare and inexcusable condition in domestic animals today, we now see nutritional deficiencies that are more subtle and difficult to diagnose.

Domestic animals are dependent on the feed we offer them, and the science of animal nutrition has become extremely important. Any successful animal husbandry manager must have a good understanding of the nutrient needs of the animals he feeds. Many good textbooks are available for the serious student of animal nutrition. The National Academy of Sciences has a series of booklets on the nutrient requirements of all the major animal species. These booklets (called the "Nutrient Requirement Series") are concise, current, and contain everything the husbandry manager needs to know about the nutrition of his or her animals. These are available at nominal cost by writing the Printing and Publishing Office, National Academy of Sciences, 2101 Constitution Avenue, N.W., Box 285, Washington, D.C. 20055 or calling 1-800-624-6242.

Without some understanding of nutrition, it's not easy to be sure animals are being properly fed. For example, dairy cattle maintained on a diet of the best looking alfalfa hay will have serious problems with milk fever or post-parturient paresis. The reason for this is that alfalfa is very high in calcium but low in phosphorus. The cow must have adequate amounts of these minerals in a ratio of about 1.5:1. An imbalance in this ratio leads to milk fever. Alfalfa is an excellent feed but it must be supplemented with phosphorus to prevent this disease.

Trace Minerals and Vitamins

Animals grazing on land with a high molybdenum content may develop a copper deficiency because molybdenum ties up copper, making it unavailable to the animal. Copper deficiency leads to anemia, causing, among other things, poor reproduction. Zinc deficiency causes a skin disease in swine called parakeratosis. Calves and lambs frequently suffer from white muscle disease, an often fatal condition resulting from a deficiency of selenium or vitamin E.

Unfortunately, deficiency diseases are insidious and slow developing although the final result may be dramatic. White muscle disease may cause sudden death of the healthiest looking calf, and the comatose cow with milk fever is a real emergency. But the conditions leading to these conditions prevail over a long period of time. Once a diagnosis is made, further problems in the herd can usually be prevented by varying the diet and, if necessary, adding mineral supplements. Commercial interests have capitalized on the latter by marketing complicated mineral mixes at exorbitant prices for the unwary buyer. Generally speaking, if herbivorous animals are offered a diet of good quality mixed hay and grain to which has been added 1 percent dicalcium phosphate and 1 percent trace mineral salt, no additional supplementation is necessary. Exceptions are dairy cattle and animals not fed grain. These should also have free-choice access to a mixture of equal parts of dicalcium phosphate and trace mineral salt.

Parasitism

Parasitism is a third common cause of disease in animals that ranges from dramatic to innocuous. Animal parasites vary from single-celled coccidia to more complex organisms such as worms and insects. Some are free-living part of the time, others are totally dependent on the host animal for survival. Many have intricate life cycles that are absolutely fascinating to the biologist.

One of the more interesting parasites is the common horse bot, *Gasterophilus intestinalis.* The adult bot fly deposits its eggs on the hair, particularly on the front legs and shoulders. These eggs have a yellowish color and are about the size of pinheads. There they remain until, stimulated by the animal's licking, they hatch. The larvae then enter the mouth, where they penetrate the tongue and oral mucosa and eventually migrate to the stomach, where they attach themselves to the wall, sometimes in very large numbers. They not only damage the wall but may also cause indigestion. After a developmental period of eight to ten months, they pass out in the feces to the soil where they pupate. In about a month an adult fly emerges to repeat the cycle.

Knowledge of parasite life cycles often presents the opportunity for control programs not dependent upon drugs. For example, liver flukes, which affect most animal species, must spend a part of their life cycle in the snail. Since snails must have moisture to survive, a simple control procedure is to keep animals out of wet areas.

Parasitologists debate the merit of attempting to maintain internal parasite-free livestock. The relationship of many parasites to their host is commensalistic, that is, the parasite derives benefit from the host without harming the host. If it were otherwise, the host would die and the parasite would be homeless. Also, some parasites such as *Haemonchus spp.* in sheep and hookworms in the dog produce a degree of immune response, and modest infestations stimulate enough immunity so that overwhelming infections normally don't occur. However, when the animal has no immunity or is debilitated from other causes such as malnutrition or stress, overwhelming infection will occur, leading to death of the animal.

Proponents of limited infection argue it is necessary for immunity. Those of the opposite school argue that with eradication or even control with medication, reinfection will not be a problem and immunity then is inconsequential. The practical course seems to lie somewhere between and is based on control through good sanitation and maintaining animals in a healthy state as well as interrupting parasite life cycles when feasible. **Parasite control through medication alone is a continuing expense without lasting benefit** that frequently doesn't work and in some cases may not even be necessary. Internal parasitism is generally a problem primarily of the young and the debilitated especially when coupled with unsanitary housing and feeding conditions or malnutrition.

External parasitism, most often found in animals that are debilitated or kept under unsanitary housing conditions, presents a different problem. The principal external parasites of farm animals are ticks, lice, and mites. While ticks cause some discomfort and they do suck blood from the unlucky animal or man to which they become attached, they are chiefly important as vectors or carriers of disease-producing organisms. The tick *Boophilus annulatus* was the vector of a serious cattle disease in the Southwest called piroplasmosis or Texas fever that caused losses running into millions of dollars. Once this vector relationship was recognized, the disease was eradicated by eradicating the specific tick that carried it. Ticks are still responsible for transmission of diseases such as Rocky Mountain spotted fever, equine piroplasmosis, tularemia, and Lyme disease.

Lice are divided into two groups: biting and sucking. The biting lice feed on cellular debris on the skin surface and cause intense itching. Sucking lice, on the other hand, suck blood from the host. Severe infestations can cause fatal blood loss. Adult ticks and lice are visible to the naked eye and frequent grooming of the animal may be sufficient to control them.

Mites are microscopic in size and are the cause of mange, or scabies, found in almost all species. This condition, which can become severe, causes itching and loss of weight. Psoroptic mange in sheep causes the wool to fall out in patches, which is a direct economic loss.

Where external parasites are a problem, the only effective control measure is the use of insecticides on the animal as a spray, dip, or powders. Some insecticides may be given orally, by injection or by the pour-on method for systemic effect. However, the use of many of the best insecticides is severely restricted by the federal and state governments because of environmental contamination. Restrictions are even greater if the compound is to be used on food-producing animals, especially lactating dairy cattle because of possible residue in milk or meat.

Hereditary and Congenital Defects

Sixty-four hereditary defects have been identified in cattle alone. The influence of relatively few bulls on large numbers of offspring through artificial insemination has made hereditary defects in cattle a matter of concern. Two of the most common are umbilical hernia, recognizable at birth, and spastic syndrome, which doesn't appear until the animal approaches maturity.

Congenital defects are those which result either from developmental accident during the embryonic stage or from the influence of a toxic or infectious agent during prenatal development. The former are uncontrollable accidents. The latter have an external cause and are preventable if one knows the contributing factors. For example, consumption of a weed *Veratrum californicum* by the ewe about the fourteenth day of pregnancy results in birth of a high percentage of deformed cyclopian lambs. Knowing this, the shepherd can prevent it by keeping ewes out of pastures where the weed grows during early pregnancy or he can eliminate the weeds in the pasture with herbicides.

Infection with bovine virus diarrhea during early pregnancy has been shown to cause cerebellar hypoplasia and cataracts in calves as well as abortion in some cases. This can be prevented by vaccination of the dam at least thirty days prior to breeding.

It's vitally important, regardless of species, that developmental defects or diseases that may be hereditary in origin be reported to the appropriate breed associations. Identification of hereditary defects is always retrospective and dependent on large numbers of reports. Just as we keep careful production records on purebred animals and plan matings to improve the breed, so should we keep good records of matings that result in offspring detrimental to the breed. Fortunately, most hereditary defects are lethal or at least render the animal uneconomical to raise to maturity. But not all of them are and we need to identify those individuals that carry the genes leading to defective offspring so they can be removed from the population or at least neutered. Too many breeders adopt the opposite approach and go to great lengths to conceal the birth of defective offspring. Such conduct is irresponsible to say the least.

The Human Contribution

Thus far in this chapter a number and variety of agents contributing to animal disease have been described. To these, people are often the unwitting accomplices in myriad ways. Accident and injuries are not uncommon and frequently they are our fault. It's easier to clean a smooth barn floor so we trowel the concrete smooth and wonder why the cows slip and fall, sometimes breaking a leg. The problem of spraddle-legged pigs is directly attributable to slippery floors. We build barbed wire fences because it's cheaper than woven wire and call the animals that get tangled in it "stupid." And when the wire gets chopped up in the hay baler and the resulting pieces pierce the cow's stomach we call it bad luck.

Barns are expensive, so in the name of efficiency, we crowd in as many animals as possible. This improves the opportunity for disease transmission and the problem is compounded during cold weather when, because we don't like to work in the cold, we shut the barn up tight. This raises temperatures and particularly humidity, fostering the production of ammonia from manure and urine. The respiratory tract irritation this causes is one of the leading factors predisposing young animals to pneumonia. From a health standpoint, they would be better off outside with an open shed for shelter. **All too often we design animal housing with our own comfort and convenience in mind rather than that of the animals.**

Every animal harbors pathogens to which it has become immune but which are transmissible to other animals in the herd. But it's a rare buyer who insists on a complete physical examination or immunization record of the animal he buys. And it's an even rarer individual who isolates a purchased addition from the herd to be sure it isn't in the incubation period of a contagious disease before putting it with the others. If you have young children you are familiar with the outbreaks of head colds, etc., that occur soon after school starts. The situation is the same whether people or animals are brought together in close confinement.

Exhibiting at Fairs

A special word of caution is in order for people who exhibit animals at fairs and shows. This is an ideal place for transmission of contagious diseases. Not only is a large group of animals (and pathogens) brought together from a variety of areas but the animals are also under stress from trucking, a strange environment, and often a complete change of diet. This makes them much more susceptible to infection which in turn spreads to the rest of the herd when they are returned. The prudent exhibitor will minimize stress as much as possible, will immunize his animal against every disease for which safe reliable vaccines are available, and will isolate the animal from the herd for two weeks after the show is over.

If after reading this far you have gotten the impression that animal health and disease is highly complex, the chapter will have served its purpose. **Nothing is absolute in medicine, be it human or veterinary.** Each animal is unique in its response to extraneous influences as are the pathogens which affect its health. **The variables are infinite and the line between health and disease is easily breached.** It behooves us, and in fact it's our obligation, to do everything possible to maintain our animals in good health.

Fortunately, medical research has made tremendous gains in techniques for disease control and prevention. What has been lacking generally in veterinary medicine is the application of that knowledge on the farm to prevent animal disease. Your veterinarian and the information in this book can help you correct that deficiency. Remember that animal disease is not always bad luck; it's more often a reflection of bad management and fully 90 percent of the animal health problems we encounter could have been prevented.

Nutrition and Health

IT GOES WITHOUT SAYING that a well-fed animal is more likely to be a healthy animal. The question is, "What is a well-fed animal?" What does well-fed mean? There is no simple answer because nutrient requirements vary with age, body weight, stage of gestation, and, for the dairy cow, level of milk production. Extensive research has produced guidelines that help, but they are guidelines only. Feeding cattle or other animals is part science and part art because of individual variation. Animals respond much like people to nutrient intake and at a given level some get thin, some stay the same, and some get fat. A good herd manager recognizes the individual variations in the herd and adjusts feed intake accordingly.

Cattle

Good cattle nutrition begins with the newborn calf. There are some differences between the dairy and the beef calf that will be pointed out as we go along. As a rule of thumb, young calves should receive 10 percent of their body weight daily of whole milk equivalent. For example, a 100-pound calf should have ten pounds of milk or about five quarts daily.

A note of caution for the dairy calf should be injected here. The cow's first milk, or colostrum, contains about twice the total solids of whole milk and the dairy cow will yield colostrum far in excess of the needs of her calf. If allowed to nurse at will, the calf is likely to overeat, causing digestive upset. In fact, **overeating is one of the important causes of indigestion and diarrhea in young calves.** Colostrum intake therefore should be about half that of whole milk. From a health standpoint, it's far better to keep calves a little bit hungry than to give them all the milk they clamor for. Calves are much like children and they will beg for more milk just like children will beg for candy, but that doesn't mean it's good for them.

The situation differs with the beef calf and it's customary to leave them with their dams to nurse. Overfeeding problems generally don't occur because most beef cows don't produce milk significantly in excess of need. In fact, beef breeders usually select for cows with extra milking capacity so they will have enough milk to raise a good calf.

Don't Waste Colostrum

While the dairy cow gives more colostrum than her calf needs, the excess need not be wasted. It can be diluted 50 percent with water and fed to other calves or can be stored. It can be frozen and kept indefinitely or stored at room temperature and fed as sour or "pickled" colostrum. It can be held this way about three weeks and, while it doesn't look or smell the greatest to us, calves like it and thrive on it.

Where dairy calves are held in group pens, another health consideration related to feeding enters in. Young calves will instinctively suck after they are fed and will suck each other's ears and udders if given the opportunity. They should be tied after each feeding for about an hour or until the sucking urge disappears. While sucking ears is not especially harmful, wet ears will freeze if it is below freezing where the calves are housed. Sucking udders may introduce infection which will flare up as mastitis when the udder begins to develop. Equally important, the sucking habit may become fixed as a lifelong habit and it's not rare for cows to suck their own udders or that of a willing neighbor. This is a vice carried over from calfhood that makes the animal a liability.

Before leaving the subject of feeding milk to calves there is one recurring question that should be answered. Dairy farmers often ask if it's all right to feed milk from cows with mastitis to calves. Nutritionally it's probably satisfactory and economically it makes sense but, in my opinion, such milk should not be used, for two reasons. First, it is usually teeming with pathogenic organisms that caused the mastitis. From a health standpoint, it doesn't make sense to expose the calf to these and at the same time spread them to other areas of the barn. Second, if the infected quarters have been treated with antibiotics and milk from them is fed to calves, the calves will absorb some of the antibiotic and have tissue residues of these antibiotics for varying periods of time thereafter. In the case of streptomycin it may be over a month and it's illegal to market veal containing drug residues.

Milk Replacers

Purely for economic reasons, it's sometimes advantageous to use commercially prepared milk replacer rather than whole milk for calves. These powdered products, when reconstituted with water, make a satisfactory milk substitute. Many companies market milk replacer and they vary widely in price — and quality. All of them indicate on the label the composition analysis in terms of protein and fat. But the quality of the protein, for calves, is equally as important as the amount. The cheaper ones use vegetable sources such as soybean oil meal as the protein source while the better ones use milk by-products. Very young calves do not utilize vegetable protein well, and calves maintained on this type of diet are often stunted and unthrifty. With milk replacers, as with most things, you get about what you pay for.

Frequency of feeding apparently has little significant effect on overall growth of calves. The nursing calf, of course, will get a little milk whenever he feels like it, which is the way nature intended it and which perhaps must be considered the ideal. But it has been explained why ad libitum nursing for dairy calves is undesirable. Hand feeding is almost a necessity for dairy calves and this creates a labor problem. Most dairy farmers feed their calves twice daily, but research at Cornell University indicates that calves do about as well when fed only once a day. Similarly, it seems to make little difference whether the milk is fed warm or cold. However, feeding the total daily intake in one meal of ice cold milk may cause chilling and stomach cramps.

Sanitation

Whatever method is used — once a day, twice a day, warm or cold — sanitation is important. Whether you use ordinary pails, nipple pails, or automatic feeders, these should be scrubbed and sanitized after each use. Milk is the most nearly complete food and this attribute, which is desirable for young animals, also makes it suitable for bacterial growth. Any amount of milk left in the pail at room temperature becomes a thriving bacterial culture in a few hours. If these happen to be pathogenic such as some of the *Salmonella* species, every calf that subsequently drinks from that pail is likely to get sick. Always remember that the calf has virtually no immunity at birth and is vulnerable to every pathogen it encounters. The health of your calves will be proportional to your success in reducing that exposure.

At the age of one week, calves will begin to eat a little grain and hay. The hay offered should be early cut and of high quality. Consumption will be insignificant at first but will gradually increase to a major part of the diet at the end of a month. The amount of milk being fed can be reduced commensurately as grain and roughage consumption increase. Calves can usually be weaned from milk at four to six weeks of age but it's part of the art of husbandry to tell how fast and how soon. The nutritional problems of the calf, once weaned, become similar to those of the mature cow. The important thing is to keep calves growing and gaining weight steadily. **An animal in a weight-gaining condition is more likely to be a healthy animal.**

Clean Water

In addition to whatever it eats, whole milk or milk replacer, the growing calf needs clean water. The ideal way is to have a supply of fresh water available at all times. However, where physical conditions won't permit this, additional water must be hand-fed by adding it to the milk or separately. A good way to wean calves as they get older is to add increasing amounts of water to a constant amount of milk. Eventually the solution gets so dilute that when the milk is stopped, they hardly miss it.

A complete discussion of the nutrition of the growing and mature cow is beyond the scope of this book. For a concise summary, the reader is referred to Nutrient Requirements of Dairy Cattle and its counterpart for beef cattle, both published by the National Academy of Sciences, 2101 Constitution Avenue, N.W., Box 285, Washington, D.C. 20055, 1-800-624-6242. In it one will find the recommendations for protein, energy, minerals, and vitamins for growing and mature cattle in various weight ranges. For mature cattle a basic amount is given for maintenance and to this must be added an increment for advanced pregnancy and for milk production at various levels.

Balancing the Ration

Also given are examples of how to balance a ration using readily available feedstuffs. Ability to balance a ration is a must for the serious herd manager who wants to feed the animals adequately at minimum cost. Also given is the average nutrient composition of several hundred feed ingredients. These can be used as a guide in formulation of rations but it's much more reliable to have a forage analysis done on your own hay and silage and, using that as a base, figure out how much additional grain is needed to balance the daily ration.

TABLE 2-1

Daily Intake for Dairy Cow

	Total Protein (Kg)	TDN (Kg)	Calcium (g)	Phosphorus (g)
For maintenance and pregnancy	1.0	6.3	39	30
For milk production	1.48	0.6	52	38
Total	2.48	6.9	91	68

Analysis of forage is a laboratory procedure that, in most states, can be arranged by your Cooperative Extension agent, your D.H.I.C. technician, your feed dealer, or a commercial laboratory. Analyses are usually reported in terms of percentage of total digestible nutrients (TDN) and total or crude protein (C.P.). Mineral and some vitamin analyses can be obtained as well, but usually at added cost.

To illustrate how this information is used, let's assume we have a 700 kg (1540 lb.) dairy cow giving 20 kg (44 lb.) of 3.5 percent butterfat milk daily and due to calve in two months. Her daily intake, according to the N.R.C. standards, should meet the amounts outlined in Table 2-1.

Let's further assume that we have available good-quality mixed alfalfa-brome grass hay to feed this cow. How much will she need to eat to meet her nutritional needs? Looking first at TDN in the feedstuff composition tables, we find that this mixed hay will average 55 percent TDN on a dry matter basis but it is only 82.5 percent dry matter with the balance moisture. Our cow needs 6.9 kg of TDN daily. By simple arithmetic we find that 15 kg (33 lbs.) of hay daily will meet her energy needs, but will it supply enough protein? The same hay is composed of 16.2 percent total protein on a dry matter basis. By multiplying we find that 15 kg contains 2.4 kg of protein. But, since the hay is only 82.5 percent dry matter, the actual total protein is only 2 kg, or 0.4 kg less than recommended. While the cow would undoubtedly survive with this modest protein deficiency, her milk production would be less than she is capable of producing.

Mineral Components

Let's take a look at the important mineral components in this all-hay diet. This hay averages 1.03 percent calcium (Ca) and .3 percent phosphorus (P), both on a dry matter basis. Fifteen kg of this hay calculates out to 127 gm of calcium and 37 gm of phosphorus daily. This is more calcium than the cow needs and considerably less phosphorus than she requires. Furthermore, the Ca:P ratio is wide, being 3.4:1. With a phosphorus-deficient ration and a wide Ca:P ratio, the cow on this diet would be very likely to have parturient paresis (milk fever, hypocalcemia) when she calves. This is an example of how nutrition influences health.

Well, we have all this good alfalfa-brome hay on hand, which incidentally, is higher in protein and energy than most hay. What can we do so it can be used and still give the cow an adequate diet? Depending on available feeds, several things can be done. Corn silage can be substituted for part of the hay. This will narrow the Ca:P ratio but also reduce the protein. To balance the diet using this hay, some mixed grain dairy ration containing 1 percent dicalcium phosphate or liquid protein supplement will have to be used.

The same procedure can be used to determine adequacy of other essential minerals and vitamins. If all the mathematics scares you or you don't feel confident trying to balance a ration yourself, your local Cooperative Extension agent or feed dealer will be glad to help.

The purpose in all this discussion is to demonstrate that feeding the dairy cow adequately is not a hit-or-miss proposition and that nutrition does have an important bearing on health. Just how important can be seen from the following table compiled by Hillman and Newman at Michigan State University:

TABLE 2-2

Nutrients and Their Functions

Nutrient	Function	Requirement	Deficiency Symptoms
Energy (glucose, fats, fatty acids)	Muscle and nerve activity, growth, fattening, milk secretion.	Variable with size, rate of growth, milk production, and milk fat percentage.	Low milk production; slow growth rate; poor body condition; silent estrus (heat). Lowered protein content of milk. Energy in excess of requirement: Fattening, high blood fat levels; fatty liver; tendency for depressed appetite and ketosis post-calving; Unsaturated fats in tissue and fat deposits; tendency toward low resistence to infectious diseases, retained placentas and metritis; sudden increase causes lactic acidosis, death.
Fiber	Stimulates rumination and secretion of saliva, helps maintain rumen pH near neutral ±6.8; partially fermented to short chain fatty acids for energy and synthesis of milk fat.	Minimum 15% of ration dry matter for lactating cows; higher with finely chopped feeds.	Rumenitis, founder, rumen stasis; tendency toward displaced abomasum post-calving; Low milk fat test; higher unsaturated fats in tissue fats; may contribute to poor muscle contractility.
Protein	Cell formation, muscle, hair blood proteins, enzymes; Milk protein secretion.	11–15% of ration dry matter depending on age and rate of production; Proportional to energy intake.	Emaciation (poor body condition), retarded growth, low milk production. Reduced digestion of feed, poor conversion of feed to growth, fat or milk, lower blood protein, and possibly immune fractions. Underdeveloped reproductive organs possibly due to retarded growth.

Nutrient	Function	Requirement	Deficiency Symptoms
Salt Sodium (Na) and **Chloride** (Cl)	Acid-base balance; nerve and muscle action; water retention; hydrochloric acid.	2–3 grams/cwt/day; Estimated 0.18% sodium or 0.45% salt (NaCl) in dry ration.	Lack of appetite; unthrifty; low production; craving for salt, appetite for soil, clothing, licking objects, drinking of urine from other cows during urination.
Calcium (Ca)	Skeletal growth and milk production; muscle quiescence.	Maintenance 10–15 g/day plus 1 g per lb. milk; 0.3–0.4% in dry ration for lactation.	Bones and teeth easily broken. Low calcium content in bones.
Phosphorus (P)	Energy metabolism, skeletal growth, milk production.	Maintenance 10–15 g +0.75 g/lb. milk; 0.25–0.3% in dry ration.	Lack of appetite, irregular estrus (heat periods) depraved appetite for bones, wood, bark, etc.
Vitamin D	Absorption of Ca and P; reduced excretion of P; mobilization of Ca and P from skeleton.	300–400 IU/cwt/day; D2 or D3, 5000–15,000 IU/head/day.	Rickets, enlarged joints, wobbly gait, lack of appetite, stiff legs, arched back, swelling of pasterns, lameness; calves deficient in Ca, P, or vitamin D.
Magnesium (Mg)	Muscle irritability; electrolyte balance; enzymes.	Calves: 0.4–0.6 g/cwt/day; or 0.15–0.20% in the dry ration of milking cows.	Grass tetany (or grass staggers), twitching of the skin, staggering or unsteady on feet, down. Common with cattle grazing rapidly growing, succulent pasture, or similar green chop and occasionally stored feeds. May be aggravated by high nitrogen and potassium levels in feeds.
Potassium (K)	Acid-base balance in intracellular fluid. Osmotic pressure, activates enzymes, heart, muscle tone.	0.6% of dry ration for growth of lambs; 0.7% suggested for cattle, more for high producing cows.	Overall muscle weakness, loss of appetite, poor intestinal tone with intestinal distension; cardiac and respiratory muscle weakness and failure.
Iron (Fe)	Formation of hemoglobin.	Growth, 150 mg/cwt/day for growth, 100 ppm; in adult ration 2 grams per day.	Anemia — particularly in calves maintained on milk. Seldom in adult cattle.

Nutrient	Function	Requirement	Deficiency Symptoms
Iodine (I)	Thyroxine synthesis; metabolic rate.	0.1 ppm in dry ration (for non-lactation, 2 mg/head daily). 0.8 ppm for pregnancy or 8 to 12 mg. More may be required when soybean meal or other goitrogenic feeds are fed heavily.	Goiterous (big neck) calves frequently dead or hairless. Failure to show estrus, high incidence of retained placentas in mature cows.
Fluorine (F)		Small amount appears to prevent dental caries.	Toxic above 10 ppm. Deformed teeth and bones.
Manganese (Mn)	Growth, enzymes.	Cows: 20 ppm in dry ration for normal reproduction and offspring. Normal growth at lower levels.	Newborn: Deformed bones, enlarged joints, stiffness, twisted legs, shorter humeri (foreleg), general physical weakness of newborn calves. Deficiency could occur in cattle fed high-grain, low roughage rations where symptom could be ataxia (uncoordinated movements).
Copper (Cu)	Respiratory pigments of blood, some enzymes.	5 ppm dry ration, 6–8 ppm suggested. Increases with high molybdenum intake.	"Coast disease" or "salt sick" in Florida. Anemia, stillbirth of young, loss of wool in sheep, incoordination of hind legs, sudden death in cows due to heart degeneration. Baby pig "thumps" due to Cu and iron deficiency.
Cobalt (Co)	Microbial synthesis of vitamin B_{12} in rumen.	0.1 ppm in dry ration (2 mg/day).	Loss of appetite, anemia, emaciation, low appetite for grain. Calves unthrifty, poor appetite, first to exhibit symptoms because low vitamin B_{12} content of milk.
Vitamin B_{12} (cobalamin)	Energy metabolism, maturation of red blood cells.	Calves 1.5 mg/cwt/day.	*See above.*

Nutrient	Function	Requirement	Deficiency Symptoms
Selenium (Se)	Muscle integrity.	Uncertain: believed 0.05 ppm minimum.	Nutritional muscular dystrophy; high calf and lamb mortality; retained placentas increased; liver necrosis (degeneration) in pigs. Toxic above 3 ppm.
Sulfur (S)	Synthesis of S-amino acids, Co-enzyme A.	0.2% in dry ration; 1 S to 10 parts N in high NPN rations.	Lowered production, poor nitrogen utilization. Cellulose digestion and conversion of lactate to propionate.
Zinc	Enzyme systems.	Calves: 9 ppm in ration was adequate for normal growth and appearance. About 20 ppm may be desirable for lactation.	Itch, hair slicking, stiff gait, swelling of hocks and knees, soft swelling above rear feet, rough and thickened skin, dermatitis between rear legs and behind elbows. Undersize testicles in bull calves and low fertility in cows have been attributed to zinc deficiency.
Vitamin A	Growth, differen-tiation and health of epithelial tissue; especially of eyes, alimen-tary tract, and respiratory mucosa.	3000 IU/cwt/day or 6 mg carotene/cwt/day; no lactation require-ment except for health of animal.	Night blindness, bulging and watery eyes, muscle incoor-dination. Bronchitis and coughing may progress to pneumonia. Chronic symptoms: roughened haircoat, emaciation; hairless or blind calves if dam deficient; edema or swelling of the brisket and forelegs (anasarca); abor-tions. Young calves, weak-ness at birth, susceptible to pneumonia and digestive infections, watering of the eyes, cloudiness of the cornea, protrusion or "bulging" of eye followed by permanent blindness and death.

Nutrient	Function	Requirement	Deficiency Symptoms
B Vitamins	Synthesized by organisms in normal functioning rumen to meet requirement.	Calves to weaning; contained in milk.	Deficiency symptoms produced only with abnormal restricted diets. May occur in calves with prolonged severe scours or fed artificial milk diets.
	Niacin, Nicotin or Nicotinamide.	Energy metabolism enzymes.	Dermatitis and necrotic lesions in mouth.
	Thiamin B_1	Prevented by 0.65 mg thiamin-HCl per kg of liquid diet or 0.065 mg per kg live wt.	Polioencephalomalacia. Necrosis in the gray matter of the brain. Muscular incoordination, tremor, grinding of teeth, convulsions. High blood and urine lactate and pyruvate.
	Riboflavin B_2	Calves <0.075 mg/ kg live weight or 0.65 ppm in liquid diet.	Lesions around the corner of the mouth, eyes and nose, damp haircoat, loss of hair, copious salivation, and lacrimation.
	Biotin	0.01 mg/kg liquid diet; 1.0 ug/kg body wt.	Paralysis of hind quarters.
	Pantothenic acid	<1.3 mg/kg liquid diet.	Lack of growth and emaciation. Scaly dermatitis around eyes and muzzle, susceptible to respiratory infection.
	Folic acid	0.39 mg/kg liquid prevented in lamb.	Lack of growth and emaciation, leukopenia (low WBC).
	Vitamin B_{12}	0.34–0.68 microgram (ug) per kg live weight.	Lack of growth and emaciation (see Cobalt).
	Pyridoxine	<0.065 mg/kg wt.	Lack of appetite, epileptiform fits, demyelination of peripheral nerves.

Nutrient	Function	Requirement	Deficiency Symptoms
Choline		260 mg/kg liquid promoted recovery.	Extreme weakness, labored breathing within 6–8 days.
Vitamin C (Ascorbic acid)	Synthesized in tissue of calves and adult bovines.		Other species — scurvy, loosening of teeth, subepithelial hemorrhage and other problems related to faulty collagen formation.
Vitamin E (alpha-to-copherol)	Antioxidant, muscle integrity.	Calves: less than 40 mg/day. Adults not established.	Nutritional muscular dystrophy; white muscle disease in calves; stiff lamb disease; stiff legs; sudden death from heart muscle degeneration. Heart, dia-phragm, and intercostal muscles show light streaking.

Water

Last, water is the most important constituent of the cow's diet, although it is seldom thought of as such. The cow can go several days without feed but one day without water will cause a precipitate drop in milk production, two days without will make a very sick animal, and three days without will likely kill the animal. Adult cattle consume water in proportion to the amount and moisture content of feed consumed, level of milk production, and environmental temperatures. An average cow eating 20 kg of dry matter daily and producing 20 kg of milk will consume about 120 liters or approximately 30 gallons of water daily. Milk production will be higher if water is available free choice.

Digestion in Cows

From a health standpoint there are some other important factors about cattle nutrition to keep in mind. The first is the nature of the beast. Cattle are ruminants, as are sheep and goats, with a digestive system that differs markedly from simple-stomached animals such as the horse, the pig, and man. The cow's stomach is divided into four distinct compartments designated in order of progression as rumen, reticulum, omasum, and abomasum. The rumen is basically a large fermentation vat where the action of bacteria and other microorganisms begin the digestive process by converting fiber into usable energy forms. It's this capacity to utilize fiber that makes the cow unique.

We hear a lot these days about how cattle compete with man for available grain thereby contributing to the world food shortages. Nothing could be further from the truth. Even under our system of finishing beef cattle in feedlots less than 20 percent of the animal's lifetime feed intake is grain. Most of it comes from grass which humans couldn't digest even if they could swallow it. In terms of food resource utilization alone, beef is a real bargain.

The cow doesn't have upper incisor teeth and eats grass more by pulling it off than biting it off as a horse does. Similarly, a cow will take a mouthful of hay and chew it very little before swallowing it. Most of her jaw motions when eating are directed toward mixing the hay with saliva, wadding it into a bolus and swallowing it. It's this failure to chew that contributes to the cow's propensity for swallowing foreign objects, especially pieces of wire that are tangled in hay. These eventually gravitate to the lowest part of the digestive tract, the reticulum, where they sometimes perforate the wall, causing peritonitis.

Ingested feed in the rumen is churned by rhythmic contractions which normally occur two to four times a minute. The fermentation and digestion process, aided by rumen microorganisms, is going on constantly. When the cow is at rest she voluntarily regurgitates part of the rumen contents, chews it a while, and swallows again. The process is called rumination, and the regurgitated ingesta is called a "cud." Most of the cud when swallowed passes into the reticulum.

Metal found in a cow's rumen.

Occasionally a cow will drop a cud out of her mouth, and it was a favorite old wives' tale that losing a cud would make a cow go off feed. There is no truth in this. However it is good therapy to give a cud from a healthy cow to one that has been or is off feed. When you see a cow chewing, simply open her mouth and remove the cud she is chewing on. Then put it in the mouth of the cow that has been off feed. This has the effect of inoculating her rumen with normal rumen microorganisms, which will frequently restore digestive function and improve appetite.

Rumination and Health

Normal rumination is a good indicator of the animal's health. Rumination is absent in such diseases as traumatic gastritis, milk fever, and most digestive disorders. Rumen activity will be greater than normal in diseases causing diarrhea. Because digestion in the cow is first a fermentation process she is subject to some problems rarely seen in non-ruminants. Radical changes in diet such as excessive amounts of grain change the rumen pH from slightly alkaline to acidic which is not desirable for rumen microorganisms and they die. This leads to incomplete digestion and rumen stasis, the results of which can be fatal. Fermentation with evolution of gas is a normal digestive function. However, if the cow eats large amounts of lush green pasture, especially clover or alfalfa, excess gas will be trapped in a froth causing bloat which can be rapidly fatal.

If the cow is sick and not eating, important alterations in rumen digestive activity take place that have a bearing on her recovery. Without a daily addition of nutrients to the rumen, protozoa decrease almost to zero, bacteria decrease to 10–25 percent of normal and the balance between bacterial species is altered. All of these changes reduce fermentation activity which reduces the animal's energy supply in both quantity and quality, cuts off the supply of water soluble vitamins, and increases susceptibility to acidosis and other digestive disturbances.

An important consideration in restoring the sick animal to health is the restoration of normal rumen activity. Poor quality hay high in fiber and poor quality silage should be avoided. Rather, the best quality hay available should be selected and grain intake should be increased gradually as appetite improves.

Although some absorption of nutrients takes place in the rumen, most occurs further along in the digestive tract. From the reticulum, ingesta passes to the omasum and then to the abomasum. From the abomasum down through the intestinal tract the digestive process is comparable to that of simple-stomached animals. The difference is primarily one of size. The gut is subject to the same ailments seen in other animals.

Feed for animals should not be placed on the ground. Fecal contamination leads to internal parasitism.

Two Systems

Ruminant nutrition really concerns two biological systems, the microorganisms in the rumen and, of course, the animal itself. The feed offered must be conducive to proper microbiological metabolism and the end product must meet the nutrient needs of the animal. Since digestion is dependent on rumen microorganisms, it follows that their activity must be the first concern. Abrupt changes in diet are often detrimental. The most common example is what happens every spring when cows are put on pasture for the first time after a winter diet of perhaps dry hay, corn silage, and grain. If they are turned out directly on pasture without being fed some hay first, a few cows will bloat in a matter of a few hours but almost all will have diarrhea in twelve hours or less. This is not so much because fresh grass has a laxative effect, which it does to some degree. It occurs primarily because the rumen organisms are not adapted to it. After a week or so at pasture, the cows' manure will return to a normal consistency.

The matter of rumen microorganism adaptation is especially important when alternate protein sources are used. Protein is usually the most expensive ingredient in the cow's diet and it is frequently advantageous to use a substitute.

Urea is the chemical usually used and the cow can derive up to 30 percent of her protein needs from it. It may be added to the grain or to the silage as long as it is thoroughly mixed. Urea itself has no nutritional value whatsoever. But in the rumen it breaks down to its component elements and the rumen microorganisms utilize the nitrogen ion to synthesize amino acids, which are protein precursors used by the cow. If too much urea is accidentally fed or it is fed at too high a level for cows not conditioned to it, death may result. This happens because the nitrogen is not utilized fast enough by the rumen organisms and an excess of ammonia, fatal to the cow, is produced. Urea, not exceeding 3 percent of the grain ration, can safely provide 30 percent of the cow's protein needs once the rumen flora have been adapted to it. The majority of formula dairy feeds contain some urea and it is commonly used in liquid protein supplements.

Vitamins and Minerals

Although the chief concern in cattle nutrition is with energy, protein, and the minerals calcium and phosphorus, attention must be given as well to vitamins, trace minerals, and salt. The B vitamins are largely synthesized by rumen microorganisms so that supplementation for the healthy cow is generally not required. The fat-soluble vitamins, A, D, and E, are more of a concern. Vitamin A is the most important of the three. It and its precursor, carotene, are found in green feeds and grain so that supplementation is not required when cows are on pasture. However, it oxidizes rather rapidly in storage so that hay that was high in vitamin A when cut will have very little after six months in storage. If stored hay or silage is a major part of the diet, vitamin A supplementation, in the feed or by injection, is usually necessary. Vitamin A is routinely added to most commercial grain mixes.

Vitamin D plays an important role in calcium metabolism and is sometimes used prophylactically in high doses prior to calving for the prevention of milk fever. It is synthesized by specialized cells in the skin under the action of sunlight. Deficiencies are unlikely to occur in adult cattle except where cattle are housed indoors constantly. Deficiency in calves causes rickets and this vitamin is usually added to milk replacers to prevent this possibility. Vitamin E plays a role, with selenium in muscle metabolism. A deficiency of either leads to a sometimes fatal condition in calves and lambs called white muscle disease. This is more likely to occur on an all-milk diet, which is a reason for getting some grain and hay into the diet as early as possible.

The need for the essential trace elements and salt can be met by giving cattle free access to trace mineralized salt (sometimes called "blue" salt). The addition of an equal part of dicalcium phosphate will help to maintain an adequate calcium and phosphorus intake. The mixture should be put in a container protected from rain and placed in an area where the cattle have daily access.

Horses

With the advent of the tractor and automobile, horse numbers declined precipitously during the 1930s and 40s to a point where immediately after World War II many people believed the future of the horse was very limited. As a consequence, most colleges and experiment stations discontinued equine research and husbandry programs. However, with the unpredictable resurgence of interest in the light horse, it is evident, with the advantage of 20/20 hindsight, that this was a mistake.

One result of the temporary decline of interest in the horse is a lack of good research data on equine nutrition. Only within recent years has this important area begun to get the attention it deserves and there is still much to learn. Until this time, equine diets have been largely a matter of trial and error, unfounded opinion, and even superstition. There are horse owners today who believe the only safe and satisfactory diet for horses is timothy hay and oats. This opinion has been thoroughly discredited but there are factors about the horse and diet that have a profound influence on health.

Although the horse is an herbivore like the cow, its digestive system is entirely different. The horse has only a simple stomach comparable to the fourth compartment of the cow's stomach. It has limited capacity, and the horse, although it needs some roughage, cannot handle the volume the cow does to meet its energy requirements, especially when heavy work is required. If fed enough, the horse can survive on hay alone, but the volume required frequently results in chronic abdominal distention referred to as "hay belly" which is undesirable, particularly for a show animal. The horse doing heavy work must get most of its energy needs from concentrates.

The energy requirements of the horse are comparable in some ways to those of the gasoline engine. The greater the power output required, the greater the fuel consumption. As a rule of thumb, the horse needs 1½–1¾ pounds of good quality hay per 100 pounds of body weight to maintain his condition. In addition, if he is doing light work he needs ¾–1½ pounds of grain per hour of work, and for heavy work, this need goes up to 8 pounds of grain per hour of work. Like the cow, the mare during advanced pregnancy or during lactation has an additional requirement for energy ranging from 1½–1¾ pounds of grain per 100 pounds of body weight. While these figures are good guides they are not absolute, and the horse owner must feed according to the needs of the individual animal. **The most common error in feeding light horses is overfeeding.** The resulting obesity contributes to lack of stamina, liver disease, and leg problems, as well as foaling complications for the mare.

Which Grain?

A variety of grains can be used to meet the energy needs of the horse. Oats are traditional and good. They are higher in fiber and lower in energy than corn and wheat and therefore overfeeding is less likely to have health repercussions. Many horse owners feel that corn is "too hot" for the horse and will cause indigestion and even laminitis. This is not true if the corn is fed on an energy equivalent basis. It's common practice to feed grain to horses on a volume rather than a weight basis as used with other species. If, for example, you are feeding six quarts of oats twice a day to a working horse and decide to use shelled corn instead, the same measure will provide almost twice the energy needs because corn weighs 1.7 times as much as oats. Cut the volume in half and you will have no difficulty, but make any feed change gradually over a period of several days because the horse is particularly sensitive to radical changes in diet. **Abrupt change frequently causes indigestion and colic.**

The protein requirement of the mature horse is much less critical than that of the dairy cow or dairy goat. The horse needs protein at the level of about 8–10 percent of the total ration and this is readily met by a combination of hay

Feeding hay from a rack reduces waste and prevents fecal contamination.

and grain. The requirement increases during pregnancy and lactation and can be met by switching to mixed hay with a higher percentage of legumes or to a grain mix formula that includes a higher percentage of protein. The weanling needs considerably more high-quality protein than the mature horse. To provide the 14–18 percent of protein needed in the weanling's diet, creep feeding is usually necessary.

Quality of Feed

A word of caution should be given about hay. Any grass or legume hay of good quality is satisfactory from a nutritional standpoint but **never feed moldy or "smoky" hay to horses.** Mold spores and dust are largely responsible for the chronic lung disease pulmonary emphysema or "heaves" in the horse. Moldy grain is equally hazardous from the standpoint of mycotoxicosis. The horse, the pig, and the chicken seem to be particularly susceptible to poisoning by the toxins that some molds produce. Both of these problems can be avoided largely by paying attention to feed quality.

Grain for the horse (and in fact for all livestock) should be coarsely ground or pelleted. Finely ground grain is less palatable and dusty but, more important, when swallowed it may lodge in the esophagus, causing the animal to choke. This is a serious condition requiring prompt professional attention.

Although the specific nutrient requirements of the horse have not been investigated as thoroughly as those for the cow and pig, enough information is available so that some valid recommendations can be made. If you know the composition of your own hay from forage analysis or use the average composition from feed analysis tables, the following recommendations will be useful.

TABLE 2-3
Requirements Expressed as Percentage of Diet

Category	Protein	Calcium	Phosphorus
Weanling	14–16	0.7	0.4
Mature	8–10	0.35	0.25
Late Pregnancy	11–12	0.4	0.3
Lactating	13–15	0.6	0.35

Note that the calcium and phosphorus requirements for the weanling as a percent of daily intake are much higher than for the mature horse. This is to meet the need for rapid skeletal growth. Calcium and phosphorus are the two most important minerals for the horse. Grains are rich sources of phosphorus, and if the horse is being fed relatively large amounts of grain, phosphorus is likely to be consumed in excess in proportion to calcium unless legume hay is also being fed. Over a period of time this imbalance will cause a demineralization of bone and a disease called nutritional secondary hyperparathyroidism or "big head." To avoid this condition, additional calcium must usually be added to the diet.

The horse also has a relatively high requirement for salt, especially when sweating from hot weather or strenuous exercise. The mature horse needs 50–60 gm (2 ounces) of salt daily and considerably more when sweating. The need for salt and extra calcium can be met by free-choice feeding of dicalcium phosphate and trace mineralized salt as recommended for cattle. When salt is first fed free-choice, be sure an ample amount of fresh water is available in case the horse eats too much. Once his initial craving for salt is satisfied, he will consume only enough to meet his needs.

Swine

Of all the farm animals, the dietary needs of swine most nearly parallel those of humans. Pigs are omnivores — that is, they can utilize energy and protein from both vegetable and animal sources to meet their requirements. This ability, coupled with economics, for years made garbage feeding a part of many swine enterprises. From a disease control standpoint, however, feeding garbage is hazardous because pathogenic organisms may be present in the meat scraps that will infect pigs. The last outbreak of foot and mouth disease in this country occurred this way in 1929, and many outbreaks of hog cholera have occured since then. Because of the disease transmission hazard, feeding raw garbage to pigs has been made illegal, and some states have banned the feeding of cooked garbage as well. Undoubtedly, many people who keep one or two pigs for their own use continue to feed their own household garbage because it reduces the feed costs and helps to solve a disposal problem. There is nothing wrong with the practice provided raw meat scraps are not included. But for all practical purposes, garbage feeding as a commercial enterprise is no longer a consideration in swine nutrition.

The question, then, is what to feed for maximum economical rate of gain and for a minimum of nutrition-related disease problems. Perhaps because of its rapid growth rate and small stomach capacity compared with the ruminant, the pig seems more susceptible to disease conditions resulting from vitamin, mineral, or amino acid deficiencies. There is a wealth of information available as a result of intensive research on these conditions that, with a few exceptions, is beyond the scope of this book. It is important to the professional swine nutritionist responsible for formulating commercial rations. Most of the land grant universities have good bulletins available on swine nutrition for those needing more detail, and there are a number of good texts on the subject.

Formula Feed

If you are raising just a few pigs as a hobby or for your own use, probably the easiest way to avoid nutritional problems is to use a formula feed prepared by a reputable milling company for the class of pig you are feeding. Most companies have rations available as pre-starters for pigs one to four weeks old, starters for pigs one to four months of age, finishers for pigs four months to market weight, and maintenance rations for sows and boars. Although perhaps not the cheapest, in the long run this may be the simplest course to follow.

However, if you have some homegrown feed available, it certainly can be used if a few basic nutritional needs of the pig are kept in mind. Pigs have a very limited capacity for roughage, and total fiber in the diet for young pigs probably should not exceed 7 percent. For sows there is some advantage to increasing this to 15 percent to keep them from getting too fat and to reduce the problem of constipation so common when sows are put in crates at farrowing time. Good-quality alfalfa or other legume hay can provide up to 20 percent of swine diets. This can be in the form of pasture or as alfalfa meal in the ration with the balance being grain.

The general need of swine for diets containing 75–80 percent energy and 16 percent protein (higher for young growing pigs) dictates that most of the diet must be grain when both composition and economy are considered. To avoid deficiency disease problems, a combination of grains should be used.

Corn is an excellent source of energy for pigs. It is usually the cheapest and is commonly equated with fattening. Whenever we think of high-quality meat we usually think of "corn-fed" pork or "corn-fed" beef. Over the short finishing period a high percentage of corn **can** be used without difficulty. But if corn makes up most of the diet for the pig's lifetime, disease problems will occur because corn is deficient in the amino acids, lysine and tryptophan, as well as calcium and total protein. Without supplementation, pigs maintained on a

Pigs can make good use of pasture.

corn diet will suffer stunting and skeletal disease problems such as osteo-dystrophy. Using a mixture of grains will reduce this possibility.

Of course, the various amino acids, fatty acids, vitamins, or minerals that may be deficient in a diet can be supplemented. But, how much and what to add is a job for the professional nutritionist. Compared with the herbivores, such as cattle and horses, the pig is much more sensitive to dietary deficiencies because much less of the digestive process is done by microorganisms, which, in the cow for instance, synthesize the B vitamins the animal needs.

Health Problems

There are a few nutrition-related health problems in addition to deficien-cies that should be mentioned. Moldy feed should never be fed to pigs because they are very sensitive to the toxins that some molds produce. *Gibberella zeae,* a common grain mold, produces a toxin that has the same effect on the pig as female hormones. Sows and gilts fed diets contaminated with this mold have lowered conception rates and sometimes reddening and swelling of the vulva as well as enlargement of the mammary glands. The condition is reversible when the contaminated feed is removed but it may take several months for normal fertility to be restored.

Baby pigs frequently suffer from iron deficiency anemia. This is because they are born with little iron reserve and sow's milk is very low in iron. Symp-toms generally appear one to three weeks after birth and include listlessness and failure to grow. Perhaps the most dramatic symptom, aside from possible sudden death, is the spasmodic contraction of the diaphragm and simultaneous expansion of the rib cage, from which the disease gets the name "thumps."

Fortunately the condition is readily preventable by several methods. Feed-ing additional iron to the sow has no value because it is not passed through in the milk. One of the early and still widely used practices is to put a few chunks of sod in the pen where the baby pigs can root around in it and even lick or eat some of it. A second method is to swab the udder of the sow with a ferrous sulfate solution (one pound in three quarts of water), so that when the piglets nurse they also get some iron. Perhaps the most certain way to be sure they get adequate iron supplementation is by intramuscular injection of iron dextran when they are two or three days old. A number of preparations are commercially available for this purpose. Once piglets begin to eat some starter ration, their iron intake usually will be adequate to prevent further problems.

Use of Dairy Rations

Some people raising just a few pigs for their own use will feed them dairy rations or even horse feed. The pigs will usually do all right on it, but a note of caution should be injected regarding the use of dairy ration. Many formula dairy feeds contain urea that, we have explained, the cow's rumen bacteria can convert into protein components. Pigs don't have this capacity and if dairy ration is their only feed, protein deficiency may result that will cause poor growth rates. If, for example, the tag on a 16 percent protein dairy ration feed bag says something like "contains 3 percent protein equivalent from non-protein nitrogen sources (NPN)," it means that the feed actually contains only 13 percent natural protein. This would be too low for optimum long-term maintenance of swine. Urea by itself has no nutritional value and it is also a highly toxic chemical when consumed in excess. It could easily kill a pig.

Salt and Water

Last, in addition to the usual nutrients, pigs need salt and a good supply of clean water at all times. On a comparative weight basis, pigs will consume twice as much water as dry feed. In hot weather their consumption will double. Young growing pigs may drink water equivalent to 20 percent of their body weight daily but as they get older this amount declines to about 7 percent. In any case, the water should be fresh, preferably from fountains or drinking cups. If you must water them by hand, don't just add to what is left in the trough or pan. Empty it out and give them a clean supply daily because any feed rinsed off their mouths when they drink will settle to the bottom, where it not only sours but provides a good place for pathogenic bacteria such as *Salmonella* spp. to grow. For the same reasons, a mud hole is not a healthful water supply for pigs.

If you are using some homegrown grains to build your own swine ration, I'd strongly advise you to get some professional help in making up its formulation. Your local Cooperative Extension agent can help or steer you in the right direction to get some help. Because you will need some supplements, your feed dealer can help, too. Making up a swine ration on a "by-guess-or-by-

PHOTO COURTESY OF WARREN BRANNON

Flocks should be observed frequently for signs of illness.

gosh" basis will sooner or later lead to deficiency disease problems, especially if your pigs are raised in total confinement where they must depend solely upon you for a balanced diet.

Sheep and Goats

Some goat enthusiasts will no doubt take offense at having their favorite species lumped together with sheep in this brief discussion of nutrition. Let me assure them now that this is purely for pragmatic reasons. Very little work has been done on the specific nutrient needs of the goat. Anatomically and physiologically, as far as diet goes, their needs are essentially the same as the cow and the sheep for proportional body weight.

Goats are unique in only one respect. For its size the goat can consume substantially more forage than the cow or the sheep. Their ability to consume twice the volume makes it possible for goats to survive and produce milk on marginal pastures where a cow would starve. It does not, however, confer on them the ability to recycle tin cans, as some people seem to think. For a dairy goat to be productive it must have adequate good pasture or hay to meet at least half its needs, with the balance coming from concentrates such as dairy ration. As a rule of thumb the milking doe should get about a half-pound of dairy ration daily for each quart of milk produced, in addition to as much pasture or hay as she wants. Between lactations, pasture or hay alone will usually suffice. When fed in this manner with a clean water supply available, a goat will have a minimum of nutrition-related health problems.

The nutrient needs of sheep have been extensively studied. In fact, because of its size and economy, the sheep has served as the experimental model for most of the basic nutrition research that has subsequently been extrapolated to the cow. From this you can correctly infer that the needs of the sheep are the same as those of the cow in proportion to its body weight.

For the person who keeps a few sheep as a hobby with costs secondary to the pleasures of ownership, this knowledge simplifies the feeding problem. Good pasture or hay supplemented with some dairy ration during advanced pregnancy will usually free the animals of nutritional problems. Commercially, however, the situation may be quite different. Sheep not only have a relatively low unit value but the margin of profit is also small. Because feed costs make up about 75 percent of the cost of production, this is where the greatest savings can be made. Unfortunately some growers try to save too much, and the end result is poor fertility, small lamb crops, reduced rate of gain, and a variety of disease problems — not the least of which is sometimes plain starvation.

The Right Combination

Sheep get along well on combinations of pasture, hay, silage, and grain. The possible combinations are almost infinite and the choice will depend on available feeds and their cost. No single combination can be said to be the best but the serious sheep grower can find guidance in the NRC recommendations referred to earlier or the *Sheepman's Production Handbook*, published by Sheep Industry Development, Inc., American Sheep Industry Association, 6911 South Yosemite St., Englewood, CO 80112-1414.

While it's important to maintain sheep on an adequate diet, it's also important from a health standpoint to recognize that individual animals respond differently to the same nutrient intake and that nutritional needs vary depending on the status of the animal. With most species the owner's eyeball is usually the best diagnostic tool to determine whether the animal is getting enough to eat. If your sheep look thin, feed them more; if they look too fat, feed less. Except in the head of the experienced shepherd, however, the eyeball is not nearly as useful to determine the status of sheep, because of the wool covering. I have seen sheep that were actually emaciated and yet the owner was unaware of it. To determine body condition on a sheep one has to feel down over the shoulder and loin with the fingertips. If all you feel is bone, better feed them more. Conversely if you have trouble feeling bone through the fat, feed them less.

Always remember that while we may have good data on the protein and energy needs of animals, the numbers given are only averages, not absolutes. Judgment must be used. Economically, it's important to feed sheep the minimum needed, recognizing that minimum needs change. For example a 140-pound dry ewe early in gestation will get along on about 3½ pounds of alfalfa hay daily without supplementation. The same ewe during the first months of lactation will need 5 pounds of alfalfa and ¾ pounds of corn daily and even then will probably lose some body weight. Like cows, most sheep cannot consume enough feed to replace the energy lost through high milk production. Especially in ewes with twins or triplets, this negative energy balance is largely responsible for "pregnancy disease" or ketosis. This common metabolic disease is largely preventable by keeping ewes on a minimum maintenance diet early in gestation to prevent obesity and then raising energy intake during the last four to six weeks of pregnancy and during early lactation.

Loose Salt

Like other livestock, sheep and goats need salt in addition to the usual nutrients. This should be fed as loose salt rather than in salt blocks. They are more inclined to bite a block rather than lick it like a cow or horse, and in so doing may break their teeth. Depending on diet, they usually need additional calcium and phosphorus. The best way to provide all three is to feed a mixture of equal parts of dicalcium phosphate and trace mineralized salt. This may be fed free-choice. However, as a management technique for sheep at pasture it's a good idea to hand-feed the mixture in a feed trough about once a week. This not only gives you a chance to observe the flock at close quarters, but also keeps the sheep accustomed to people in the pasture, making them easier to handle when the need arises.

Feeding Orphan Lambs

Orphan lambs, unfortunately, are a common part of the sheep business and how to keep them alive presents a problem. Sometimes a ewe with adequate milk and only a single offspring can be persuaded to adopt them. But more often it's a bottle feeding proposition best delegated to one of the

Creep feeding lambs for maximum growth rate.

PHOTO COURTESY OF WARREN BRANNON

children in the family. Cow's milk or milk replacer can be used with the lamb bottles and nipples commercially available or with a baby bottle. The orphans always should have colostrum early in life from their dam or another ewe. If calf milk replacer must be used, select one formulated for veal calf production that has a fat content of 25 percent or more. Older (three to four weeks) lambs usually can be taught to drink from a nipple or from a conventional pail.

An ample supply of clean fresh water is important for all livestock. But it has added importance in preventing the common problem of urolithiasis, seen in wethers and rams. This condition results when stones composed of precipitated mineral salts form in the urinary bladder and are flushed down the urethra where they may lodge in the urethral process of the male. Because of anatomical differences, urolithiasis rarely happens in the female. Especially in wethers on full feed these calculi may plug several centimeters of the urethra. This makes urination difficult or impossible and a ruptured bladder is the usual fatal sequel. Increased water intake to reduce the concentration of dissolved salts in the urine effectively reduces the prevalence of this condition. In the lamb feedlots where this condition is seen most frequently, it is common practice to encourage water consumption by adding additional salt up to 10 percent of the daily ration.

Summary

A great variety of nutrients is available to feed livestock. The ruminants, cattle, sheep, and goats, have similar needs as far as dietary components are concerned and, generally speaking, the amounts needed vary only according to body weight and stage of lactation. The horse is closely related, although its energy needs are higher when working and its stomach capacity is less. The pig is quite different in its needs.

Remember that good nutrition is fundamental to good health. Deficiency diseases are usually insidious and slow in onset and the response to correction of a deficiency in most cases is not dramatic. Diagnosis is often difficult. Help, if you need it, is available from your veterinarian, your Cooperative Extension agent, the animal science departments of the land-grant universities, and most of the larger feed companies. If you suspect a problem, don't hesitate to seek their advice.

To prevent problems, use only good-quality nutrients undamaged by weather or spoilage in recommended amounts and keep a supply of fresh clean water available at all times.

Proper feeding of livestock has become a much more scientific process than it was at one time. There is a wealth of good research information available from the animal science departments of the land-grant universities pertaining to nutrient requirements and composition of feedstuffs. It remains for the herd manager to utilize this information to best advantage.

Even the process of ration formulation has been simplified. It is possible to buy computer programs for use in your personal computer that, when your data are fed in, will do all the calculations for you. The same type of service is available from most feed companies, animal science departments and, in the major livestock production areas, from private nutrition consulting firms.

Remember, though, that nutrition recommendations are averages, not absolutes. No two animals respond alike and the best scientific information available will not totally replace the judgment of the good herd manager.

Housing and Health

Cattle

THE ENVIRONMENT IN WHICH THE COW IS KEPT plays an important role in health. If survival is the only consideration, shelter requirements of cattle regardless of temperature are minimal. If they have enough to eat they get along very nicely with nothing more than an open shed to provide shade in summer and protection from wind and freezing rain in winter. In fact, this is the way most beef cattle are kept. Range cattle manage to get along with nothing except perhaps a grove of trees as a windbreak. It's when humans intervene that health problems related to housing are more likely to arise. Keep in mind, however, that when cattle are outside in cold weather, they utilize more energy to maintain body heat and must be fed accordingly.

Without exception, dairy cattle housing is designed to facilitate materials handling, to make milking more convenient, or to comply with sanitary codes, and always to provide the owner with a way to handle cattle with minimum effort and maximum comfort. There is nothing wrong with these objectives provided the health of the cow is considered, too. But when people build facilities for their cows, they often overlook or subordinate the cows' needs to their own comfort.

The Traditional Barn

The traditional dairy barn in northern climates has a concrete floor with the cows confined to stanchions or tied in stalls. The barn is tightly enclosed in winter and body heat keeps it warm. High density of cows per square foot not only keeps construction costs to a minimum but also keeps the barn warmer. This sounds logical and efficient, but what does it imply for the cow?

The sanitary codes governing commercial milk production require that barn floors be constructed of impervious material and kept clean. Concrete is really the only choice and troweling the concrete smooth when installed facilitates cleaning but makes the floor so slippery it's a real hazard for cows walking on it. Even if it isn't smooth when installed it soon gets that way from constant cleaning and scraping.

To avoid falls, better footing must be provided for cows. Some dairy farmers scatter superphosphate on the barn floor to improve traction. In theory this is good because it is also a valuable fertilizer when later spread on the land with the manure. In practice, it's poor because many of the superphosphate prills are round, making it somewhat like walking on marbles. Calcite, which is finely crushed limestone, provides excellent traction but the particles are sharp and get ground into the feet and cause lameness. Ground limestone is better but tends to be slippery when wet. **There is probably nothing better than sand or gravel lightly spread where the cows walk.** A few wood shavings or sawdust add to the appearance and help keep the floor dry. Mechanical grooving of the floor is helpful and some contractors provide this service.

Another health detriment inherent in the stanchion barn is lack of exercise. This contributes to rapid hoof growth and the need for more frequent hoof trimming and, equally important, loss of muscle tone. When total body weight is considered, the dairy cow is not heavily muscled. In fact, the description of "a big bag of guts supported by four posts" is not inappropriate. When there is loss of muscle tone due to physical inactivity the stage is set for difficulties at calving time. Some of the so-called "downer" cows following calving are that way because they don't have the strength to get up unassisted and often injure themselves trying. Entirely too many cows are unnecessarily lost this way.

The Stall Bed

The stall bed must be considered, too, because that's where the cow must stand or lie day and night. Particularly in stanchion barns the size of the stall is critical for the cleanliness, comfort, and health of the cow. Short stalls force the cow to stand with hind legs in the gutter, long stalls mean manure in the stall and on the udder, and narrow stalls increase teat injuries. Concrete stalls must be padded or bedded in some manner to protect her from the constant bruising and irritation that concrete causes. This becomes especially apparent on the hocks and knees. Adequate amounts of straw, dry shavings, sawdust, or shredded paper are satisfactory but because they are a recurring expense many dairy farmers use heavy rubber mats designed for the purpose or even indoor-outdoor carpet. Either is a help but the cows will stay cleaner if some additional bedding is added. Green sawdust or shavings and especially bark chips are not recommended for bedding because they may be contaminated with a bacterium, *Klebsiella spp.*, which may cause mastitis.

Ventilation

Ventilation is another problem directly influencing health. Most barns have a combination of windows and forced ventilation to provide air circulation and frequently the combination is inadequate. Inadequate ventilation leads to high humidity, condensation on ceiling and walls, and accumulation of stale air — an ideal environment for pneumonia to start in the herd. With an outside temperature of 50°F, for example, a ventilation rate of 174 cubic feet per minute is required per 1,000 pounds of animal housed to maintain the inside temperature at 60°F. From a health standpoint, an inside temperature of 50°F in winter is preferable. The agricultural engineering departments at most of the land-grant universities have excellent technical bulletins on barn construction and ventilation available at nominal cost. Anyone contemplating barn construction should take advantage of their advice.

Avoiding Drafts

Another point should be emphasized with respect to ventilation and health. Cold is not harmful to the cow, but drafts can be deadly. In winter the cow stanchioned next to a broken or open window with cold air pouring in is almost certain to get pneumonia. If allowed to move, cows will always avoid these situations. I was called some years ago as a consultant to investigate what was reported to be an unusual outbreak of calf pneumonia. It was mid-winter and on this farm calves three months old and up were consistently getting pneumonia. The mortality rate was very high. It didn't take long to confirm that the calves were dying from pneumonia; several had obvious signs of pneumonia when I was there. Nor did it take long to figure out the underlying cause.

This dairy farmer made it a practice to move calves to a separate barn after they were weaned. His "calf barn" was an old, former dairy barn oriented north and south on a hillside. One side of the barn was below grade and on the other, westerly side, he had built five box stalls, each large enough to hold five calves. Windows extended the whole length of the west side. Doors were located at the north and south ends and the south door was open. So far, so good! But windows adjacent to three pens were broken and the prevailing westerly wind at 10°F was whistling through those openings, with a velocity that must have approached 30 mph, directly on the calves in those pens. Even with a heavy coat on, I was uncomfortable examining the calves in the pens.

The answer to the problem was simple: Replace the broken glass in the windows to stop the draft! This was done and the mysterious pneumonia outbreak came to a rapid close. Ironically, this man's veterinarian had given him the same advice a month previously but he couldn't believe the answer was that simple. As he told me, "I thought fresh air was good for calves." It is, but not in a wind tunnel.

Economy and simplicity in dairy cattle housing. Free stalls in an open shed in New England.

Free-Stall Barns

One of the reasons for the rapidly increasing popularity of free-stall barns, aside from construction economy, is improved herd health. In these the cows are free to move about at will, the stall beds are elevated, bedded usually with deep sand and sawdust, and the cows lie in them as they choose. The slippery floor problem remains and, in fact, is worse, but because the cows move about at their leisure, falls are less frequent. They get some exercise and drafts are not a problem because the cow can move. In fact, in the "cold" system of free stall housing with no ceiling in the barn only natural ventilation is required, if the design is right, to get an adequate change of air. Most dairy farmers with free-stall barns report improved reproductive performance because more pronounced signs of estrus make it easier to detect.

Teat Injuries

Another housing-related health problem is the matter of teat injury. This occurs with both housing systems but is more prevalent in stanchion barns particularly when the stall beds are narrow or when the cows are fidgety because they have lice. Cows are not especially bright, are certainly clumsy, and seem to have a great propensity for stepping on each other's teats. Sometimes they even step on their own when they get up. A teat caught between concrete and the foot of an animal weighing over a half a ton suffers a variety of injuries ranging from amputation to, at the least, a severe bruise. In any case, it makes milking difficult and frequently leads to mastitis. This type of accident is more common when cows are spaced too close together. For the larger breeds such as the Holstein, stall beds should be at least four feet wide, and a partition between cows is helpful. A curb of concrete in stanchion barns or plank in free stalls at the bottom of the partition helps to keep the cow's feet away from her neighbor.

A word of caution about partitions, especially in free-stall barns. These should be designed so that cows can't get caught underneath them. Many cows suffer fractured legs or backs when they are caught under a partition and struggle to get up.

Without belaboring the point, it should be obvious by now that with a little forethought a lot of potential health problems can be eliminated by proper building design. If you are building a new barn or remodeling an old one, visit some newly constructed barns in your area to get some good ideas. And talk with your veterinarian. In practice all of us see accidents to animals that could have been avoided, and we pick up ideas in the many barns that we visit in the course of our daily work.

Shade Needed

If you are concerned only about the family cow or live in the South, discussion of construction and housing is moot. The family cow usually survives in whatever shelter is provided, although the same consideration should be given to ventilation, drafts, and floors. In warm climates the shelter requirement is reversed and the prime necessity is shade. Similarly, the housing requirements for beef cattle are minimal. All they need is a dry place to lie down and protection from driving rain or snow. An open shed facing south in a well-drained area is quite adequate. A few translucent fiberglass panels in the shed roof let some sunlight in, making it more comfortable for the cattle.

Calf Housing

Housing probably has a greater influence on the health of dairy calves than any other class of cattle. Several surveys have shown that 15 percent of the calves die before two weeks of age, and environmental factors play an important role in this excessive mortality. Because of their vulnerability to infectious diseases, ideally they should be kept isolated from each other and from other animals. Unfortunately, this adds to housing costs and labor requirements but some practical compromises have been developed.

The system of having a pen in the barn in which calves are kept loose and new ones added as they are born is most likely to lead to disease problems. Most commercial dairy farmers are moving away from this housing method as rapidly as possible. The typical history of calf pens is that for the first year or so, health problems were minimal. But in the second and ensuing years they increased to a point where every calf put in the pen would develop diarrhea, septicemia, or pneumonia and die. The reason for this is that calf pens are difficult to keep clean and dry. They are often located in a section of the barn that is difficult to ventilate. These problems are compounded if sunlight is not available. These factors create an ideal environment for pathogens to survive and when new susceptible calves are constantly added to the group, the level of pathogens such as *E. coli* and *Salmonella* spp. increases rapidly and they infect every calf. Any factor which then lowers resistance results in disease.

Use in Rotation

It's well established that, to use this housing system successfully over a period of years, more than one pen must be available and they must be used in rotation. If a pen can be vacated, thoroughly cleaned and disinfected, preferably with steam, and left vacant for six to eight weeks, pathogens in it will die and it can be used again.

A modification of this system that works well is the elevated calf stall in which the calves are kept tied until weaned. These are often built in units of four on skids so that the whole assembly can be moved outside for cleaning and left out in the sunlight to kill any pathogenic organisms. This system has the advantage of preventing direct contact among calves. It makes it easier to observe individuals for signs of illness, gives calves a dry place to lie down, and cleaning the floor underneath is easier. This system is widely used in commercial veal production.

From a disease control standpoint, probably the best innovation is the calf hutch. This is a small open shed, usually made with 3½ sheets of 4 ft. x 8 ft. exterior plywood, and has a small exercise area attached designed to accommodate one calf. If the budget permits, fiberglass calf hutches are commercially available. Hutches provide isolation, ventilation, and sunlight, all of which are important. Furthermore, they can be moved easily to clean the ground before the next calf is brought in so pathogen build-up is not a problem. Of course, it

Elevated stalls keep calves clean, dry, and separated from each other.

Typical elevated calf stall.

Cross section layout plan for elevated calf stall.

Plywood calf hutches.

is cold in the winter, but this is only a problem for the person feeding the calves. With ample bedding, calves in hutches tolerate below-zero temperatures very well, and in fact, will be far healthier than in a warm barn. It should be noted, however, that calves' feed (energy) requirement increases up to two to three times normal during extended below-zero temperature periods and that they should be fed accordingly. Choice of the optimum housing system for dairy calves is a trade-off between disease risk for the calf and labor-saving convenience for the operator. No system rates highest in both categories except perhaps the old method of putting three or four calves with a good motherly nurse cow and turning them loose. Economically, even that has disadvantages.

Maternity Pens

A word should also be said here about the use of maternity stalls or pens. For a variety of reasons, not the least of which is comfort of the cow, it's common practice to put cows into box stalls just prior to calving so they have ample room to move at will when parturition is imminent. A dimension of roughly 10 ft. x 10 ft. is adequate and it's a good idea to have a strong ring fastened to the ceiling to which a sling can be attached to help the cow to her feet after calving, if necessary. Ideally, for reasons which will become apparent, the walls and floors of the maternity pens should be constructed of impervious material that is easily cleaned and disinfected.

There is little doubt that, on many dairy farms, problems with metritis and mastitis in the cow as well as navel infection, septicemia, and diarrhea in newborn calves can be traced directly to contaminated maternity pens. When the same pens are in constant use a buildup of pathogens occurs that makes infection inevitable. The pens must be cleaned and disinfected thoroughly after each use. Construction with smooth impervious material makes the job easier, especially when the floor slopes toward a drain so that ample water can be used.

Check Electrical System

Last, be sure your electrical system is in good repair and properly grounded. There is nothing more disconcerting than seeing a whole row of cows drop to their knees because of electric shock when the milking machine pump or the water pump is turned on. While that is an extreme which doesn't happen often, a low-voltage tingle, called stray voltage, which makes them very uneasy is fairly common. It can originate anywhere on the line and it may require the help of a master electrician and the power company to find the source. If the cow associates the tingle with the milking machine, a precipitous drop in production is likely to occur.

Horses

Housing for horses generally is more dependent on the desires of the owner than the needs of the horse. In terms of need, horses are akin to beef cattle, and an open shed or other windbreak is adequate. In fact, it is not unusual to see horses, if they have a choice, out in a pasture on the most inclement winter day pawing through the snow to reach a bit of grass even though there is hay in the shed under cover where they could be. We are talking, of course, about the minimum needs of the horse that has grown a winter hair coat and is being left to his own devices. The horse that is kept groomed and ready for the show circuit all year is a different matter. This horse requires warmer housing and, in very cold weather, blanketing as well.

The show horse usually is kept in a box stall and perhaps put in an exercise yard during the day. The type of barn in which the stall is located is limited only by the imagination and financial resources of the owner. Nevertheless, the same need for fresh air in a draft-free environment prevails for the same reasons given in the section on cattle housing.

Flooring

There are some peculiarities of the horse that influence the choice and design of housing for health. Fortunately, the sanitary codes that require impervious flooring for dairy cattle do not apply to horses because concrete is perhaps the least desirable flooring material for the horse. Clay or a mixture of clay and sand covered with a bedding material of some sort is very good. Clean, bright straw makes a good absorbent bedding but some horses will eat it. This provides the opportunity for worm infestation when it is contaminated with manure but, more important, it takes the place of the nutritious hay which the horse needs. The horse which makes a habit of filling up on straw will gradually lose weight because the straw is high in fiber and low in both protein and digestible energy. For horses that eat straw bedding, something less palatable such as wood shavings can be used. Keep an eye on your horses bedded with shavings, though. Some of them out of curiosity will eat enough shavings to cause indigestion.

Accidents related to housing conditions are probably more common with horses than any other species. Horses tend to be quick in their movements and are more inclined, with a quick toss of the head, to break unprotected light bulbs or windows. This may cause serious lacerations. For the same reason the stalls and areas where they walk should be free from projecting nails or sharp protrusions of any kind. This also applies to the fencing around the exercise yard. The horse has a thin skin that cuts very easily. At best a laceration probably will leave a scar, at worst it may lead to tetanus and death. With a little care on the owner's part, this type of accident is easily preventable.

Cribbing

Some horses, out of boredom, develop a habit called *cribbing*, in which they will bite and chew on the edge of a board, and at the same time arch the neck and swallow air. This leads to indigestion, colic, an unthrifty horse, and an unsightly stall. To reduce this possibility, build or alter the stall so that insofar as possible there will be no edges to grab. Where an edge can't be prevented, such as the top edge of the gate or door, sheathing the top four to six inches with sheet metal will help.

Lastly, be sure the stall is strong enough so the horse can't kick a hole in it. This is more likely to happen when horses are kept in adjoining stalls. The average horse easily can kick a hole in a one-inch board and, in fact, can knock down a whole wall constructed of such light material. In so doing it is very likely to injure its legs. To avoid such injuries the lower four feet of the stall should be plank, preferably oak, two inches thick.

Hauling Horses

One more thing, although not directly related to housing, has bearing on it and that is the trailers and trucks used to haul horses. One of the factors contributing to the popularity of the horse is the ease of mobility using modern trailers. It's not at all unusual to put a horse in a trailer behind the family car and travel 100 miles to take part in a show and return the same day. **Before you load your horse in a vehicle be sure that vehicle is strong enough to carry the load.** I think the most pitiful sight I ever saw was a horse who had one foot fall through the rotted floor of a trailer. The foot was caught and dragged there until it was worn off by the pavement up to the coronet. All I could do was put the suffering horse to sleep, and I was sorely tempted to do the same with the owner. Such accidents are not bad luck. They are the result of carelessness and stupidity.

With regard to health and housing for the horse, perhaps the best rule of thumb to keep in mind is that what can go wrong probably will. Granted, horses shouldn't kick holes in the wall, get tangled in the wire or step in the hole, but sooner or later they do, and injury results. Perhaps because of the closeness that develops between horse and owner, we tend to attribute a measure of intelligence to them that is undeserved. When it comes to accidents, the behavior of the horse is perhaps the least predictable of the large domestic animals. It's up to us to foresee the potential hazards and eliminate them before accidents occur.

Swine

The nature of the beast and the business tends to make several aspects of swine housing unique from a health standpoint. Separation or isolation of susceptible individuals is a valid fundamental of disease control that must be compromised in the swine operation, first, because pigs come in litters rather than singly and, second, because profitable swine production is a high-volume business. To the hobbyist with only one or two pigs, this is less of a concern but even then the need for good sanitation and management prevails.

The housing needs of different age groups of pigs vary with the farrowing house being most critical. Because of the need for good sanitation, ventilation, and environmental temperature control, the commercial farrowing house is usually a specialized building used for that purpose only. In fact, it is possible to buy prefabricated farrowing houses that outwardly resemble mobile homes. When moved to the site and when utilities are connected, they are ready for operation. With liquid manure handling, forced ventilation, automatic feeders, electric heat, and other conveniences installed, these farrowing houses are a delight to behold, but baby pigs will die in them just as fast as anywhere else if you forget the basics of disease control.

Preventing Infection

Preventing spread of infection by separation of susceptible individuals is one of the basics of disease control. But how do you separate newborn pigs that come a dozen or more at a time and all have to nurse the same sow? Obviously modifications have to be made.

Two things are important. One is to prevent introduction of contagious disease, and as a part of this effort related to housing, a conspicuous sign on the door of the farrowing house asking visitors to stay out is helpful. Some swine diseases can be carried from farm to farm on clothing and equipment, in addition to those such as influenza which are shared by man and animals. The other thing that helps to cut down disease spread is scrupulous cleanliness in the farrowing house, paying particular attention to feeding equipment, floors, and farrowing crates. The risk of spreading disease will be reduced further if separate cleaning equipment, shovels, brooms, and buckets are kept in the farrowing house and not used anywhere else.

I recall some years ago being asked to investigate a long-standing problem of high baby pig mortality. For several years half or more of every litter born would be dead within a week, despite the use of all kinds of medication. Diarrhea, lack of appetite, weakness, and death were commonplace and a major contributing factor was obvious. The farrowing area was incredibly filthy, with sour feed in the troughs and manure not only built up on the floor but spattered to the ceiling. Ironically this was on a state prison farm where, considering the cost and availability of labor, the place should have been spotless. The manager simply didn't recognize the importance of sanitation and was an advocate of the popular fallacy that pigs are inherently dirty animals. Nothing could be further from the truth. **Given the opportunity, pigs will be as clean or cleaner than most other species.**

Protecting Baby Pigs

Apart from the need for good sanitation, there are some other specialized requirements in the farrowing house. One of these is heat in the colder climates. Baby pigs are born with virtually no hair and little if any body fat to insulate them from the cold. Chilling is a common cause of death. To prevent it, supplemental heat to provide a temperature of about 85–90°F at floor level is necessary for the first two or three days, after which it can be reduced gradually. Heat lamps are used for this purpose, but a word of caution is in order, especially if you use heat lamps on a temporary, makeshift basis. **Be sure the wiring is adequate to carry the load and be sure, too, that the lamps are far enough away from combustible bedding,** such as straw, so you don't end up with barbecued pigs instead of warm pigs. The ideal way to warm the floor is with hot water pipes or hot air ducts buried in the concrete.

Another consideration in the farrowing house is a means of protecting the baby pigs from their mother. A clumsy 300-pound sow lying down can flatten a two-pound piglet. This kind of accident happens too often, especially when the sow and piglets are in a pen or box stall. One way of reducing the risk when a pen is the only farrowing place available is to fasten a strong rail around the inside of the pen six inches out from the wall and about eight inches above the floor. This provides an avenue of escape for the piglet that might otherwise be crushed against the wall. A better device used almost universally by commercial hog producers is the **farrowing crate.** This is a steel framework which gives the sow freedom to eat, drink, stand, or lie down but keeps her in one place, reducing the opportunity for her to lie on the pigs. Except when nursing, the piglets will stay alongside the crate under the heat lamp or brooder, whichever is provided.

Every precaution must be taken to avoid introducing infectious diseases into the farrowing house. This begins with preparation of the sow. Sows should be immunized against the common diseases such as erysipelas and leptospirosis, of course. But beyond that they should be scrubbed thoroughly with soap and warm water before being put into the farrowing house. This removes dirt and manure that usually is teeming with bacteria and frequently with worm eggs as well. A preparation room adjacent to the farrowing house where washing can be done with a reasonable degree of convenience and comfort for both sow and operator, regardless of the weather, is a necessity for a farrowing operation of any size.

Farrowing House Floor

Some attention should be given to the farrowing house floor. Concrete is most satisfactory for ease of cleaning, but very smooth, slippery floors are a major contributing factor to the condition known as "spraddle-legged" pigs. New concrete should not be troweled smooth, nor should it be brushed to leave it rough because the roughness causes abrasions on the piglets' knees and legs. Once over with a wooden float is about right. If you are stuck with an existing facility that has a glass-smooth floor it can be mechanically roughened or you can use bedding on the floor. Some people use wooden floors successfully in the farrowing house, but they are difficult to clean and sanitize. However, they are warmer and more comfortable for the pigs.

Once the piglets are weaned, usually at four weeks of age, they can be separated from the sow and grouped together in another building. What happens to them thereafter depends on the type of swine operation. In some cases they will be sold as feeder pigs at about forty pounds body weight. In other cases they will be fed to market weight (200–220 pounds) on the original farm.

Vulnerable to Heat Stroke

In any event, housing for the older pigs is much less critical from a health standpoint as long as sanitation and ventilation are adequate. Inside temperatures should be above freezing, preferably about 50°F in winter and no warmer than outside air temperature in summer. The latter can be a major problem on a hot day. The body heat of a large number of pigs in a building dependent on forced ventilation can quickly raise the inside temperature well over 100°F on a summer day if the electric power goes off. Pigs have a dismal cooling system and are very vulnerable to heat stroke. Therefore, if you are operating a confinement raising system, a standby generator is a worthwhile investment.

One innovation that has made total confinement finishing systems practical has been the use of slotted floors and liquid manure handling systems. In these the pigs trample manure down through slots in the floor to a pit underneath. This eliminates the need for manure removal in the pens, greatly reducing the labor requirements. However, a means of ventilating the manure pit should be provided. As manure decomposes, methane gas is produced. It is highly explosive. In Iowa some years ago, a spark ignited methane in a manure pit and the resulting explosion blew finishing house and pigs sky high.

Sheep and Goats

One of the factors leading to the current popularity of the goat and one making sheep raising economically feasible is that housing requirements are minimal. Except for the very young, a good windbreak or shed to provide protection from severely inclement weather is all that is required. However, the dairy goats will produce a little more and it's certainly easier for the milker if they are housed in a stable in winter, but the health-related housing requirements are not unique.

Sheep require extra attention at lambing time, and a lambing shed in the North is a necessity not only for the comfort of the ewe but for the survival of the lambs. Sheep tend to be seasonal breeders and lambs are usually born in early spring when weather is likely to be the worst. The lambs are wet and often weak when born, so supplemental heat for a short period is usually a necessity. For the small flock, heat lamps are probably the most practical heat source. Check adequacy of wiring and proximity of combustible bedding. Don't set the shed on fire with them.

Cleanliness Essential

It's not unusual for ewes and sometimes does to require assistance when giving birth. This means that you will need clean warm water available to thoroughly scrub the vulva and surrounding area before putting a hand in to straighten out a twisted lamb or kid. And you will need water to clean yourself up after you get through. Cleanliness is absolutely essential to prevent uterine infection following lambing, and the clean-up job will be more thorough if the materials to do it are readily at hand. Therefore, a washroom with ample hot water available should be part of the lambing shed. I might add that you may find your veterinarian more responsive to a call for help with parturition problems if he knows you have a decent place where he can clean up before he goes on to the next call.

Summary

A few suggestions have been presented in this chapter that will help to prevent some of the housing-related health problems that veterinarians and livestock owners see. Keep in mind, however, that there is no one best system and that livestock housing frequently must be governed by circumstances unrelated to animal welfare.

But, regardless of the constraints imposed by finances or whatever, keep the comfort and safety of your animals uppermost in mind. **Be safety conscious!** Pick up the loose wire, junk, machinery, and other obstacles in the pasture. Pull out the projecting nails or other sharp objects in the barn where animals move. The injuries these cause are easily avoided if you look ahead and anticipate what might happen.

Above all, keep the animal quarters clean. All it takes is a little ambition and energy and if you don't have that, you shouldn't have animals. It's heartbreaking to see the conditions under which some people keep their livestock and the needless health problems this causes. If you have any doubt about the adequacy of your facilities, ask yourself this simple question, "Even if I had a fur coat, would I be comfortable living in there?" If the answer is no, some changes are in order.

Animal Reproduction

WHILE IT MAY SEEM STRANGE to include reproduction in a book on animal health, veterinarians get more questions about reproduction and infertility than any other single entity. And nothing else is more vital to a profitable livestock enterprise and the nutritional well-being of the world population. While we could survive without meat and milk, most of us would find vegetables and grain a rather dull diet. Furthermore, cattle, sheep, and goats can convert otherwise useless roughage into high quality protein and energy to supplement the world food supply so it's important that we keep them producing and reproducing.

Reproduction is truly a remarkable process that, for many people, is also a mystery. In the next few pages we will try to take some of the mystery out of it by describing the reproductive functions common to all species and then pointing out differences that make the various livestock species unique. At the risk of criticism from the women, I'll start with the male, the most important individual in livestock breeding (and often the most neglected). Why the most important? First, because the traits of the herd sire will appear in all the offspring in the herd whereas the dam will influence only her own progeny. Second, if the herd sire is sterile there will be no herd offspring. If the dam is infertile, she is the only one affected.

Male Anatomy

The primary sex glands of the male are the two **testicles.** During embryonic and fetal development the testicles are formed within the abdominal cavity. Just prior to or soon after birth they descend through the inguinal canal into an external pouch called the **scrotum.** Each has its own nerve and blood supply and a duct called the vas deferens connecting to the urethra. Spermatozoa are transported through the vas deferens and a section of it is removed in the sterilizing operation called a vasectomy. Occasionally one or both testicles fail to descend, leading to a condition called cryptorchidism. A cryptorchid animal will have the external sex characteristics of a male but will be sterile if the testicles are within the abdomen. If they are near the external inguinal ring the animal may or may not be fertile. If only one testicle is undescended, the animal will be fertile.

Cryptorchidism sometimes presents a dilemma when castration to control aggressive behavior or render the animal sterile is a consideration. Removal of only the descended testicle will not change behavior and may or may not make the animal sterile. But it greatly complicates the surgical procedure if a decision is made later to go in and find the other one because there is usually no way to tell which side it is on. Castration of the monorchid should be done completely the first time to avoid confusion later on. Castration of the cryptorchid is a major surgical procedure requiring general anesthesia and aseptic technique.

Two Functions

The testicles serve two primary functions. They are the source of the male hormone, **testosterone,** which gives the male his secondary sex characteristics, larger size, heavy shoulders, and deeper voice. It also influences aggressive behavior and sex drive or libido. The testicles also produce sperm cells or **spermatozoa** in a gradual developmental process called spermatogenesis. As the animal reaches sexual maturity, or puberty, mature sperm cells are produced constantly by the millions. Fertility of the male is governed primarily by the numbers of live sperm cells produced and libido. Sperm count is influenced by general health and frequency of ejaculation. It declines during prolonged illness, periods of fevers, and, strangely enough, periods of high environmental temperature.

Nature has provided a way to maintain the testicles at a temperature slightly below body temperature for maximum fertility. On a hot day, involuntary muscles relax, allowing the testicles to drop further from the body in the scrotum. Conversely, on a cold day they will be drawn close to the body wall. The "short scrotum" method of castrating bull calves destined for the feedlot capitalizes on this phenomenon. With this technique the testicles are left intact but the lower half of the scrotum is removed so that the testicles are held tightly against the body wall where the higher temperature inhibits spermatogenesis. The advantage claimed is that testosterone production continues, resulting in a larger animal with improved rate of gain.

The secondary sex organ of the male is the **penis.** It has a rich blood supply which becomes important in erection. The penis must be fully erect before copulation can occur. The mechanisms by which this occurs is a simple problem in hydraulics. Blood comes in under arterial pressure and returns, in part, through spongy cavernous tissue. When the animal is sexually aroused, the return blood flow is restricted by smooth muscle contraction. Pressure then builds in the cavernous tissue. The penis becomes extended, enlarges some in diameter, especially in the horse, and becomes rigid. This change is completely involuntary and cannot be controlled by the animal. It is the result of external sex stimuli such as sight and smell coupled with libido or sex drive. The latter is most marked in young animals and sometimes leads to aberrant behavior such as mounting other males or masturbation. With young healthy animals, except boars, libido is rarely absent. Some young boars, especially if exposed to an aggressive domineering sow, have to be taught what their function in life is.

Female Anatomy

While the anatomy and physiology of the male reproductive system is quite uncomplicated, that of the female is considerably more complex. This complexity probably accounts for infertility problems, which are more frequent in the female. The primary sex glands of the female are the two **ovaries** located, roughly, behind the kidneys and supported in the broad ligament attached to the uterus. Like the testicles, the ovaries serve a dual role, production of germ cells called **ova,** and hormones. Unlike the male where new sperm cells are constantly developing, the female is born with all the ova in her ovaries that she will ever have. They are released in a precisely orchestrated sequence of events controlled by several interacting hormones. This sequence is called the **estrous cycle** and although its length varies in different species, the events are the same.

The Estrous Cycle

The estrous cycle is initiated by a portion of the brain called the hypothalamus acting through the pituitary gland located at the base of the brain. The pituitary gland produces follicle-stimulating hormone (FSH). This hormone brings about the development of a **follicle** on the ovary. These normally occur singly in the mare and the cow but are multiple in the sow and are frequently in pairs in the ewe and doe. The follicle in the cow resembles a large blister on the surface of the ovary, and when mature will be about half the size of the ovary. The follicle contains an ovum and is lined with specialized cells that produce the estrogenic hormones, estrone and estradiol. These hormones have a twofold effect. In animals they bring about the period of sexual desire called **estrum** or **heat,** and they initiate changes in the cellular lining of the uterus to prepare it for attachment of a fertilized ovum.

Through a feedback mechanism, as estrogen levels peak and the follicle reaches maturity, further production of FSH is inhibited and in its place, luteinizing hormone (LH) is produced by the pituitary. LH brings about rupture of the follicle, release of the ovum, and counteracts estrogen to terminate signs of heat. It also initiates development of a corpus luteum or yellow body at the site of the ruptured follicle. The corpus luteum, through its production of progesterone, plays an essential role in the attachment and maintenance of the fertilized ovum. It also overrides or counteracts further FSH production temporarily. If the animal becomes pregnant, additional progesterone is produced by the placenta that prevents resumption of the estrus cycle for the duration of the pregnancy. If pregnancy does not occur, FSH levels again increase and the entire cycle is repeated.

A Complex Process

Numerous physiological changes take place during the estrous cycle that we haven't yet mentioned. To give the reader an appreciation of the complexity of the reproductive process some of these will be mentioned in the sequence of the estrous cycle segments:

Proestrum — the period during which the follicle is enlarging. Concurrently there is an increase in the growth of cells and cilia lining the oviduct, in the blood supply to the uterine lining (endometrium), and in the amount of mucus produced in the vagina. In the sow, the vulva swells slightly and in all species there is increased muscular activity of the oviduct and uterus. Estrogen levels are increasing and the corpus luteum from the previous cycle is rapidly getting smaller.

Estrum — the period during which the female is receptive to the male and will stand to be mounted. The uterus is contracted, the cervix is dilated, and mucus in the vagina is copious. Ovulation or release of the ovum occurs soon after the period of estrum.

Diestrum — a period of several days during which the corpus luteum is developing and producing progesterone. This hormone brings about what might best be described as a return to the status quo. The estrogen level drops rapidly and the uterus becomes soft and relaxed. In the cow there may be some capillary bleeding from the endometrium with blood visible at the vulva or on the tail about 48–72 hours after signs of estrum have passed. This can be a very useful indicator of the stage of estrous. Some cows, especially high-producing ones, do not show strong signs of heat and it's difficult to know when to breed them. If you see blood on the tail you know a heat period has just passed. About half of them will conceive if you breed them artificially eighteen days later whether they show signs of heat or not.

Anestrum — best described as a resting place during which little uterine or ovarian activity takes place. Anestrum is prolonged in the mare during the late fall and early winter and in the ewe and doe during the late spring and summer. These species are called **seasonally polyestrous,** since they cycle seasonally. The cow and the sow on the other hand cycle the year around and are called **polyestrous.** The mare is polyestrous except in late fall and early winter.

While the foregoing discussion has outlined the principal hormonal activity and its effects in the female, the thyroid and adrenal glands play a role as well. Other factors are important, too. An animal that is well fed will reach sexual maturity earlier and will cycle regularly. Those whose energy intake is low often fail to cycle. **As a general rule of thumb, fertility will be best when the animal is in a weight-gaining condition.** But this, of course, can be carried to an extreme and obesity is also a cause of infertility.

Sight, sound, and smell play a less well-defined role, but it is well known that putting a boar near a pen of gilts or a stallion near a mare will often initiate signs of heat. Hours of daylight influence the onset of the estrous cycle in the mare and the use of artificial light will often advance the time of first estrum in the spring. Extremes of temperature, especially heat, induce a stress that interferes with reproduction and is a major problem for dairy farmers in southern climates. With so many factors involved in the estrous cycle alone, it's remarkable that reproductive failures are not more frequent.

Conception

Assuming all systems are functioning normally, the follicle ruptures, marking the end of estrus or standing heat, and the ovum is released. It is trapped in the open, fimbriated end of the oviduct and is worked down in the oviduct toward the horns of the uterus. The oviduct is a tubelike structure (about the diameter of a pencil lead in the cow) that leads from the ovary to the tip of the uterine horn. It is lined with ciliated cells and mucus-producing cells whose action and secretion help move the ovum to its final destination in the uterus. The trip requires about three days in the sow and five in the other domestic species.

The **uterus** is a "Y"-shaped organ in domestic animals consisting of two horns and a body. It has a capacity for tremendous distention during advanced pregnancy and a very rapid return to normal size following birth of the fetus. The normal nonpregnant uterus in the cow and mare can easily be held in both hands and is proportionately smaller in other species. It has a rich blood supply and a cellular lining, the endometrium, that responds to hormonal influence. The fertilized ovum develops to maturity in the uterus. The uterus is separated from the vagina by the **cervix,** a firm muscular band that during pregnancy remains tightly closed. It relaxes slightly during estrus and during parturition dilates to a point where it is almost imperceptible. Incomplete dilation makes parturition difficult, if not impossible, and may lead to tears or lacerations which occasionally cause complications such as scar tissue or incomplete closure which impairs subsequent fertility. The cervix opens into the vagina, which in turn is open to the outside world at the vulva.

Copulation

During copulation the male mounts the female and thrusts the erect penis into the vagina, a process called **intromission.** Intromission, or copulation, terminates with ejaculation of semen at the cervical opening. The female seeks out, and in fact will tolerate, this procedure only during the period of estrum or standing heat. Depending on the libido of the male, copulation will take place several times during the heat period. Frequency, duration of coitus, and volume of ejaculate vary with different species. Keep in mind, though, that simply because the male goes through the right motions doesn't mean he is fertile. He can look and act entirely normal and be sterile. **For that reason,** test matings or fertility examination of the male prior to the breeding season is a good investment.

Sperm cells have the capacity of independent movement with the aid of a long tail or **flagellum** that swishes back and forth to propel them through the copious mucus which is always present during estrum. This, coupled with capillary action and muscular contractions in the uterus and oviducts, transport spermatozoa through the genital tract quite rapidly. Bovine spermatozoa have been found at the ovarian end of the oviduct two to four minutes after deposition at the cervix. Despite this rapid transport, attrition of spermatozoa enroute is high. Although millions are deposited during ejaculation only a few hundred get into the oviduct where fertilization takes place and they rarely remain viable more than twenty-four hours. Similarly, the fertile life of ova is short — only about twelve hours. Timing of the mating, therefore, becomes very critical except, of course, when the animals are left to their own devices and nature takes its course. Then repeated copulation removes the element of timing chance.

Fertilization

Only one active sperm cell is necessary for fertilization to take place, but it must be at the right place at the right time. With frequent natural breeding during the heat period, spermatozoa will be in the oviduct at the time of ovulation, but with artificial insemination, the timing may not be as precise, leading to conception failures. Fertilization takes place in the oviduct, at which time a single sperm cell will penetrate the ovum and all others will be blocked out.

Each germ cell, sperm and ovum, contains half the normal complement of chromosomes for the species. The cow, for example, has 60 pairs of chromosomes. Each chromosome contains the genes that determine the physical characteristics of the offspring. At fertilization, these combine in a random manner so that no two offspring of the same mating will be identical but each will have some of the characteristics of both parents. Cell division commences immediately following fertilization and about three to five days later the aggregation of cells, at this time called a zygote, arrives in the uterus. At this point the corpus luteum has formed and progesterone from it has brought about the changes in the uterine lining necessary for attachment and further development of the embryo.

In animals such as the pig, a dozen or more ova are fertilized at the same time but otherwise the process is the same. As a matter of interest, if the sow is bred to more than one boar during the heat period, as is commonly done, spermatozoa from different boars will fertilize different ova so that the piglets, although born at the same time, will be half-brothers or half-sisters genetically related to each other only on the sow's side.

Twinning

In animals such as the mare and cow that normally have single births, twinning, if it is going to occur, is determined at this time. Twins can form in two different ways. The most common is when two ova are released from the ovary and fertilized. In this case the twins will not be identical since there is a different combination of genes in each zygote. Identical twins result when a fertilized ovum divides into two independent cells that then continue to develop in the normal manner. While identical twins may be considered a developmental accident, there is some hereditary predisposition to multiple ovulation in some individuals and families.

In uniparous animals (having a single offspring) the embryo develops in the uterine horn on the same side where ovulation occurred, whereas in multiparous species such as the pig, the zygotes will be spaced throughout both uterine horns. Development of the zygote to an embryo is by cell division and differentiation. Without going into all the details of embryology, suffice to say that different cell types form that develop into muscle, bone, nerve, tissue, and so on, in a coherent manner that ultimately terminates in a functional animal at the time of birth. Occasionally, cellular differentiation and organization gets disorganized, resulting in a fetal monster. This can be caused by some chemicals and poisonous plants.

Some of these cells become the **placenta,** a membranous three-layered sac within which the fetus develops. It is attached to the uterine wall and is filled with fluid. On the fetal side, it is, for descriptive purposes, an outgrowth of the umbilical cord. The umbilical blood vessels branch out through it to the point of uterine attachment. The type of attachment varies in different species from 60–70 isolated structures called cotyledons in ruminants, to complete attachment called diffuse placentation in the pig. Function is the same in any case and it is through the placenta that the fetus gets nutrients from the dam and eliminates the waste products of cell metabolism. **There is no direct interchange of blood between the dam and the fetus,** the only exception being when as a result of rare injury there is some bleeding from the uterine lining. The placenta is a very important structure for the well-being of the fetus, and anything that disrupts it may result in abortion. It is a common site of infection by bacteria, viruses, and fungi. Diseases causing abortion, such as brucellosis, affect the placenta primarily.

Rate of Growth

Because fetal development takes place by cell division in geometric progression, rate of growth accelerates throughout gestation with the greatest increase in size coming during the last third of pregnancy. Allowance must be made for this in the feeding program or the dam will lose weight during late pregnancy. It's a marvel of nature that with an inadequate diet the pregnant animal will utilize all her stored reserves of energy, protein, vitamins, and minerals for fetal nourishment at her own expense and can be at the verge of death from starvation before any adverse changes in the fetus occurs. This is not as true in humans, where protein deficiency in the maternal diet has been linked to some types of mental retardation in the newborn.

When all goes according to plan, pregnancy terminates in parturition or birth of the young. This is often a time of anxiety for the novice animal owner but it need not be if you know what to expect and are prepared. The most elementary thing is to note the date of breeding so you know when to expect parturition. Although the length of the gestation period is not always precise, it does fall within a narrow range of days, so you shouldn't be taken by surprise.

TABLE 4-1

Gestation Periods

Species	Average Gestation Period
Cow	280 days
Mare	340 days
Sow	114 days
Ewe	145 days
Doe	150 days

In all species there will be some premonitory signs of impending parturition. A few days before, the udder begins to get distended with milk. The ligaments around the tailhead will relax to give a sunken appearance, although this may not be noticeable in swine. Concurrently, the vulva may become distended and relaxed and some sticky tenacious mucus may appear. Just before labor begins the animal may be restless, may seek out an isolated area, and may refuse feed. Of course, with animals such as sheep that are pasture bred and kept in flocks, these signs usually will not be observed even though they occur. That's why it's advisable to pen them up in a lambing shed about 140 days after the ram is put into the flock.

Most, but not all, animals will lie down when giving birth. In fact, as the onset of labor begins, they may act very restless, getting up and down several times before getting on with the business at hand.

The Birth Process

Normally, the young will be born front feet first, followed by the head and shoulders. The placenta usually will appear first and, since it is filled with fluid, it exerts a cushioning effect as it is forced against the cervix by uterine contractions. This helps to dilate the cervix and as the feet and nose follow along, the cervix is dilated even further to permit birth of the animal. As the feet enter the vagina, strong abdominal contractions begin that hasten the whole process. As the intensity of contractions increases, the placenta frequently ruptures, releasing its fluid contents. This is not a cause for concern when everything else is normal and, in fact, helps to lubricate the birth canal. The duration of labor is generally longer in animals giving birth for the first time and varies considerably in different species, ranging from as little as fifteen minutes in the mare to six to eight hours in the sow until the last piglet is born.

Is Assistance Needed?

People frequently ask if it's necessary to assist an animal giving birth by pulling on the fetus. Generally speaking, assuming the dam is healthy and the presentation is normal, the answer is no. Millions of animals have been born without help, and forced extraction of the fetus may actually precipitate the complication of retained placenta. But the decision when to intervene is a matter of judgment that improves with experience. The cow that labors over an hour with the front feet and nose of the calf showing and no signs of further progress would certainly appreciate a little help. The cow that labors over an hour with nothing showing obviously needs help.

With the front feet showing and the head started, it's a simple matter to apply traction by pulling on the front legs of the calf. That traction should be gentle, however, and should coincide with abdominal contractions. This is not a time for brute strength and determination. I have seen dairy farmers go at the job as if it had to be done right now at all costs, even to the point, one time, of hooking a tractor to the calf and trying to pull it out. Such brutality is uncalled for and frequently results in a dead calf and a paralyzed cow.

Assuming the presentation is normal and the feet are out where you can reach them, there is no reason why you cannot give the animal some help if necessary. But, remember that presentations are not always normal and that's when your veterinarian should be called. If labor continues more than an hour, it's quite possible that the presentation is something other than normal and the possibilities are numerous and often quite difficult to handle. For that reason, these are best left to a person with training, experience, and the equipment to handle the situation. The drawings on pages 70–71 illustrate some of the unusual positions the fetus can be in. In all species the **anterior,** front feet first, presentation is normal and most common. The next most common is the **posterior** or hind feet first position, and it's easy to tell the two apart even if the head isn't visible. If the soles of the feet are on the down side toward the dam's feet, the presentation is anterior; if they are up toward the dam's tail, the presentation is posterior. While this rule of thumb is not infallible, it is true at least 99 percent of the time and it's helpful early in the game to know what kind of problem you may be getting into so you can make an early decision whether to call your veterinarian. He can do you more good at the early stages than after you have struggled with the situation for a couple of hours, exhausting yourself and the dam. Those of us in practice encounter this circumstance all too often and the end result is usually a dead fetus, sometimes a dead dam, and always short tempers all the way around, especially when the owner gets the bill for what has unnecessarily become a salvage operation.

How to Help

But if it's a normal anterior presentation with only a little added traction necessary you can handle it. You will find the legs slippery to handle and, in the larger species, attaching a clean rope or, better yet, an obstetrical chain makes the job easier. Be sure that this is placed above the fetlock joint. If it's attached lower it may slide off when you pull, tearing the hoof wall. The direction of pull should be outward and downward, coinciding with the dam's abdominal straining. Having an assistant rotate the fetus slightly back and forth each way on its longitudinal axis at the same time will often facilitate matters. The dam's pelvic canal is longer in the vertical axis than the horizontal; therefore the fetus must be in the vertical position with its backbone next to the dam's.

There may be times when, for whatever reason, you can't get a veterinarian to help with a complicated delivery. For those in this unenviable circumstance, the following will be a little guidance. But, I hasten to add, whenever possible **get a veterinarian to help with the complicated cases** because the outcome is likely to be far better.

Cleanliness is very important when assisting with a delivery. The uterus is very susceptible to infection, especially following the trauma of birth. The first step is to get the dam on her feet and then thoroughly scrub the vulvar area with soap and water and do the same with your hands and arms. Next, lubricate one hand thoroughly using soap solution or, if available, a neutral lubricant such as K-Y jelly or even mineral oil.

Gently put your hand in the vagina and try to ascertain what is wrong. If the cervix is not dilated, just wait awhile longer and try again. But any number of other malpresentations may be encountered. Before delivery can be accomplished, the fetus must be in the anterior or posterior position.

In attempting to correct malposition it might be useful to list what can't be done so you don't waste time trying.
- You can't change a posterior to an anterior presentation or vice versa — there isn't room.
- You can't deliver an anterior presentation unless both legs and the head are started through the cervix. Sometimes only the legs come through

and the head turns to the side. The head must be straightened around before the fetus can be delivered.

- You can't make a delivery when three or more legs are through the cervix. They may all be from the same fetus or from two. In any event, the proper two legs have to be sorted out and the other pushed back out of the way.
- Only rarely can you deliver a fetus when just the head is through the cervix. It must be pushed back and the forelegs brought through first. If the head is swollen, and it usually is in this case, it frequently must first be amputated to make room to get the legs through.
- Another impossible situation seen more commonly in the sow is when the fetus lies across the cervix and extends into both uterine horns. It must first be slid one way or the other to place it in an anterior or posterior position before it can be delivered. With limited space available this is easier said than done.

In fact, none of these procedures is as easy as it may sound. In all animals, space is limited and in the mare and cow you may be working at the limit of your reach. Also, your arm in the vagina stimulates the animal's straining reflex and working conditions are not the best, to say the least. Add to this that with an animal that can't get up, you, too, may have to lie on your belly to reach as far as necessary. I think you can visualize a difficult situation.

Torsion of Uterus

The last impossible situation, encountered most frequently in the cow, ewe, and doe, is **torsion of the uterus.** This condition is simply an accident in which the uterus becomes twisted on its long axis. The end result is analogous to a bag, the opening of which has been twisted until it is partially or completely closed. A 180° rotation is most common and it is enough to constrict the cervical opening so that birth cannot occur until the twist is reversed. The diagnosis is not difficult but correction sometimes is. Generally, with a uterine torsion the early signs of parturition, restlessness, perineal relaxation, and leaking milk, will appear but the state of true labor will not and, in fact, in a few hours the animal may act entirely normal again — but this is transitory. A uterine torsion, if uncorrected, will ultimately lead to death. When the hand is placed in the vagina, spiral folds reflecting the direction of the twist can usually be felt.

Two methods commonly are used to correct a torsion. If it's only a partial torsion and one or two feet can be reached, it is often possible to rotate the fetus longitudinally in a direction opposite from the twist. The uterus will rotate along with the fetus to relieve the condition. The other method is to roll the entire animal sideways in a direction opposite from the twist. If the animal is rolled fast enough, inertia will hold the uterus in place long enough so that the twist unwinds.

Anterior presentation, forelegs flexed. For delivery, the head must be pushed back and the legs pulled to an extended position.

Anterior position, hind legs in the pelvic canal. Hind legs must be pushed back out of the pelvic canal while maintaining traction on the forelegs.

Normal anterior position.

Anterior position, one foreleg retained. Head and foreleg must be pushed back while retained leg is flexed and brought into position.

Head deviated to the side. Push forelegs back to get room and bring the head into position.

Head deviated ventrally. Push head and shoulders back and bring head up into position.

Anterior position, head and neck deviated to the side. Head must be brought into the pelvic canal. Difficult to handle. Sometimes requires fetotomy or Caesarian section.

Breech position. While applying forward pressure to the rump, bring the hind legs into the pelvic canal.

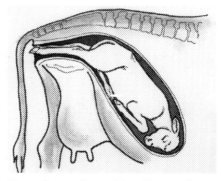

Posterior position, one leg retained. Push forward on the leg presented and bring the retained leg into position.

Normal posterior position. Frequently requires traction for delivery.

Anterior position, fetus upside down. Rotate 180° and the normal delivery follows.

Anterior position, head and legs flexed. Rotate 180°, bring head and front legs into pelvic canal for normal delivery.

A modification makes this somewhat more successful in the cow. If, for example, the cow needs to be rolled on her right, lay her on her right side (see the chapter on restraint) and place one end of an eight-foot plank on her belly with the other end on the ground to her left. Have an assistant stand on the plank. This helps to hold the uterus in place. Then roll the cow over quickly. It may be necessary to repeat this several times but re-examine the cow each time first or you may overdo it. If neither technique succeeds, a Caesarian section is the only recourse. In the ewe and doe, with less weight to move, torsions can usually be corrected manually.

While there is much satisfaction to be derived from successful correction of a difficult birth (dystocia), in the large animals it is physically hard work that can be exhausting. Occasionally a dystocia may be such that the fetus cannot be manipulated to accomplish a normal delivery. When this is the case there are only two alternatives. One is a **fetotomy** in which the fetus is cut up and removed piece by piece; the other is a **Caesarian section.** Either technique is a job for the veterinary surgeon.

Except for the impossible situations described, correction of a malpresentation is mainly a matter of mechanics, common sense, and hard work. **Remember to be clean and be gentle.** Not only is the fetus delicate, but the uterine wall is thin in advanced pregnancy and lacerates easily. Small tears may cause enough hemorrhage to be fatal, but even without that complication, peritonitis and death may result. So be careful in straightening out a fetus and in the application of traction when necessary. And, if at all possible, get veterinary help for the complicated cases, especially for the mare. They are in a class by themselves when it comes to complications but fortunately they have complications less frequently than other species.

The Offspring

Immediately following parturition there is a second animal to contend with and what you do in the few minutes after birth may determine whether the offspring lives or dies. Remember that up until the moment of birth the young animal was in a completely protected aquatic environment at a constant temperature, well protected from infection and totally dependent on its mother for survival. Consider the stress to which the newborn is subjected! It is pushed and squeezed through a very narrow opening and at the moment it reaches the outside world, depending on where and when it is born, the environmental temperature may be 100°F lower. At the same time it is cut loose from oxygen via the umbilical blood supply and immediately must begin to breathe.

Care of the Newborn

Normally, the dam will lick the newborn vigorously after birth to help dry it and stimulate respiration. This is instinctive in animals with good "mothering" ability but sometimes they are either physically unable to or simply will ignore their offspring. I have seen young heifers and ewes that actually seem to be afraid of their first-born. In any event what they can't or won't do you may have to do if the newborn animal is to survive. First, be sure all the mucus and fluid is out of the nostrils so the airway is clear. If a lot of mucus is present, suspending the animal by the rear legs for a few minutes may help drain it out. Tickling the nostrils with a straw initiates sneezing which also helps. Once the air passages are clear the animal will usually breathe on its own, but rubbing it vigorously with a cloth will help the process and at the same time dry the animal so it can better withstand the temperature change.

Once breathing is established, the next step is to dip the navel in tincture of iodine. It should be literally dipped rather than just swabbing some on the outside. This has two purposes. It kills any bacteria present, which could travel up the umbilical vessels to establish a septicemic infection, and the astringent action of the alcohol in tincture of iodine helps to close the ends of the umbilical vessels so bacteria can't enter. Frequently with horses and less frequently with other species, the umbilical vessels don't rupture at birth. When this happens, wait a few minutes to let the foal recover as much blood as possible from the placenta, then tie the cord and cut it.

Colostrum

By the time all this has been done, the animal is usually strong enough to stand and be introduced to the dairy bar for its first meal of colostrum, important in establishing disease immunity as well as for nutrition, as explained in the Chapter 1. If for any reason the animal doesn't nurse during the first hour, colostrum should be milked from the dam by hand and fed to the newborn. This will do much to insure that the newborn animal survives the rigors of the outside world.

The importance of animal reproduction has fostered intensive research throughout the world. This has been highly successful and new knowledge is still being gained, much of it applicable to human reproduction as well.

Artificial Insemination

Perhaps the single most important development in animal reproduction has been the technique of **artificial insemination.** While used to some degree in all species, it has thus far found greatest application in dairy cattle. Over half the dairy cattle in the United States are now bred to bulls they never see. With this technique, semen from a single ejaculate is collected and extended with a diluent usually about a hundred times. Thus instead of siring a single calf per ejaculation, the bull can sire a hundred. The genetic advantages are obvious. Bulls with superior milk production transmitting capability or conformation can now sire thousands more calves than they could by natural service. In fact, the average sire in A.I. service produces 40,000 breeding units annually and some go as high as 60,000. Economically, it means the individual dairy farmer can have the use of superior sires that he could never otherwise afford. For the person with a small herd, it is cheaper now to breed cows artificially than it is to keep a bull. The technique has proven so successful that there are many companies and cooperatives whose sole business is the production of high quality semen from superior sires for use on the farm by their own technicians on a fee basis or for direct sale to the farmer who wants to do his own insemination.

Although genetic improvement and economics are important advantages for artificial insemination, disease control is equally important. Bulls in the A.I. studs are not put into service until they have had extensive examinations to be sure they are free of contagious diseases, especially venereal diseases such as trichomoniasis. Similarly, every batch of semen is carefully evaluated and then standardized for number of spermatozoa. And their genetic potential is proven by test matings before their semen is offered for sale. When all things are considered, the advantages of artificial insemination are substantial.

Although the technique is feasible in other species, it has not been as widely accepted as it has for dairy cattle. It is being done more frequently in swine and beef cattle but the need for individual handling increases the labor requirement, thus reducing the economic advantage. Conception rates in mares bred artificially are somewhat less than in cattle and the extended semen is not as stable. But it's probable that additional research could overcome this deficiency if there were sufficient demand. However, the concept has not been accepted enthusiastically by the industry. When top stallions can command stud fees of $10,000 or more it isn't hard to see why.

Initially, extended bovine semen was stored and used in a liquid state and its life was limited. Further research led to techniques for freezing it and semen stored in liquid nitrogen remains viable for years. In fact, calves are being born today from sires long since dead. Frozen semen is regularly being shipped now to all parts of the world.

Technique Not Difficult

The technique of inseminating cows is not difficult, although proficiency certainly improves with practice. Most of the A.I. organizations conduct periodic training schools for farmers who want to do their own insemination. Although artificial insemination has advantages, it does place an added burden on management. Because the cows are usually inseminated only once, timing becomes critical so that sperm and ova meet at the right time. In the absence of a bull, heat detection is a major problem for the dairy farmer and more time must be devoted to watching the herd for signs of heat.

Planned Matings

Research has led to another significant development that is a useful management tool. Sometimes it is desirable to plan matings within a short time period. By feeding synthetic progesterone to a group of females it is possible to synchronize their estrous cycles so that all of them will come in heat about forty-eight hours after the drug is withdrawn. I had the opportunity as a practitioner years ago to participate in some of the early clinical trials of this technique and I'll never forget the sight of about 400 beef cows in heat at the same time. It was like a three-ring circus.

The same technique is applicable to other species and, as a matter of interest, forms the basis for the oral contraceptives used by women. Heat synchronization is most applicable in special situations where it is desirable either to shorten the breeding season such as breeding range cattle by artificial insemination or to have all offspring born within a short space of time. Needless to say, where large numbers of females are in heat at the same time, artificial insemination is a must.

More recent endocrine research has centered on the effect of a unique class of compounds called **prostaglandins.** Prostaglandin $F_2\alpha$ will reliably induce ovulation about forty-eight hours after administration to animals that are cycling normally. Its use is most applicable where a precisely timed mating is desirable. Neither technique will correct major infertility problems.

Embryo Transfer

The success of artificial insemination, particularly with the advent of frozen semen, has had a major impact not only on the economics of animal husbandry but also on genetic improvement of livestock. But the rate of improvement was limited by the length of the gestation period because, even though bred to a superior sire, a cow still could have only one calf per year.

Improvement in the technique and reliability of embryo transfer during the 1980s brought about change that would have been considered science fiction not many years before. Transferable embryos are obtained by inducing the donor animal to superovulate through the use of hormones. The many ova that are released are then fertilized by artificial insemination. At the same time, recipient or surrogate animals are given hormones to synchronize their estrus cycles with that of the donor.

Fertilized ova (embryos), generally five or six in each cow, are collected by flushing them from the uterus of the donor cow. They are then examined microscopically for viability and, if satisfactory, are transferred to the surrogate or frozen in liquid nitrogen for transfer at a later time. This technique is being used in all livestock species although swine embryos do not withstand freezing well. The technique is not widely used in horses because the major breed associations don't favor it, just as they oppose artificial insemination. With the technique of embryo transfer, genetic improvement of the breed can proceed more rapidly than before. A single cow, for example, could theoretically produce 25–30 calves per year. Obviously, the technique requires specialized skills and is not inexpensive but costs are coming down and the procedure is being more widely used.

With the ability to examine living embryos in vitro well established, related procedures are on the horizon that present some potentially frightening prospects. For example, using microsurgery it is possible now to split a single embryo into two, producing identical twins. It's conceivable then that one of these embryos could be stored frozen and later transferred to its twin, so that a cow could give birth to her genetically identical twin. And if one embryo can be divided into two it won't be long before two will become four, four eight, and so on. Perhaps in the 21st century, we will see entire herds of genetically identical animals (clones).

A bit further down the road, but not far, is the application of gene splicing techniques to determine the sex of the embryo and, by modifying its genetic make-up, to "engineer" an animal more suited for a particular purpose. Perhaps we can remove genetic weaknesses and genetically add disease resistance to create a more healthy and productive animal. These achievements are all possible but they must be produced by responsible scientists with due regard for the welfare of the species as a whole.

To this point, we have been discussing embryo transfer in animals but what is truly frightening is that the same techniques are applicable to the human species. It was reported in 1993 for example that a group of British scientists propagated cloned human embryos *in vitro* to the 60 cell stage before allowing them to die. Think what a moral and ethical dilemma this type of research presents!

Let's look now at some of the reproduction characteristics that make the various species unique.

Cattle

Cows are polyestrous, normally coming into heat or estrus every twenty-one days from the onset of puberty. Some individuals will have estrous cycles a couple days shorter or a few days longer but as long as the cycle is consistent it doesn't matter. Onset of puberty in the heifer is governed more by physical size than chronological age. Well-fed, rapidly growing animals may show signs of heat as early as four months of age. Conversely, those grown on a marginal diet may not come into heat until they are almost two years old. Young bulls will show signs of sexual activity at four months and are usually fertile at six months. They certainly should be separated from the females by that time.

When to Breed

Since calving difficulties are inversely proportional to size, heifers should not be bred until they are big enough, but should be bred when they reach optimal weight. Proper breeding weight varies with the breed, but 800 pounds is considered the optimum for Holsteins, with others in proportion. Holstein heifers should reach 800 pounds at about fifteen months of age and, given an adequate diet, will continue to grow during pregnancy until they reach their definitive weight. The gestation period of the cow is 280 days, so heifers bred at fifteen months will calve at two years old.

There is great controversy over the merit of breeding heifers to bulls of smaller breeds to yield a small calf the first time so that there are fewer calving complications. Geneticists argue that this causes a wasteful lose of genetic potential since the resulting crossbred offspring have limited value for milk production. Most veterinarians, myself included, who have seen too many good heifers injured by oversized calves will argue that the loss of any genetic potential is more than offset by the reduced injury or death loss at calving time and the increased milk production during the first lactation as a result of less calving stress. It's the breeder's choice, but fewer calving complications occur when dairy heifers are bred to beef bulls such as Aberdeen Angus, and when beef-type heifers are bred only when they are big enough or to bulls of smaller breeds.

Changes in Behavior

Signs of impending estrum in the bovine are generally marked by well-defined behavioral change. The lactating cow may have a transitory decline in production lasting about a day. Concurrently there will be restlessness, occasionally bawling, and usually some clear mucus discharge from the vulva. The most definitive sign is standing to be mounted by other cows, the period of standing heat. When a bull is placed with a cow in standing heat there is very little foreplay involved. The bull will usually sniff the vulva once or twice, curling his upper lip in a very characteristic manner. Smell seems to increase libido and the bull very quickly gets an erection and mounts the cow. The whole procedure is accomplished very quickly and the interval between intromission and ejaculation averages about seven seconds. Depending on the vigor of the bull, ejaculation occurs at the moment of a violent thrust during which the bull's hind feet actually leave the ground. It's important, therefore, that the bull and cow have good footing during copulation. Heavy bulls can easily knock down a small cow or heifer during breeding. Similarly if they slip, injury may result, making them useless for further service. To avoid injury, mating should not take place on a slippery floor.

Using a Breeding Rack

When a heavy bull must be used on a small heifer or cow, the use of a breeding rack is advisable. This is basically a stanchion in which the cow is placed that on each side has a strong plank extending from the stanchion frame at the level of the cow's shoulders back to the ground at her hind feet. When the bull mounts, his weight is supported by his front legs on the plank rather than by putting all his weight on the cow. The risk of injury can be eliminated entirely, of course, by artificial insemination. More will be said about that later.

Intromission terminates in ejaculation of 3–10 cc. of semen containing up to a billion spermatozoa. Volume and concentration declines somewhat with frequency of mating. Copulation will usually occur several times during the heat period. For that reason if a single bull is turned out with a herd at pasture and several cows come in heat the same day, conception rates may be lower than anticipated. Controlled mating, sometimes called hand breeding, will conserve bull power and generally yield higher first service conception rates.

Keep Good Records

For good breeding efficiency, it's vitally important that records be kept of dates of heat periods, breeding, and calving. In addition, all cows should be examined by a veterinarian about thirty days after calving to be sure the uterus is normal and no infection is present, and this should be a part of the record. Examination of the ovaries at the same time will indicate whether the cow is cycling normally, as she should be at this time. Most cows begin to cycle two to three weeks after calving although they may not show standing heat. Examination at thirty days allows time for correction of any abnormalities before sixty days post-calving, which experience shows is about the best time to breed the cow again.

All this information should be recorded for each individual in the herd. A variety of commercially prepared forms is available for the purpose, but human nature considered, the simplest is the most likely to be used. Reproduced here (Figure 1) is a facsimile of a simple individual health and breeding record. It is based on one used by the author and further refined in collaboration with the late Professor A.M. Meek in the Department of Animal Science at Cornell University. These 5-inch X 8-inch cards are available at nominal cost from that department and well over half a million of them are currently in use. A binder is available that holds the cards in an overlapping manner so that the names or numbers of up to ten cows can be seen at a glance.

The front has space for the identifying name and number of the individual cow, her sire and dam, and the dates of vaccination for the more common diseases. Dates are important for vaccines such as leptospirosis, which must be repeated annually. The remainder of the front has space for five years of breeding history in columnar form.

| Reg. Name and Number | Ragapple Annie | 516280 |

Birth Date 1-1-75
Sire Big Apple
Dam Maude
R. Ear Tag 21AN2146
L. Ear Tag CY31850
Purchase Date 3-1-75
Purchase From
John Doe

VACCINATION DATE
Brucel-
losis 3-15-75

Lepto-
spirosis 6-15-75

I.B.R. 6-15-75

B.V.D. 6-15-75

Other

Barn Name or Number
98

BREEDING HISTORY

YEAR	1976	Sire	1977	Sire		Sire		Sire		Sire
Jan.			30							
Feb.	28		20							
Mar.	20		(13)	1005						
Apr.	(11)	1153								
May										
June										
July										
Aug.										
Sept.										
Oct.										
Nov										
Dec.										
Date Due	12/26									
Date Fresh	1/1/77									

GENITAL EXAMINATIONS | **GENERAL HEALTH RECORD**

Date	Cervix	Uterus	Right Ovary	Left Ovary	Breeding Date or Treatment	Date	
1/1/76	N	N	CL	N			

Produced by Animal Science Extension, Cornell University, Ithaca, New York

Figure 1. Health and breeding record, front (top) and back (bottom).

To illustrate how the cards are used, the example Ragapple Annie was born on New Year's Day, 1975 and purchased from John Doe on March 1 of that year. She was vaccinated on the dates indicated and was observed to be in heat on February 28, 1976, and again twenty days later. Her next heat period was on April 11 at which time she was bred to bull number 1153. Breeding is indicated by circling the date. She was examined for pregnancy by a veterinarian fifty days later and found to be pregnant. Her due date was recorded as 12/26/76 and she actually calved on 1/1/77. Due date is not entered until the pregnancy is confirmed. She came in heat again on January 30 and the condition of her reproductive tract was determined by veterinary examination on February 3. The cervix, uterus, and ovaries were found to be normal with a corpus luteum (C.L.) on the right ovary. Her next heat periods were on February 20 and March 13, at which time she was again bred. If any abnormalities had been found at the time of post-calving examination, these would have been noted together with treatment given. Similarly, if she had failed to show a heat period after February 3, 1977, and a subsequent examination revealed a C.L. on the left ovary, this would be positive evidence that she had a heat period although it was not observed.

A majority of reproductive problems are hormonal in origin and since there is no practical field test for hormone levels, diagnosis must be retrospective and based to a considerable extent on what changes have occurred. Without good records of reproductive history and results of prior examination, the diagnosis is frequently more difficult and less reliable. Although there are other systems equally good, none is more simple or economical. When coupled with a heat expectancy chart for barn use, it provides about all the information needed. Under general health, on the reverse side, there is space to record in abbreviated form any major disease episodes the animal experiences.

The importance of management in cattle reproduction cannot be overemphasized and the economic importance of reproduction is obvious. Unless the beef cow has a calf every year her production is zero, and despite extensive research and some claims to the contrary, no feasible method has yet been devised to consistently induce dairy cattle to give a profitable quantity of milk without the stimulus of parturition.

Pregnancy Examinations

It behooves the cattle owner, therefore, to learn all possible about reproduction and to apply it diligently. One management tool that should be employed is pregnancy examination. There is no need to wait up to nine months to see whether a cow is pregnant. An experienced veterinarian can diagnose pregnancy, or the lack thereof, with a high degree of accuracy beginning about thirty-five days after breeding, simply by rectal examination. With first-calf heifers, the diagnosis can even be made a few days earlier. Most theriogenologists, however, recommend that the examination be postponed until forty-five days after breeding. Until that time the placental attachment to the uterus is quite tenuous and manipulation may induce abortion. This hazard is greatly reduced after forty-five days, which is still early enough, as a practical matter, to initiate treatment of the nonpregnant cow to get her with calf in a reasonable length of time. The more advanced the pregnancy is, the easier and more accurate the diagnosis will be.

Early diagnosis is not made on the basis of palpating the embryo but on a combination of factors. Record of breeding is one, of course, but beyond that, disparity in size of uterine horns with a corpus luteum on the side of the larger is one indication of pregnancy. In addition, if an amniotic vesicle, the sac within which the embryo lies, can be felt, the pregnancy is confirmed. After forty to forty-five days the fetal membranes can be "slipped" between the fingers and after sixty days the fetus itself usually can be felt.

Cattlemen often ask if they can't save some money by doing pregnancy examinations themselves. The technique can be learned by anyone of reasonable intelligence but accuracy comes only with practice. And cattle owners simply don't have sufficient practical opportunity to become proficient. Whereas a veterinarian in cattle practice may average over 100 pregnancy examinations in a week, very few cattle owners will have the opportunity to do that many in a year. Since accuracy of diagnosis is essential and inaccuracy is useless, it seems to me that the herd manager's time could be used more profitably in other endeavors that only he can do best.

Milk Progesterone Assay Test

The advent of hormone assay for pregnancy may make this argument moot. Serum progesterone levels increase during pregnancy and some of the excess is eliminated in milk. Based on this, a relatively simple milk progesterone assay test has been devised for pregnancy diagnosis. It is not quite as reliable as a rectal examination done by an experienced veterinarian and is somewhat more costly, but further refinements are sure to come that may make the test both reliable and competitive.

In any event, pregnancy diagnosis is an important management tool for optimum cattle reproduction that should be used more extensively. If coupled with all of the fruits of reproduction research on the farm, cattle reproduction would not be nearly as much of a problem as some cattle raisers report it to be.

Abortions

Once a viable pregnancy has been established and confirmed it's just a matter of time until the calf is born — if an abortion doesn't occur. Abortion may occur at any time and there are many possible causes. If you have a cow that aborts, don't attribute it to bad luck and forget about it. There is always a reason and any money and effort spent to find the reason can pay big dividends even if you only have one cow. If the abortion is due, for example, to brucellosis, that cow will shed *Br. abortus* organisms in her milk. If she is your only milk supply there is thus a possibility of your getting undulant fever unless the milk is pasteurized. For the protection of the rest of the herd it's vitally important that a diagnosis be made.

At the very least, segregate the aborting cow from the rest of the herd until a diagnosis has been made because her vaginal discharge may be teeming with pathogens. Put the aborted fetus in a plastic bag and hold it in a cool place until your veterinarian can get there to do a necropsy and collect samples for laboratory diagnosis. Last, thoroughly clean and disinfect the area where the abortion occurred to reduce the risk of spreading infection.

Calving

Where to have the cow calve often presents a dilemma. An 8 feet x 10 feet or larger box stall can be ideal — or it can be a disaster. If it is clean, well bedded and left vacant for a couple weeks after the cow calves it is ideal. But if it must be in constant use with one cow right after the other, it can be a disaster because the resulting build-up of pathogenic organisms will infect a majority of the cows and calves using it. This will show up as a frequently fatal septicemia in the calves, and metritis, mastitis, or both in the cows. The only way to break this cycle is to stop using the maternity pen — even if it means the cows must calve outside.

The approach of parturition in the cow is characterized by udder enlargement and relaxation of the pelvic ligaments, giving the tail head a raised appearance. Frequently the vulva lips become puffy and distended and a string of gummy mucus will be seen extending from it. The cow will act restless and often will refuse feed for twelve hours prior to calving. Once true labor begins, the calf usually will be delivered in an hour or so.

Complications: Retained Placenta

The cow is unique from other species in the frequency with which parturition-associated complications occur. One of these is **parturient paresis,** or **milk fever,** which will be described in more detail later. The other is **retained placenta,** which may affect 10 percent or more of the cows in the herd. For a variety of reasons, some known and others not, the cotyledons and caruncles fail to separate as the calf is being born. Retained placenta is more frequent when twins are born and usually ensues when forced extraction of the fetus is necessary.

If infection is not present, retained placenta by itself is not a serious complication. It will eventually loosen up and fall out. Unfortunately, it acts as a wick along which bacteria can travel to set up a serious uterine infection called **metritis.** Also, once the calf is born, circulation to the placenta is cut off and the tissue dies and decomposes. Decomposing placenta has a very characteristic foul odor and it may be a month before all the bits and pieces have liquified and been discharged. Medicating the uterus may help to prevent serious infection but does little to hasten placental expulsion.

A substantial majority of veterinarians, myself included, feel that a retained placenta should be manually removed. This is a job best left to the veterinarian because it must be done carefully. Otherwise injury to the uterus may result which, if nothing else, will delay the next conception.

If an unusually high percentage of retained placentae occurs in the herd, some attempt should be made to find the cause. This isn't easy and usually ends up as a trial procedure. Malnutrition is a factor that can be eliminated by balancing the ration. Lack of exercise during the dry period also seems to play a role in all calving complications. Vitamin A deficiency has been considered a factor, although scientific evidence is lacking. Because the incidence of retained placenta is unpredictable, it's hard to design a controlled study. I do recall a herd in which administration of one million units of Vitamin A intramuscularly during the dry period seemed to reduce the prevalence from over 30 percent to less than 5 percent.

More recently selenium deficiency has been incriminated as a cause, and as with the vitamin A, injection during the dry period reduced the prevalence. Selenium is known to be an essential trace element but in large doses it is also carcinogenic, so its availability is controlled by law. There are undoubtedly other factors such as hormone imbalances and miscellaneous infections which contribute to retained placenta. It's a problem that needs more study.

Prolapsed Uterus

The last major complication of parturition in the cow is prolapsed uterus. This condition in which the uterus turns completely inside out is one of the few true emergencies in farm animal practice that is most prevalent in cows but certainly not rare in sheep and goats. This condition requires veterinary assistance without delay. It's a rare occasion when a prolapsed uterus can be replaced without medical assistance because it invariably swells. Attempts to push it back in stimulates a straining reflex, and in a contest of push against strain the cow always wins.

The best thing to do is to restrain the cow so she can't walk around, thereby injuring the uterus. Then wrap it in a clean cloth such as a large towel or even a bedsheet and keep it moist with warm water until the veterinarian arrives. And, in the interest of veterinarians everywhere, I would add, be prepared to help with the job at hand. Replacing a prolapsed uterus can be physically demanding work, taxing the strength of the strongest individual.

Surprisingly, most cows survive the ordeal if the prolapse can be corrected before many hours elapse. Many will even become pregnant again. However, when it happens once it is likely to occur again at the next calving and for that reason it is probably not advisable to keep the cow in the herd.

Horses

The mare is classified as seasonally polyestrous, that is, she will show signs of heat on a regular basis only during certain seasons. This seems to be a function of hours of daylight and the mare will usually cease cycling in late fall and early winter, beginning again as the days get longer. In the northern latitudes, the mare will usually begin to show signs of heat every sixteen to twenty-five days in March and will continue on into the fall if she is not bred.

The onset of estrus can be hastened by artificial light and by a management technique called "teasing." This is controlled daily exposure of the mare to the stallion without allowing direct contact. On breeding farms, mares and stallions are brought together this way once or twice a day but with a strong board fence between them and under hand control so injuries don't result. This procedure heightens libido in the stallion and accelerates onset of estrus in the mare.

When to Breed

Breeding mares as early as possible in the spring has importance in the racing industry, but because it is counter to the normal reproductive pattern, it leads to more frequent reproductive failures than occur when mares are bred in May or June.

Early breeding is important in the racing industry because somewhere in antiquity it was decided that a horse's age would be decided by calendar year of birth rather than by date of birth. Thus horses born on New Year's Day and those born on December 31 of the same year are reckoned to be the same age. Since the normal gestation period of the mare is eleven months, it is most desirable to get them bred in early February and to have them foal soon after January 1. From a physiological standpoint, this is the poorest time to breed them. However, the advantages to the owner are obvious. In a race for two-year-olds, for example, early in the season, a horse barely two and one almost three would qualify. Since the older horse is likely to be larger and stronger, the odds favor his winning the race. Don't bet on it, though, because genetics and training are still important factors.

The duration of standing heat in the mare is usually about five days and will be evident for the first time at around eighteen months of age although it may appear as early as ten and as late as twenty-four months, depending upon such things as heredity, plan of nutrition, and season of the year. Unlike the cow, ovulation in the mare takes place about one to two days before signs of heat subside. The optimum time to breed, therefore, is generally about the third day of estrum. The possibility of conception failure due to faulty timing can be reduced somewhat by breeding twice during the heat period if conserving the stallion is not important. The use of prostaglandin $F_2\alpha$ to induce estrus and ovulation in otherwise fertile mares has taken some of the guesswork out of timing the breeding. Use of hormones such as this should be considered a supplement to, and not a substitute for, good management. Careful rectal palpation will often detect imminent ovulation.

Estrus Harder to Detect

Detection of estrus in the mare is not as simple a matter as it is in the cow because mares rarely exhibit the homosexual behavior of standing to be mounted by other mares. Daily teasing and noting changes in attitude toward the stallion are the most reliable. The mare not in heat will resist the overtures of the stallion by squealing and kicking. The latter can cause serious injury if the stallion is not protected by a strong barrier. Gradually, as the heat period approaches, her attitude will soften and she will actually seek out the stallion, turning her hind quarters to him. Coincident with this she may show other signs such as squatting, frequent urination, "winking" of the clitoris, and rapid tail switching.

Breeding Management

Conception rates can vary tremendously on different breeding farms due to season (lowest in February and highest in July) and management. Good managers provide mares and stallions with ample exercise and maintain them on a balanced, nutritious diet. They also start planning for the breeding season several months ahead of time by having mares and stallions examined for fertility in late fall by a veterinarian. Mares are particularly susceptible to uterine infections, which, if detected early, can be treated successfully by the time the mare is ready to breed.

Hygiene

Because of susceptibility to infection, good hygiene at the time of breeding is essential. The mare's tail should be bandaged and her hindquarters thoroughly scrubbed with soap and water and then rinsed. Similarly the stallion's penis and sheath should be scrubbed and rinsed prior to breeding.

To prevent injuries, good restraint, depending on the disposition of mare and stallion, may be needed during breeding. To prevent injury to the stallion, breeding hobbles are often put on the mare (see section on restraint in Chapter 5). These should be tight enough to prevent a well-directed kick but, at the same time, loose enough so she won't lose her balance and fall when the stallion mounts.

Some stallions have a habit of biting mares severely when they mount, necessitating use of shoulder pads on the mare. If the stallion is overly large for the mare he is breeding, possible vaginal injury can be prevented by placing a stallion roll over the erect penis to control the depth of penetration. If necessary, one can be improvised by holding a roll of cotton between the penis and the belly wall as the stallion mounts.

Handling Precautions

Breeding should be done on ground where footing is good because concrete or plank floors are often dangerously slippery for horses. Both mare and stallion are restrained in halters and the person controlling the stallion must be particularly alert to any untoward moves that might result in injury. The stallion is brought alongside the mare and, after a period of foreplay during which the penis becomes erect, the stallion mounts and intromission takes place. Manually directing the penis into the vagina precludes the possibility of false entry into the rectum. Copulation in horses lasts five to seven minutes and terminates with ejaculation of 50–100 cc. of semen. As with other species, volume is determined to a large degree by frequency of use.

When the stallion dismounts he should be put back in the stall. Young vigorous stallions may want a second chance but it serves no useful purpose at this time.

Some older mares have vulvae that tip inward, allowing fecal contamination of the vagina with subsequent extension of infection to the uterus, followed by early abortion. It has been shown in mares with this condition that suturing the upper two-thirds of the lips of the vulva together (a procedure known as a Caslick operation) immediately after breeding will improve conception rates. The vulva must then be surgically opened, of course, prior to a subsequent breeding or foaling.

Artificial Insemination

Artificial insemination in the mare has had limited application for a number of reasons. First, fresh horse semen does not remain fertile much beyond eight hours, although techniques have been developed for freezing it to keep it viable much longer. Second, the difficulty of detecting mares in heat makes the timing of insemination too much a matter of luck. Third, the objections of several breed organizations have tended to discourage research. At present, the best application appears to be where two or more mares are to be bred to the same stallion on the same day. Semen can be collected using a "breeder's bag," or condom, or, preferably, an artificial vagina. The semen thus collected from a single ejaculate can be extended 1:1 and used to breed several mares.

Tests for Pregnancy

Pregnancy diagnosis is perhaps more important in mares than in cattle because of the relatively short breeding season. The teasing schedule should be maintained for at least three weeks after breeding to see if the mare returns to estrum. Failure to return to estrum is not positive evidence she is pregnant, although odds favor it, but it does provide a logical basis for a rectal examination for pregnancy a couple of weeks later. A small percentage of mares may show signs of heat three weeks after breeding, but it is usually of short duration and can be differentiated from a true heat period by rectal palpation.

Although several biological tests for pregnancy in mares are available, none is superior to or can be done earlier than rectal palpation by an experienced veterinarian. Those who do such examinations frequently become sufficiently skilled to detect pregnancy as early as seventeen days after breeding, but thirty to forty days after breeding is probably more realistic. In the hands of a skilled operator, ultrasonography is reliable for pregnancy diagnosis. A diagnosis of pregnancy made very early during gestation should be confirmed by a second examination a couple of months later, since early embryonic deaths occur in about 5 percent of equine pregnancies. When this occurs, the mare may not return to heat that season and the breeder blissfully assumes that she is pregnant. It pays to confirm the pregnancy!

Biological Tests

The biological tests for pregnancy rely on the changes in hormone concentration, especially chorionic gonadotropin and estrogen that occurs during the pregnancy. All of them are laboratory procedures and none is superior to careful rectal palpation. The Acheim-Zondek test or the Friedman modification of it are commonly used. These depend on gonadotropin in the mare's blood serum, which peaks at fifty to eighty days of pregnancy. Serum from a mare at this stage injected into rats, rabbits, or toads will produce readily recognizable changes in the reproductive organs of the test animals. The test has no value prior to forty days of pregnancy and its accuracy declines rapidly after eighty days. An immunological test accurate from 40 to 120 days of pregnancy that also relies on the presence of gonadotropin has been developed and is commercially available. A chemical test for estrogen in urine, the Cuboni test, is accurate from 120 to 290 days of pregnancy. However, at 120 days of gestation and beyond a rectal examination for pregnancy can be done with equal accuracy in less time than it takes to collect a urine sample.

Rectal Examination

Rectal examination of the mare is not a job for the novice, if for no other reason than that it can be dangerous. Some mares take violent exception to a hand in their rectum and will lash out with both hind feet with disastrous results if they are on target. Leave it to your veterinarian! He knows what to expect and what measures to take to prevent the worst from happening.

Outward Signs

The outward signs of pregnancy are not nearly as evident in the mare as they are in the cow, in some cases almost right up to foaling. Some increased distention of the mare's udder may be noticed, beginning about three to six weeks before foaling. It becomes filled with colostrum about two days prior to foaling and some leakage called "waxing" may be noticed on the teat ends. None of these time estimates is absolute, but waxing of the teats is an indication that preparation for foaling should not be delayed. Mares prefer peace and quiet when they foal and seem to have an uncanny ability to delay parturition until no one is around. When foaling is imminent they should be put in a clean, well-bedded box stall and watched discreetly. Sometimes observation through a knot hole is the best way. It's not uncommon to have an anxious owner stay up all night watching a mare due to foal only to have the foal born while the owner is in the house getting some breakfast.

First Signs of Labor

Perhaps the first signs that labor is beginning are slight sweating in the flanks and refusal of feed. These are followed by restlessness and evidence of abdominal discomfort. The mare will get up and down frequently until finally she stays down and begins to start some straining. The chorio-allantois or water bag usually breaks about this time, and the foal gets his first look at the world usually within the next half-hour. Strenuous labor beyond that time with no evident progress is a cause for concern and an indication that the mare needs some professional help. The foal can get into any of the malpresentations we described earlier, but because of the heavier abdominal musculature of the mare compared with other species, their straining effort makes correction somewhat more difficult. Also the uterine wall ruptures more easily and the uterus is more susceptible to infection than the cow's. For these reasons professional help is strongly recommended. If no veterinarian is available in a reasonable length of time, do the best you can, but remember that cleanliness and gentleness are essential.

The equine placenta differs from that of the cow. At the moment of birth 10–15 percent of the foal's blood supply may be in the placental blood vessels. Don't be in a hurry to cut the umbilical cord. Wait fifteen minutes or so, then tie the cord three or four inches from the belly, using umbilical tape or a piece of sterilized cotton string. Cut it on the placental side of the tie. Spread the placenta out and examine it to see that it is all there. Retained placenta is not as common in the mare as in other species, but sometimes torn pieces will be left in the uterus. Pieces or an entire placenta retained in the uterus is a complication that needs correction without much delay. This is not only an ideal medium for bacterial growth, but decomposing placenta in the uterus can cause a severe endometritis and laminitis (founder).

Care of the Foal

After the umbilical cord has been cut a few other procedures for the foal are recommended. The navel should be dipped in tincture of iodine. Unless the mare has been previously immunized, the foal should receive a dose of tetanus toxoid or antitoxin. Horses are very susceptible to tetanus and the stump of the umbilical cord is an ideal place for the bacterium *Clostridium tetani* to gain entrance.

Normally a foal will be on its feet within an hour after birth and looking for his first meal. He should be helped if necessary. If for any reason the foal can't get up to nurse, bottle feed it with colostrum milked from the mare. Lastly, many foals require an enema within six to twelve hours after birth to remove the hard lumps of meconium that would otherwise cause constipation and all the complications that implies.

The majority of mares will come into heat within a week after foaling. This is the so-called "foal heat" and if the delivery was uncomplicated and everything else is normal they can be bred back at this time. However, conception rates on this first breeding are generally not as good as they will be at the next heat period.

If you have gotten the impression that horse breeding is a complicated procedure with frequent disappointments you are right. And you might well ask why. Certainly bands of wild horses have no trouble reproducing themselves. The answer lies not with the horses but with the people who own them. Most wild mares are bred during June and July at the peak of fertility, and they foal late in the spring when there is ample grass for nourishment of mare and foal. If, instead of attempting to make nature conform to our needs through artificial birth dates and other means, we would adjust our breeding procedures to simulate those found naturally, I have no doubt that conception rates would improve markedly.

Swine

Gilts will generally start showing signs of estrum at about six months of age. However, unless they are especially well grown it is advisable to postpone breeding another three months or until they reach 250 pounds body weight. They are polyestrous, having heat periods about every three weeks throughout the year except when pregnant or lactating. The period of estrum will last two or three days and ovulation occurs a few hours thereafter. The duration of pregnancy averages 114 days. If you have trouble remembering numbers, think of it in terms of three months, three weeks, and three days. As with teasing the mare, the onset of estrum can be hastened by putting a boar in an adjacent pen.

Although the sow will cycle throughout the year, conception rates fall during periods of very hot weather. Hot weather also tends to lower the fertility of the boar. If sows must be bred when it's hot, some method of cooling the barn, such as evaporative coolers or foggers, will improve conception and litter size.

Impending estrum is usually evident a couple days prior to standing heat. The vulva shows some swelling and reddening, the sow becomes restless, utters typical grunts, and sniffs at the genitals of others in the pen. This is followed by mounting other sows and finally by standing to be mounted. During the period of peak fertility most sows will stand for hand pressure on the rump and, of course, will be receptive to the boar. Best conception results when the sow is bred about twenty hours after the onset of standing heat and again twelve hours later. A second mating will increase litter size by about 10 percent. Since weaning a maximum number of pigs per litter, at least nine, is one of the keys to success in the swine business, this extra 10 percent becomes important.

Another management technique that helps to increase litter size in pigs is called "flushing." Increasing feed intake of the sow by six or eight pounds for ten days prior to breeding will increase the number of ova released, thereby increasing litter size. Reverting back to the normal daily ration a couple days after signs of heat have passed will keep the sows from getting too fat.

When to Breed

When to breed sows depends on many factors; market conditions, feed availability, housing and, for those with only one or two sows, sometimes personal preference enters in. But for the commercial operator it is important from a disease control standpoint to plan matings so that there will be a two-week period every six months when there are no hogs in the farrowing house. This allows time for thorough cleaning, disinfection, and drying, which kills off populations of pathogens that otherwise cause a constant problem with such things as baby pig scours, metritis, and mastitis.

Availability of boars presents a problem for the person breeding one or two sows as a hobby. The economics of a swine enterprise that small is questionable at best, and if one must feed a boar all year to have him available to sire two litters of pigs a year, the enterprise certainly must be considered a hobby. As a way of saving money, some people either borrow a boar when needed, or take their sow to a boar. This is an ideal way to spread contagious swine diseases and is certainly not recommended. Artificial insemination would be much more preferable, but, unfortunately, it is not generally available except in the Midwest, where the hog industry is concentrated. The technique is successful and practical, although thus far it has not been possible even with a variety of extenders to keep boar semen viable much more than thirty-six hours. Frozen semen has not produced good conception rates.

Collecting Semen

Collection of semen and insemination are not difficult procedures and once learned are probably no more time-consuming than transporting a sow or boar from one farm to another. Certainly there is less disease hazard involved and the equipment requirements are minimal. The only real drawback is the availability of a sow in heat on the farm where the semen is to be collected to stimulate erection by the boar. Even this can be circumvented with an electro-ejaculator.

To collect semen, when the boar mounts the sow, grasp and hold the penis firmly in a gloved hand and directed toward an opaque wide-mouth, sterilized, and warm pint bottle. Firm hand pressure on the penis is sufficient to stimulate ejaculation which usually takes five minutes or more for completion. The ejaculate from a mature boar will just about fill the jar but the first part of it is heavy gelatinous material which should be discarded. The balance of the semen containing the spermatozoa should be protected from chilling by wrapping the jar in paper or other insulating material. If used within an hour or so, the loss in fertility is not great and there's a good chance of conception.

Prior to use, the ejaculate is strained through sterile cheesecloth to remove any extraneous material. Although equipment has been designed for swine insemination and is undoubtedly preferable, improvision can be done by using a bulb syringe with about a half-pint capacity attached to a semi-flexible plastic pipette similar to that used for cattle insemination. The pipette is inserted carefully into the vagina and upward at about a 30° angle and gently worked through the cervix. Once the pipette is in place, the bulb is slowly squeezed until the semen has been expelled. This technique has some obvious disadvantages but these are outweighed by the reduced risk of disease transmission inherent in transporting sows or boars from one farm to another.

The same technique is equally or more useful on the large breeding farms where there is a shortage of boar power. By extending the semen up to fivefold with commercially available semen extenders or even sterile homogenized milk, one boar can be used to breed several sows in a day which would not otherwise be possible with any degree of success. Fertility of even mature boars declines if they are used more than twice a day or ten times a week. Boars less than a year old cannot be used successfully that often. Fertility of the boar has a noticeable effect on litter size and to lessen the chance of breeding a sow to a boar of low fertility, it is common practice to breed sows twice during the heat period to different boars. This puts added demands on boar power and makes adequate care and management of boars equally important to that of the sows.

Introducing New Boars

For genetic improvement if nothing else, new boars with different bloodlines are frequently added to the herd. These boars should be purchased well in advance of anticipated need and, as a disease control procedure, segregated from other swine for thirty days. If no health problems develop they can then be placed in service, but it is good practice to first test mate them to a couple of gilts to be sure they are fertile.

Sexual and social behavior seem quite different in pigs than in other animals. A strange boar put in with a pen of sows or gilts may show more concern about his surroundings than about his love life. It helps to put them in an adjacent pen for a few days beforehand to get acclimated. Similarly, a boar simply left in a pen of females sometimes gets bored with the whole procedure and ignores their overtures. Putting a second boar in the pen introduces the element of competition and, once they settle their differences, both boars will approach the situation with renewed vigor. Some young virgin boars put in a pen with a sow in heat will simply regard the sow's antics with amazement and not know how to proceed. A few have to be patiently coaxed to mount the sow until they learn their purpose in life. Once they get the idea there is usually no further problem.

Copulation is a more protracted procedure in swine than other species lasting from twenty to thirty minutes. And also, unlike other species, the slim penis of the boar passes through the cervix so that ejaculation takes place directly into the uterus. The excitement associated with sexual activity in other species is generally absent and once ejaculation begins some boars actually give the impression they are going to sleep. The only indication of activity may be just an occasional soft grunt.

Diagnosing Pregnancy

Pregnancy diagnosis in the sow is accomplished with biological tests for blood progesterone, estrone sulfate, or the use of ultrasonography. These are most accurate at about three to four weeks of pregnancy. Except in large sows, rectal palpation is more traumatic than useful. Changes in vaginal epithelial cells determined by biopsy and microscopic examination are a reliable indicator of pregnancy but these procedures are not very practical on the farm.

Farrowing

A couple of days before the sow is due to farrow she should be scrubbed clean with soap and water and put into a previously cleaned and disinfected farrowing pen or stall. These are described in the section on housing (pages 54–56). At the same time, the sow's diet should be changed to one containing more bulk. Sows tend to develop problems with constipation when they are confined in a farrowing pen. As a result they go off feed and have a reduced milk flow when it is most needed. A diet high in fiber using more ingredients such as bran or even chopped hay helps prevent the problem.

Depending on litter size, farrowing may extend over several hours, taking longer as a rule for gilts than older sows. Sometimes the first piglet in the procession will be larger than the others or malpresented and the sow will have to be helped. These usually can be reached by hand and removed with gentle traction. Remember to be clean and gentle. Anyone farrowing hogs regularly should have a set of pig forceps and/or an obstetrical snare available. When it appears that the last piglet has arrived, some swine growers routinely give the sow a dose of oxytocin. This is a prescription drug that stimulates smooth muscle contraction. It causes the uterus to contract, hopefully expelling any additional pigs that are left, and it also helps to stimulate milk flow.

Heat Needed for Newborn Pigs

Supplemental heat from a heat lamp or a brooder is necessary for the newborn pigs except during hot weather. Chilling after birth not only predisposes piglets to disease problems such as scours and pneumonia but can itself cause death. So place the piglets under the lamp as they are born and, at the same time, swab the navel with tincture of iodine.

This is also a good time to clip the needle teeth. Baby pigs have very sharp teeth that, when nursing, may irritate the sow to a point where she won't let them nurse. Only the tips of the teeth should be removed, since clipping them at the gum line may crush the tooth, leaving the piglet with a mouth so sore that he won't nurse. A Resco brand dog nail trimmer works well for the purpose.

Anemia is Common

Iron deficiency anemia is a universal problem with baby pigs that is easily prevented. Several methods are commonly used. The oldest and simplest, which is still used by many swine growers, is to put a few shovelfuls of clean sod in the pen where the pigs can root around in it. Another less certain way to get iron into the piglets is to swab the udder of the sow with a saturated ferrous sulfate solution on the theory that the piglets will lick it off when they nurse. A more certain way is to drench the individual pigs with ferrous sulfate solution (about one teaspoon) or to give each an iron/copper tablet. But perhaps the best way is to inject each pig with iron dextran within one to two days after birth and again three weeks later. This injectable form of iron is available from several companies and the dosage depends upon the concentration of the product used.

Pigs can be weaned at four weeks of age and the sow will usually come into heat and can be bred five to seven days after weaning. Those that are destined to become market hogs can be castrated at this time or earlier. Castration of males is essential for palatable meat and the earlier that this is done the less traumatic it is.

Sheep

Sheep tend to be seasonal breeders with the onset of first estrus appearing in late summer or early fall and appearing about every sixteen days thereafter until late fall unless pregnancy intervenes. However, unlike other domestic animals there is a noticeable difference between breeds. For example, the Rambouillet and Dorset may come into heat at any time of the year and usually always by June, whereas the Cheviot and Shropshire rarely show signs of heat before September. This difference is important when selecting a breed for commercial lamb production. A great deal of crossbreeding has been done in the sheep industry in an attempt to concentrate desirable traits, one of which is a short anestrous period.

The average gestation period is 147 days, with the onset of puberty ranging from five to twelve months depending on heredity, plane of nutrition, and when the ewe lambs are born. Those born early in the year will often come into heat that fall; those born later usually don't come into heat until the following year. Since it is economically desirable that a ewe produce as many lambs as possible during her lifetime there is a distinct advantage in having lambs born early in the year. Unfortunately, lamb mortality due to inclement weather in the winter tends to be higher unless special care is taken. "Flushing" the ewes with extra feed a few weeks prior to breeding will improve conception rates and perhaps stimulate more multiple ovulation.

Ovulation takes place late in the heat period but timing of mating is of little consequence, since sheep are almost invariably pasture bred, and when sufficient ram power is available copulation will occur several times during the heat period. Although libido and fertility of rams varies, a mature ram should be able to breed twenty-five ewes during the season.

Fertility

Fertility is generally better in cool weather and when the rams are not kept with the flock all the time. As with the mare, sight, sound, and smell apparently play a role in the onset of estrus. More ewes will come into heat sooner when the rams are put with them a couple weeks prior to the desired breeding season than when rams are left with them all the time. When the rams are left with the ewes all the time they become accustomed to their presence and the element of sexual excitement is lacking.

Artificial insemination of sheep, although technically feasible, has not become a common practice. It requires close observation of the ewe flocks, individual handling, and careful timing of insemination, which makes it less practical than for other species.

Estrus synchronization through use of hormones, on the other hand, is a useful management tool adopted by some shepherds. Use of synthetic or natural progesterone-type hormones given in feed or via a pessary placed in the vagina as the breeding season approaches will inhibit the onset of estrus in most cases. When the drug is withdrawn the majority will come into heat during the space of a few days. This has the advantage of shortening the breeding season and subsequently the lambing season. It also has a disadvantage. Since all the ewes come into heat at about the same time, it keeps the rams pretty busy and for maximum conception rates, more rams are needed.

Identifying Barren Ewes

Pregnancy diagnosis in sheep is important to good management. A barren ewe must be fed, just as a pregnant one must, yet without one or more lambs she produces no income. The earlier barren ewes can be identified and culled the higher the flock productivity will be. Since the unit value of commercial sheep is low, biological tests based on hormone assay are not feasible because of the labor requirement in collecting blood samples and the cost of the test itself.

However, development of other techniques has accelerated in recent years. A few people have become adept in diagnosing pregnancy at about ninety days by digital palpation of the cervix through the vagina. In the pregnant ewe, the cervix generally cannot be reached with the fingertips, while in the barren ewe it will feel dense and almost cartilaginous.

In advanced pregnancy, of course, lambs can often be felt externally but by that time parturition, or lack of it, is so near that examination is hardly worthwhile. External ultrasonography is the most practical pregnancy diagnostic tool for the commercial sheep grower. With experience it is both fast and accurate.

Avoid Confusion of Ewes and Lambs

Because of the desirability of having ewe lambs that will come into heat as early as possible and the better market for spring lambs in some areas, most shepherds prefer to have lambs born as early in the year as possible. Unfortunately, this coincides with cold weather, so a reasonably warm, protected lambing shed is a necessity. This can be the same building in which the ewes are housed but, if so, it should have a section reserved for lambing pens holding no more than one or two ewes. When the whole flock is left together at lambing time, lambs and their mothers often get separated and mass confusion results.

As lambing time approaches it's important to watch the ewes carefully for signs of imminent parturition such as engorgement of the udder with milk or "bagging." These ewes should be separated from the flock and put into the lambing area. At the same time or even sooner, it's good practice to "tag" the ewes. This expression isn't at all what it appears to be. It means clipping off the wool around the udder and perineal area. This keeps the udder and vulvar area cleaner, which makes lambing a more sanitary procedure, and also makes it easier for the lambs to find their first meal.

Multiple Births

Twins and triplets are common in sheep and in fact, multiple births are desirable. The flock that doesn't average at least 1.5 lambs per ewe per year is not likely to be profitable. In fact, one of the criteria used in select matings is twinning and mothering ability. Due in part at least to multiple births, sheep tend to have more difficulty at parturition and frequently require assistance. The good shepherd will check his lambing ewes every couple hours day and night throughout the lambing season to be able to help those in trouble while there is still time to save the lambs.

Delivery

Normally the first lamb will be born within one hour or two after true labor begins. If nothing happens by then, a careful pelvic examination is in order. With an assistant holding the ewe, scrub the vulvar area thoroughly with soap and warm water and do the same with your hands and arms. The pelvic canal of a mature ewe will admit a well-lubricated, average-sized hand. If the problem is merely a cervix that is not fully dilated, wait a little longer and try again if nothing has happened. If the problem is a malpresentation, it must be corrected before the lambs can be delivered. The diagrams shown earlier in this chapter (see pages 70–71) should help in determining the position the lamb is in and what must be done to straighten it out. Once it is straightened out it can be delivered with gentle traction. An obstetrical snare or forceps available from most instrument supply houses is a valuable aid to grip the lamb.

Frequently when dystocia (difficult birth) occurs, the ewe will be tired and her uterine musculature exhausted, or atonic, so that any lambs remaining after the first will also have to be manually delivered. Injection of oxytocin may stimulate uterine contractions but it is a powerful drug that can be dangerous. In most states it is available only on prescription. Use of oxytocin to stimulate uterine contractions without first ascertaining that the cervix is dilated and the lamb in a normal position can lead to a ruptured uterus and a dead ewe. Oxytocin is a useful drug, but it must be used judiciously.

Infection Possible

Once the obstetrical operations have been completed it's time to look toward the future. Any time an instrument or the hand is introduced into the uterus, infection called metritis is likely to ensue. This is especially true during obstetrical operations because there is always some degree of injury to the uterine lining, making it more susceptible to bacterial invasion. A variety of antibiotic preparations are available to medicate the uterus and most of them are effective when used as directed. Tablets or boluses containing sulfanilamide and urea are commonly used, and one is usually placed in each uterine horn. Other compounds of value include nitrofurazone, chlorhexidine, and a variety of antibiotics. In addition, it's a wise precaution to give the ewe 5 cc. of penicillin intramuscularly. For a valuable ewe, a dose of tetanus antitoxin as an added precaution is indicated because sheep are very susceptible to tetanus.

Care of Lambs

The lambs need attention, too. They chill rapidly and need to be rubbed dry with a towel and kept warm. Rubbing them briskly but gently also helps to stimulate circulation and respiration. Once they appear to be breathing normally, the navel should be dipped in tincture of iodine to prevent infection. The next step is to induce them to nurse, which means patiently heading them in the right direction and sometimes stripping a little milk from the ewe into their mouths until they get the idea. If all else fails, lambs can be bottle fed until they get a little stronger or a little smarter. An ordinary baby bottle and nipple will do, although commercially made lamb nipples will last longer. In any event they need their first meal of colostrum within an hour after birth, and for the first few days they will take a little milk every few hours. As they get older, the frequency of feeding can be reduced.

Despite the best effort of the shepherd, there is usually some mortality of lambs and ewes during the lambing season, resulting in orphan lambs or ewes with milk and no lambs. It's worth the effort to try to get them together so the lamb can be raised without hand feeding. Unfortunately, most ewes will not accept nursing except by their own offspring, which they identify by smell. Sometimes they can be fooled by tying the skin of the dead lamb onto the orphan. Some ewes that are heavy milkers develop swollen, engorged, and painful udders from lack of milking and mastitis may be an added complication. Milking will help, of course, but few people have the time and patience to milk a ewe regularly. Furthermore, milking actually increases the milk flow and once started will have to be continued. It's better to dry off the milk flow as rapidly as possible. Pressure in the udder helps but contributes to the ewe's discomfort. One procedure that *is* helpful is to massage the udder several times a day with camphorated oil. This relieves some of the soreness and at the same time suppresses milk flow.

Docking and Castrating

At three to five days of age all lambs should have their tails docked and males should be castrated. At this age the emasculatome is the most satisfactory instrument for castration. It crushes the spermatic cord, interrupting the blood supply to the testicles so they don't develop. It has the advantage of not cutting into the skin or causing any bleeding and thus there is no danger of infection or hemorrhage. The instrument should be in good condition and should not be used for anything else which may spring the jaws. A small emasculatome suitable for one-hand operation is adequate for young lambs.

With an assistant holding the lamb, force the right spermatic cord to the outside edge of the scrotum with the left hand and with the emasculatome in the right hand, clamp it about halfway between the testicle and body wall. Change hands and repeat on the left side. Don't try to take a short cut by clamping the entire scrotum because, with that amount of tissue to clamp, "skips" may occur. When carefully done as outlined, this method is equally as good as the use of knives or elastrator bands and is safer. The same technique works well for calves, although a larger size emasculatome may be necessary.

The emasculatome is also a good instrument for tail docking, since virtually no hemorrhage results even though the tail must be snipped off where the instrument was applied. An application of antiseptic on the stump is usually the only aftercare required. Castration and tail docking should be done in a clean area. Docking tails of filthy lambs in a filthy place may lead to serious death losses from tetanus.

Lambing time is a busy time for the shepherd but successful sheep husbandry is proportional to success of the lamb crop and merits all the time the shepherd devotes to it.

Goats

Like sheep, goats are seasonally polyestrous, usually coming into heat from August through January, with the peak months of fertility being September, October, and November. During this period does will cycle every twenty-one days with each heat period lasting two to three days. Ovulation occurs late in the heat period, therefore the second day is usually the best time to breed.

Signs of impending estrus include uneasiness, tail shaking and frequent urination, some clear mucus discharge from the vulva and, of course, receptivity to the buck.

Bucks: Smelly But Essential

The owner of one or two goats faces a problem in getting them bred. It's uneconomical to keep a buck for one or two does. Furthermore, the odor from their musk glands makes them socially unacceptable to all but a dedicated goat enthusiast — or another goat. This usually means that the doe must be transported somewhere to a buck when she is in heat. This transporting is often inconvenient and carries with it the risk of transmitting disease from farm to farm. Artificial insemination, therefore, it a logical and practical solution, but unfortunately availability is limited.

Frozen semen is available from a limited number of sources, one of which is Central Ohio Breeding Association, Columbus, Ohio. Breed association secretaries maintain lists of semen sources and perhaps the best solution for the owner of a limited number of goats is to arrange with a local A.I. technician to obtain and store frozen semen for use in the herd. With the rapid increase in popularity of the dairy goat, artificial insemination service will no doubt become more readily available. Until then, transporting the does or keeping a buck will be the only alternatives for some people.

The larger commercial goat dairies can justify a buck on economic grounds but they still have to live with his odor, which permeates everything unless he has been successfully deodorized. Even then, bucks during the breeding season have a nasty habit of urinating on their beards and then shaking urine all over. Although undesirable from many standpoints, they are essential. Fortunately, only one is necessary for a doe herd up to thirty head.

Pregnancy

Pregnancy diagnosis in the goat, at present, must be considered an inexact science. As with sheep, ultrasonography is the most reliable method of pregnancy diagnosis in goats.

The duration of pregnancy averages 151 days and, since the breeding date for goats is usually known, the time of kidding is predictable. The pregnant doe should be put into a clean box stall, at least 5 feet x 5 feet, a few days ahead of time. Signs of impending parturition include udder enlargement, relaxation of the pelvic ligaments giving the tailhead a raised appearance, and a hollow appearance in the flank. Frequently there will be a thick white discharge from the vulva for a couple of days prior to kidding. As the time draws near, the doe will act restless, changing positions frequently. The majority give birth lying down but some will remain standing.

Birth

Once labor begins, the sequence of events is the same as other species. The water bag appears first, followed normally by the front feet and head. Parturition in the goat differs in only one respect from other species. It is usually accompanied by an excessive amount of bleating. This is not an indication that the doe is in trouble, only that she is not as stoic as other animals. If no progress is made on delivery in a reasonable length of time, she should be helped in the same manner as described for the other species. Retained placenta is not common in the goat, but when it occurs it should be handled by a veterinarian. Twinning is common.

As they are born, mucus should be cleared from the nose of the kids and they should be wiped dry if the doe refuses to lick them off. They also need colostrum within the first hour just like other animals, but feeding thereafter is a matter of choice. If the doe's milk is not to be used it's probably best to begin hand feeding immediately. The longer the kids are allowed to nurse, the more traumatic the weaning experience is.

Disbud Kids Early

One thing that definitely should be done before kids are a week old is disbudding unless you are dealing with a polled breed. Dehorning of adult goats is a major and often unsatisfactory procedure. It's much easier to do with a hot electric dehorning iron when they are young. A small dehorning iron — not the large size used for calves — is the most satisfactory. The horned breeds have a whorl of hair around each horn bud but if you can't identify this, shaving the hair will expose the horn bud attached tightly to the skull. Generally it takes five to fifteen seconds' application to burn the horn bud down to the bone. This is not a job for the squeamish and the burning must be thorough or unsightly scurs will grow at the site. Better to overdo it than to do half a job.

Although it may seem heartless, using local anesthesia is of questionable value because the kids object as much to injection of the anesthetic as they do to the actual dehorning. While you are dehorning the males, slide the iron slightly to the rear and center of the horn bud. This will destroy the musk glands from whence comes the stink when they get older. When burning has been adequate, the skin will have a leathery, copper-colored appearance. If it doesn't — burn some more.

Male kids not destined to become herd sires can be castrated at the same time using the emasculatome as described for sheep. Don't neglect this important procedure, since they are precocious and some are fertile much earlier than you may realize. The result, if they are kept together, may be doelings that are pregnant long before they should be. Unless they are unusually well grown, does should not be bred until they are at least a year old.

Restraint

EVERY ANIMAL, REGARDLESS OF SPECIES, has to be restrained for some purpose at some time. The degree of restraint depends upon the reason for it. For some things a simple halter will suffice, but on occasion more severe measures are required. The important thing is to gear the degree of restraint to the need using the minimum necessary for protection of you and the animal.

Keep in mind that domestic animals are not far removed from wild and that in some cases the more confining the restraint applied, the more they will struggle. I have seen beef calves just off the range struggle so hard to get out of a squeeze chute that they collapsed from exhaustion. Being restrained can be a frightening experience for an animal and they remember it. The more traumatic their first experience is, the more difficult it will be to get them into a similar position the next time it becomes necessary. If you are dealing with just a few animals, get them accustomed to mild restraint such as a halter early in life because it will make things much easier when they are older and larger.

Never forget that cattle, horses, and even mature pigs can hurt you badly. Much as we may love them, they are animals and their actions and reactions are unpredictable. Simply because a horse has not kicked you in the past doesn't mean he won't in the future.

Last, keep in mind that our primary advantage over animals is our capacity to reason. If you surrender that advantage and look upon restraint of the large farm animal as a contest of brute strength and determination, you will certainly lose and may get injured in the attempt. Be gentle, and compassionate, know what you want to do and how to go about it, and both you and your animal will fare much better.

Cattle

When it comes to restraint, dairy and beef cattle must be considered separately. Restraint of dairy cattle is much less of a problem because they are accustomed to being handled individually and being restrained for milking. Beef cattle, on the other hand, may be confined no more than once a year for vaccination and sometimes never. As a consequence, there is considerable difference in their attitude toward being individually handled.

Everyone who keeps more beef cattle than he can conveniently train to lead with a halter should have at least a chute and headgate to handle the herd. Too many owners of beef herds neglect this important management tool. I might add they are also the ones who find veterinarians very reluctant to work for them, since every call turns out to be a mini-rodeo and takes much longer than it should. Don't expect your veterinarian to play cowboy. He doesn't have the time and you can't afford it.

Construction plans for pen, chute, and headgate layouts are available at minimal cost from the Departments of Agricultural Engineering at all of the land-grant universities. Basically, the chute is two parallel plank or rail fences leading from the holding pen and terminating at a head gate or squeeze. It should be at least five feet high and no more than twenty-eight inches wide inside. Although it may not seem so, that is adequate for a mature beef cow. Any wider than that and a few smart cows will manage to turn around and head the other way. In a chute designed for one-way traffic this is frustrating because the cows behind the smart one have to be backed out and then all of them chased in again. The length of the chute depends on how many cows you want to handle at a time but plan on about five feet per cow. If the length of the chute warrants, it's helpful to build it in a curve so that when they enter they can't see that the far end is blocked. For a procedure such as vaccination, application of insecticides, or others, crowding cattle into the chute is all the restraint necessary.

Hold in Headgate

For more detailed procedures, cows have to be held individually in the headgate. The headgate depicted in figure 1 is simply a strong wooden gate with a stanchion built in that can be pulled shut quickly from the side. When the procedure is complete, the animal's head is released and the gate opened to let her go. When herd size warrants the investment, steel squeezes are commercially available that serve the function of the headgate but, in addition, have sides which close in to hold the animal firmly in position. Smaller editions are available for calves. At least one manufacturer has modified the calf squeeze with a large hoop at each end so the whole unit can be rolled into any position with the calf firmly fixed inside.

MATERIALS

FULL DIMENSION OAK
  2 X 4
  2 X 6
  2 X 8

BOLTS - ½" MACHINE

FLAT STEEL
  ¼ X 1½
  ¼ X 2
  ¼ X 3

3' 8"

2' 8"

¼" X 1½"
FLAT HOOK

SPRING

2" X 6" TIE

2' X 6"

6" X 6" POST

HOLES

2" X 8"

¼" X 3" STEEL
RATCH RECESSED

STEEL PLATE

⅝" ROD

¼" X 2" HINGES

6"

6'

5'

GROUND LEVEL

Figure 1. A headgate is a strong wooden gate with a stanchion built in that can be pulled shut quickly from the side.

Sooner or later rope will be necessary for restraining cattle and horses. In my opinion, thirty-five feet of ½" nylon rope with a quick release honda on one end is the most versatile. Hard manila is better for throwing a loop but it is too stiff for tying and doesn't have the tensile strength of nylon. Furthermore, manila is much more likely to cause rope burn and should never be used to restrain horses because their skin is much more tender. Cotton rope is preferable for horses.

Figure 2. Steps in tying a rope halter.

Figure 3. Rope halter with ring.

Cow Halter

A halter is the mildest restraint commonly used on the cow. These are customarily made of rope, but leather or cotton webbing is just as good. If none is available, a halter can easily be improvised with a lariat as in Figure 2a, b, and c. First a noose is put around the neck; then a bight of rope is pulled through the noose and placed up over the muzzle and the running end of the rope drawn tight. With a flick of the quick-release honda, the animal can be immediately released. A rope with a ring in one end is also a very useful item and its application as a halter is shown in Figure 3.

One of the important things to remember when tying an animal with a halter is to use a knot that can be easily undone. If the head is tied and the animal

Figure 4. Steps in tying the halter tie.

When a stanchion is not available, cattle can be restrained for minor procedures by immobilizing the head against a fencepost as shown below.

struggles and falls, it may strangle unless the rope is untied immediately. Every stockman should master the halter tie shown in Figure 4a, b, c. It's quick and easy, and a tug on the free end of the rope immediately unties the knot. While the knot left as in Figure 4c will hold, it can be untied by an animal that grabs the end and pulls. This can be prevented by passing the running end through the loop as in Figure 4d. If the knot is drawn tight in this position, however, it can't be untied easily.

The Nose Lead

A more severe form of restraint for the head is the nose lead shown in Figure 5a. This not only immobilizes the head, but it also causes sufficient pain so that the animal hesitates to move in any direction. Properly used it is quick and easy to apply, but there is a right way and a wrong way. I have seen people stand in front of the cow with one side of the nose lead in each hand making passes at the cow's nose each time she swings it by. No self-respecting cow will stand still with head outstretched so you can put a nose lead in this way. The proper technique is to stand alongside the cow's head facing in the same direc-

Figure 5. (a) Nose lead. (b) A common error — tying a nose lead in place.

tion. Grasp her head under your arm and with the other hand, put the nose lead in place. This serves two purposes. It slows down head movement and blocks her vision so she can't see what is about to be placed in her nose.

Figure 5b illustrates a common mistake people make, much to their later sorrow. *A nose lead should never be tied in place* but should be snubbed and held by an assistant. If the cow in 5b were to struggle and fall to her knees, in all probability the nose lead would tear her nose, causing unnecessary pain and suffering until it healed. An assistant holding the rope can immediately slacken off if it looks as if the cow will fall.

The Bull Ring

A modification of the nose lead, permanently installed, is the bull ring — generally reserved, as the name implies, for bulls. The dairy bull, as some people learn each year, is a dangerous animal, and his disposition doesn't improve with age. Up to a year of age, dairy bulls aren't too bad to handle, although they may play a bit rough. The best way to handle them after that is to keep them in a facility constructed in such a way that you never have to be on the same side of the fence. Because that isn't always possible, have your veterinarian put in a good strong ring when the bull is eight to twelve months of age. The ring at least gives you a handle for restraint.

A bull staff, shown in Figure 6, can be attached to the ring for leading the bull. Several types are available but essentially each is a four-foot steel pole which attaches to the ring. With it you can not only lead the bull forward, but push back if he gets too friendly. And even if your back is turned, because a rigid pole is attached to him, you can detect any movement he might make.

Figure 6. Bull staff.

Another technique that increases the utility of the bull ring as a restraint device is to attach a three-foot length of chain to it permanently. This is especially applicable for bulls at pasture. Putting bulls in a pasture is not a good safety practice but if you do and he decides to run you out, the odds favor his stepping on the chain and being brought up short, giving you time to reach the fence or climb a tree.

The same precaution applies to bull rings as to nose leads. Never tie a bull solely by the ring. Use a halter or, if he has horns, put a rope around the horns, lead the running end down through the ring and then tie it. I have seen a number of older bulls with their noses torn out because people failed to heed this advice. And once the nose is torn out, the most useful avenue of restraint is lost.

Kicking and Hind Leg Restraint

Once the cow's head is secured by stanchion, halter, or nose lead the only weapons she has left are the hind feet. Unlike the horse, she can kick forward and to the side as well as to the rear almost with equal accuracy. It also seems necessary to do procedures on the cow within range of the hind feet more frequently than anywhere else. Hind leg restraint is therefore often necessary and there are several effective methods. If you have a willing assistant with a strong back, have him pick up the front leg on the same side on which you are working. The cow won't kick effectively unless she has the other three legs planted firmly on the ground.

Figure 7. This prevents kicking.

Figure 8. Some cows will resist this restraint.

Another method is to have an assistant push the tail firmly straight up over the back as shown in Figure 7. This throws the cow off balance, making her reluctant to move. For most cows, this alone provides sufficient restraint. Caution must be exercised, however, because excessive force may break the tail. A third method is to apply a squeeze just forward of the udder as shown in Figure

8. This works well on some cows but others resist it and, while they can't kick, they will hop around, making it difficult to work.

One type of kicking restraint I would *not* recommend is the hobble. Whether fashioned from rope or the commercial variety made of metal, these have the effect of tying the rear legs together at the hock. While some cows may tolerate this, others will not.

My reason for not recommending them is based on personal experience. As a young practitioner more years ago than I care to remember, I bought a set of commercial hobbles that looked like a good idea at the time. These are still widely advertised and, I presume, sold. Basically they are two metal U straps that hook over the Achilles tendon above the hock, linked together by a chain that can be drawn tight and hooked. My first opportunity to use them came with a call requiring minor teat surgery. With pride and skill I put the new hobbles in place, intending to impress the client with my skill and the marvels of modern devices. All went well until I was about half done and struck a sensitive spot. The cow jumped into the air with both hind legs and, because they were locked together, lost her balance and landed on her side — with me underneath. After getting extricated, I took them off and as far as I know, those shiny new hobbles are still on that farm. I never put them back in the car, deciding then and there that it's preferable to be kicked than crushed.

The Rope Squeeze

As a last resort, the cow can be completely immobilized and laid down flat by applying a rope squeeze, as shown in Figures 9 and 10. The half-hitch method in Figure 9 seems to work a bit better but with either method a cow can

Figure 9. Getting a cow off her feet — first method. The rope is passed around the neck and behind one leg and tied. The long end is then passed around the body in two half-hitches, and the free end pulled back straight.

Figure 10. Getting a cow off her feet — second method. The middle of the rope is draped over the withers and the free end brought back between the forelegs (a). The ends are then crossed over the back and pulled straight back between the rear legs. In either method, pulling on the rope causes the animal to fall. An assistant should hold the animal's head down as soon as the animal is down.

be gently laid down flat by pulling on the free end of the rope. The half-hitch method should not be used on bulls because of possible injury to the penis by the rear half hitch. Once the cow is down, an assistant sitting on her head can keep her that way. Needless to say, cows should not be cast in this manner on a hard floor or where the footing is likely to be slippery when they get up. This technique is not recommended for general use because it can cause complications such as torsion of the uterus during advanced pregnancy or displaced

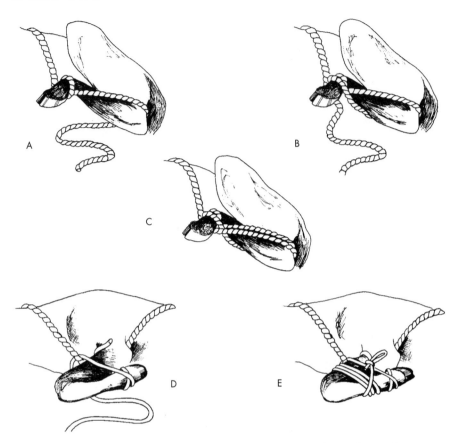

Once the animal is down, the free end of the squeeze rope can be used to tie the rear legs as shown in a, b, and c. A short piece of rope is used to restrain the foreleg, as shown in d and e.

abomasum. Furthermore, when cows are kept flat on their side very long there is a risk of bloat, regurgitation, and inhalation pneumonia.

Examining Cows' Feet

The frequency with which cows' feet need to be examined and trimmed presents a physical challenge. They simply don't stand well on three legs as a horse will. Some type of mechanical aid is usually necessary. The front feet are generally no problem; Figure 11 shows a method of supporting the front leg. The hind legs are a different story. Not only are they more mobile and lethal, but the cow resists having them picked up because they must be drawn backward and upward in order to work on the sole.

One effective method is shown in Figure 12a and b. A loop, preferably with a quick-release honda, is placed around the pastern. The running end is then

Figure 11. Supporting a front foot.

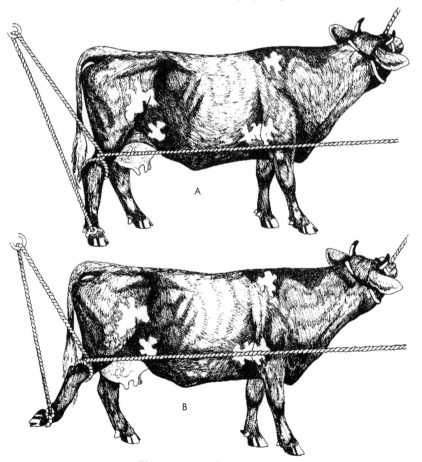

Figure 12. Rear leg gets support.

put through a ring, over a beam, or whatever is handy, brought back to form a half-hitch around the hock, and then passed forward and snubbed around something solid and held by an assistant. As the foot is picked up, the rope is tightened so that the leg is suspended with support at the hock and pastern. Once the leg is elevated to the proper position, the rope should be held in place by the assistant. It should never be tied because some cows will resist the procedure and struggle until they fall. If they fall from this position, a broken hip is a common sequel. **Always be ready to release animals from potentially dangerous restraint instantly.**

The Tail Tie

Although it restrains nothing but the tail, the tail tie shown in Figure 13 is simple and frequently useful. If nothing else it will keep a manure-soaked tail out of your face while you are milking.

As a part of good dairy herd management, extra teats should be amputated from the heifers when they are two to three weeks old. For this operation, the heifers must be restrained on their backs. Depending on the technique used, this posture may be necessary for castration of bull calves as well. Calves at this age can be pretty frisky, but it isn't hard to lay them down if you go about it right. Figure 14 shows the preferred method. Standing alongside the calf, bend over and grasp the front and rear legs nearest you and lift. This tips the calf toward you and allows her to gently slide down against your legs and you are then in position to put your knees on the calf to hold her down while you tie the rear legs as shown in Figure 15a and b. Tipping the calf the other way, away from you, not only causes the calf to fall with a jarring thump but puts you on the side where the legs will be flailing until and if you can get them under con-

Figure 13. Keeping the tail out of the way.

Figure 14. How to lower a calf to the ground.

Figure 15. How to keep the calf on the ground.

trol. Never try to throw a calf by grabbing the front and rear legs and twisting until the calf falls. This is painful for the calf and may be for you, too.

Horses

Although comparable in size and weight, when it comes to restraint, horses are much different from cows. By nature they are much less phlegmatic and more responsive to pain. Their movements are quicker and, in addition to kicking with the hind legs, they will rear and strike with the front legs and may bite when you least expect it. They are also much stronger and the potential for injury from an obstreperous horse is considerably greater than from a cow.

On the plus side, most horses today are what must be classed as companion animals. They are brushed, petted, and pampered daily to the point where a few are just plain spoiled. The frequent attention does accustom them to handling, although when the discomfort of some necessary veterinary procedure is a factor, their response may be totally unexpected.

I was called one time by a lady to vaccinate her horse for sleeping sickness. She had a beautiful two-year-old Morgan filly, born on the farm, and never handled by anyone other than herself. When I approached the filly, syringe in hand, she literally went wild. I couldn't even get into the box stall with her. After a few futile attempts, I handed the syringe to the owner and told her how to give the injection while I got out of sight. This she proceeded to do in the box stall with no restraint whatever. That's how that horse was vaccinated every year thereafter. Strange as it may seem, it turned out that the filly had never seen a man before and was simply terrified by the sight or smell or both. She just didn't like men. All of which points out that horses are different from other livestock.

Approach Quietly

Because horses are different, a little "horse sense" and judgment goes a long way in preventing injury to them and to you when restraint is necessary. Approach the horse quietly and confidently but never sneak up on him. Let him know you are there by a quiet word or two. Then put a hand on him, starting at the shoulder and working toward the area you want to reach. To avoid serious injury from a kick, incongruous as it may seem, stand in close. That way a suddenly raised leg may push you away rather violently, but you won't get the full force of the kick. Don't make the mistake of thinking you can avoid injury by standing as far away as possible and reaching to touch a sore spot or whatever. This leaves you off balance, and because the horse's leg is longer than your arm, you are certain to get hurt if the horse should kick.

The Halter

The most universal restraint device for horses is the halter and they should be introduced to it early in life. If the halter is to be used as a restraint device for a procedure the horse doesn't like, however, the lightweight show-type halter will not be strong enough. Most of them can be easily broken. A heavy leather or webbing halter will do a better job. In an emergency, a halter can be improvised with a lariat as shown in Figure 16a–c. A strong lead shank with a snap is fastened to the halter ring. A piece of ½-inch nylon rope about six feet long does a good job if properly used. The novice will often hold the lead shank near the end with one hand and try to lead the horse like a dog. This method doesn't really provide any control because, with slack in the rope, if your back is turned, the horse can reach out and bite or strike with a front foot before you realize what happened.

Figure 16. A lariat quickly tied into a halter.

The proper way to use a lead shank is to stand on the left side of the horse's head facing the same direction. Grasp the shank firmly in the right hand about six inches from the halter and hold the other end in the left hand. By holding the shank close to the halter you can detect the slightest movement of the horse and do something about it if his intentions appear hostile.

Cross-Tying

Cross-tying, illustrated in Figure 17, provides added restriction of movement. This may be all that is needed to restrain the animal for common procedures such as shoeing. Cross-tying is strongly recommended for horses being moved in trucks or trailers because it helps the animal maintain its balance when the vehicle sways, and prevents head injuries.

A variety of further restraints can be used in addition to cross-tying. Picking up one foot sometimes helps to assure that the other three will remain on the ground. Twisting an ear may provide sufficient distraction to take the animal's mind off what is being done to him somewhere else.

Figure 17. Cross-tying is used for many common procedures.

Figure 18. The chain twitch.

The Twitch

When these mild measures fail, a twitch may have to be used. A typical commercial chain twitch is shown in Figure 18. To put this on, assuming you are right-handed, put your left hand fingertips through the chain loop and spread your fingers to hold the chain near your fingertips. Then grab the horse's nose with your left hand and maintain the hold while you slide the chain loop down on the horse. Still holding the nose in the left hand, twist the twitch handle with the right until the chain tightens up, then hold the handle with both hands. While a few horses will fight a twitch, most will give up in response to the pressure applied. Use only the degree of twisting pressure required because the twitch is painful and there is no necessity for cruelty. Although the commercial twitches shown in Figures 18 and 19 will do, they are too short to provide the leverage and control sometimes needed. I prefer the homemade variety, using a thirty-six-inch hickory pick handle because it gives a little more mastery of the situation and permits you to maintain a grip and still avoid flying front feet.

In an emergency, twitches can be improvised with rope and a piece of wood or claw hammer as shown in Figure 20, but these have limited value. Although some people do it, *a twitch should never be put on a horse's ear.* Not

Figure 19. The twitch on the horse.   *Figure 20. Two improvised twitches.*

only is it acutely painful but it may rupture a blood vessel in the ear causing a hematoma which almost invariably ends up as an unsightly scar.

Other Restraints

Various other restraint techniques can be used as the situation requires. Some stallions, for example, can be difficult to control when teasing or breeding mares. A helpful technique is to use a lead shank that has a foot or so of chain interposed between the rope or strap and the snap. The snap is threaded through the left side ring of the halter, over the bridge of the nose, and attached to the corresponding ring on the right side of the halter. With this arrangement the stallion more interested in his sex life than his behavior can be brought back to reality by a sharp tug on the lead shank. The discomfort of the chain pressing on the bridge of his nose will give him something else to think about. If that is inadequate, a **war bridle** applied as in Figure 21 may help. This is simply a slip noose passed back of the poll and under the upper lip where it puts pressure on the gums of the upper incisors when tightened. It hurts, and most horses develop a healthy respect for it.

To protect the stallion from the kick of a reluctant mare during breeding, it's sometimes advisable to use **breeding hobbles.** Figure 22 shows a method of applying rope breeding hobbles. Some mares may need similar restraint for rectal palpation or pregnancy examination. The best rope to use in this manner is ⅝-inch or ¾-inch cotton. Manila and even nylon may cause rope burns,

Figure 21. A war bridle can be used on an unruly stallion.

Figure 22. How to apply rope breeding hobbles.

which are slow to heal and may leave a scar. As a word of caution, hobbles should not be so tight that the mare's movement is unduly restricted. If they are, she may lose her balance and fall, causing injury.

The **tail tie** shown in Figure 23 is sometimes useful to stabilize or control lateral movement of the rear end. It's a simple method of tying the switch to a

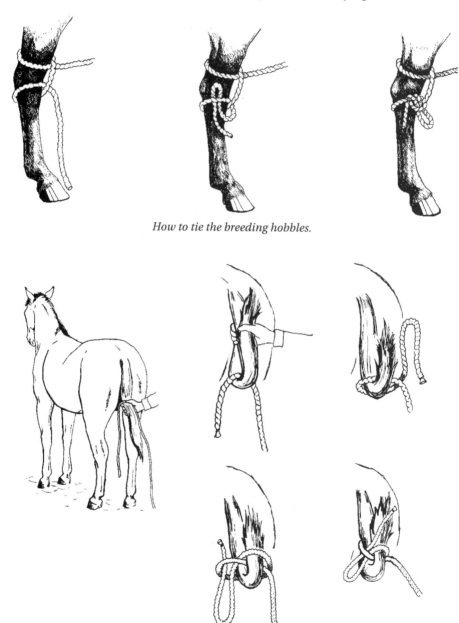

How to tie the breeding hobbles.

Figure 23. How to apply the tail tie.

rope which can be quickly released. Although it usually isn't necessary, a rope tied to the tail can be used to help support the rear leg, as shown in Figures 24 and 25. Figure 26 illustrates the use of a rope to support the foreleg.

Occasionally it's necessary to carry or restrain a young foal. Figure 27 shows the preferred method, which provides restraint yet is comfortable for the foal.

Figures 24 and 25. The tail tie can be used to support a rear leg.

Figure 26. A rope tie to support a front foot.

Figure 27. How to restrain or carry a foal.

Sheep, Swine, and Goats

With the exception of mature swine, these species are much more manageable than horses or cows because of their smaller size. Nevertheless, a few tips may be helpful.

The most difficult part about restraining a sheep is catching it. A flock of sheep will run at the slightest pretext and it's difficult to separate a single one from the flock. The only practical method is to drive the entire flock into a pen or corral to limit their movement. Then, with an assistant and a couple of portable crowding gates, you can isolate the one you want to catch. For the purpose, light gates three feet high and six to eight feet wide are very useful. When you have your sheep separated, hold it with one arm under the neck and the other under the tail. Never grab a sheep by the wool because it breaks the fibers, making the fleece less valuable. Once caught, sheep seldom struggle.

Goats, too, are not much of a problem and can be restrained easily with a collar or halter. Pigs, however, are a whole different matter. Once one reaches 100 pounds or so there is nothing much more difficult to hold than a frightened, determined pig. There are no good handles to grab and they are all muscle. Once they are cornered together, piglets and goats can be held by the hind legs for vaccination, castration, and other procedures, but larger pigs require a different technique.

Figure 28. This swine mouth speculum is used to hold the mouth open for examination or to give oral medication. The same instrument can be used on sheep and goats.

Figure 29. Use this method to move a pig backwards to where you want him.

A B C

Figure 30. This method may also work for moving a pig.

Pigs' Teeth

The only real defense a pig has is his very sharp teeth, which he doesn't hesitate to use. But he can also knock the legs out from under you if he runs into you with his solid bulk so approach with some care.

A common challenge is to move a pig from one pen to another when gates are not available. When you are trying to drive a pig he always seems to get his head on the wrong end. A good way to take advantage of this propensity is illustrated in Figure 29. Put a bucket over the pig's head and with an assistant pulling on the tail as a tiller, back the pig wherever you want him to go. A second method of dubious value is to put a noose around the neck supplemented by a half-hitch around the middle and lead — or more likely drag — the pig where you want him to go. Figure 30a–c shows the technique.

The Pig Snare

The most useful instrument for catching and holding a large pig is the snare, shown in Figure 31. This is basically a four-foot length of pipe through which a flexible cable is threaded with a loop formed in the business end. By holding the pipe in one hand and pulling the handle with the other, the loop is tightened. Characteristically, a pig trying to avoid capture in a pen will back into a corner and keep his myopic eyes on you. With a pig in this position, it's easy to put the snare loop over his snout and draw it tight. Once it is tightened he usually just pulls back and squeals. The same thing can be done with a rope, but it is a bit harder to manage (see Figure 32). With a rope, however, you have the advantage of a free end that can be tied around a hind leg, as shown in Figure 33, to immobilize the pig.

Figure 31. A pig snare, made of a pipe and flexible cable.

Figure 32. Rope can be used as a snare.

Figure 33. Rope snare looped around back leg will immobilize a pig.

Summary

Most of the restraint techniques described here along with others not described, have evolved since man first domesticated animals — a period during which there was no alternative to physical restraint. But during the past thirty years, veterinary research has developed techniques and drugs for sedation, tranquilization, and anesthesia that have made major physical restraint unnecessary in most cases. These are safer for the animal and for the operator.

Now a word on behalf of veterinarians everywhere: If you have a cow or horse that you know has an inclination to kick, tell the veterinarian before he gets in range so he knows what to expect. There are few things more maddening than the phrase all of us have heard after the fact, "I meant to tell you — she kicks." Similarly, if your veterinarian asks you to hold an animal while he works on her, do so with undivided attention. I still have a scar from a kick received when the client dropped a twitch and ran the first time the horse jumped a bit.

Finally, remember that within the context of this book on animal health you will often be restraining an animal that is sick. Be as gentle and quiet in your handling as possible because excitement and exertion will only make a sick animal worse. If the cure is worse than the disease, nothing is accomplished.

Physical Examination

ONE OF THE MOST FRUSTRATING AND DISCOURAGING ASPECTS of large animal practice to a veterinarian is the frequency with which he is called only in time to perform the last rites. Many reasons are given. "I didn't realize she was sick until this morning," or "I thought she might get better." One of the most maddening is, "Well, Doc, I knew she was a little off so I gave her penicillin, some sulfa pills, and a good laxative last week but that didn't help so I thought I'd give you a chance to see what you can do!"

All too often the animal is so far gone by then that poor Doc has no chance at all and neither does his patient. Too often the end result is that death terminates the animal's suffering and Doc gets the blame. The only benefit, if there is one, from this kind of situation is that the owner can ease his or her conscience by proclaiming to all who will listen that, "Well, I called Doc to look at her but it was a waste of money because she died anyhow. I guess he isn't too sharp."

Every veterinarian has found himself in this position many times. But the owner is right; employing veterinary service in this manner is a waste of money. The earlier a disease is recognized and properly treated the more probable a satisfactory outcome will be.

Most diseases are preventable, and if you follow the advice in this book, serious illness will be minimal. But despite everyone's best efforts, problems will occur occasionally. The effect of these can be minimized if they are recognized early and an intelligent judgment can be made as to what the condition may be and what degree of treatment may be required. If it looks as if a veterinarian may be required, don't delay calling. The oldest drug in history is tincture of time but it doesn't always work!

Watch Your Animals

Briefly defined, disease is any departure from normal function. It follows, then, that before you can recognize a disease problem you must be thoroughly familiar with the normal behavior and function of the animals in your care. Spending a few minutes every day watching your animals is time well spent. This is the only way you can learn their normal behavior and attitude and unless you know that, you won't recognize anything that may be wrong. This knowledge marks the difference between the animal husbandryman and the less experienced animal owner.

For example, are you always greeted by a whinny when you first enter the horse barn in the morning? This is typical of most horses but suppose you don't hear that whinny some morning. What does it mean? Perhaps nothing, but it certainly merits further investigation. You can be sure your horse's whinny isn't broken but he may be sick. Take time to observe his attitude. Does he hang back in the stall with head down or ears drooping? Does he seem interested in feed or not? Is he sweating or salivating? These are the kinds of things to look for and investigate further.

Watch the herd at pasture for signs of unusual behavior. Cattle, sheep and to a lesser degree, swine, tend to be gregarious and will usually stay together when grazing. Horses are a little more independent and goats are even more so, but they all tend to congregate. The animal that stays off in a corner by itself usually does so for a reason. That reason may be nothing more than aberrant social behavior if it does so consistently. But if an animal normally found with the herd seeks solitude it is usually for a reason. It may be a normal function such as imminent parturition, but it could be illness and needs to be investigated.

Common sense, a little knowledge, and your physical senses applied to examination will often reveal the problem. The important thing is to apply these in a systematic manner and not jump to conclusion.

Things to Look For

In physical examination the first thing to do is observe the animal from some distance. Look for such things as symmetry of conformation. Swellings, depending on location, may indicate an infection, an abscess, a tumor, a hernia, a fracture, a hematoma, or just a bruise.

Note the crusty muzzle and slobbering, suggestive of bovine virus diarrhea or malignant catarrhal fever.

An unusual posture like this is indicative of a lesion in the brain or upper spinal cord.

Look at the head. Does one ear droop or is one eye partially closed?

Is the animal drooling or making aimless movements with its tongue? Are the eyes bright or do they lack lustre and appear dull? Are they sunken, indicating dehydration? Although non-specific, the lustre of the eye is a good measure of an animal's well being.

Does the abdomen have a "tucked up" appearance? Note the character and consistency of the manure. Is it abnormally hard or soft? Does the animal make straining movements? Is the urine of normal color or is it coffee-colored or bloody? In the male animals does the urine flow in a normal stream or does it just dribble, or is there none at all? Is the animal thin, its haircoat rough? Is hair falling out or being rubbed off?

Watch how the animal moves. Is its gait normal, stilted, staggering? Is it reluctant to move at all or is it lame? A keen observer can learn a lot by systematic observation of an animal from a distance. Once this part of the examination has been completed the next step is to zero in at close range on those things noted by visual examination.

Preliminary Examination

Be methodical by not overlooking anything or jumping to conclusions. Where a problem is not obvious the possibilities can be narrowed down by the simple expedient of recording temperature, pulse, and respiration rate before the animal gets excited from handling. The normal ranges are given in accompanying table, 6-1.

TABLE 6-1

Normal Vital Signs

	Temperature (°F)	Pulse/minute	Respiration/minute
Cow	100.4–102.8	60–70	18–28
Horse	99.1–100.8	32–44	8–16
Pig	101.6–103.6	60–80	8–18
Sheep	100.9–103.8	70–80	12–20
Goat	101.7–105.3	70–80	12–20

Take the Temperature

The most useful diagnostic instrument an animal owner can have is a five-inch ring top rectal thermometer. These are obtainable from almost any instrument supply house or drug store. As a word of advice from one who has been there, tie a string on the thermometer unless you want to hold it in the rectum for the required three minutes or so. In the cow, especially with a relaxed anal sphincter, the deeply inserted thermometer may slip in out of sight by the time you are ready to retrieve it. The only recourse then is to go in after it — or pull the string! To prevent loss of the thermometer, tie the free end of the string to a spring-type clothespin and clip it to the tail fold. When the thermometer is attached in this manner you can proceed with the rest of the examination while the temperature is being recorded. For a little more money, instant reading electronic thermometers are available which are more convenient.

The body temperature of animals is not nearly as consistent as ours. Their heat regulatory mechanism is not as efficient, and on a cold day the body temperature will be at the low end of the range and on a hot day at the high end or even higher. Excitement will also raise body temperature, leading to an erroneous interpretation. Pigs are particularly vulnerable to hot weather and may suffer heat stroke with body temperatures sometimes exceeding 108°F. Therefore, one must use judgment in interpreting the reading on the thermometer. On a hot day, a reading slightly above the normal range does not necessarily indicate a fever.

Aside from weather influence and excitement, fever is generally indicative of viral or bacterial infection or occasionally of severe pain. Temperature will be subnormal in the cow with milk fever, for a transitory period following high fever, and prior to death. A normal temperature at initial examination of an animal off feed is usually indicative of some type of digestive, metabolic, or functional disorder. Thus, much can be learned with the aid of a simple inexpensive thermometer.

Pulse and respiration rate generally but not always parallel body temperature. Both go up, of course, in response to excitement or exertion, therefore it's important to handle sick animals quietly and carefully. The added exertion of being chased around the pen can kill the animal with pneumonia. Heart and respiratory rates will be elevated without fever in cases of anemia due to iron deficiency, blood loss due to parasitism or hemorrhage, red blood cell destruction as occurs with anaplasmosis or piroplasmosis, and in some types of poisoning as well as in response to pain or fear.

Check the Pulse

The pulse is the surge of blood through the arteries immediately following contraction of the heart ventricles. It normally parallels the heart rate and its character reveals much about the animal's condition. Pulse rate may be variously classified as regular, irregular, weak, strong, or thready. Except for regularity, these nuances will not be detected by the layperson, and, for our purposes, need not be.

In cows, the pulse is most easily detected by palpating the middle coccygeal artery on the underside of the tail about six inches down from the tail head. The easiest site in horses is where the facial artery crosses the underside of the jawbone just in front of the large muscle that forms the cheek. In goats and sheep, the heartbeat can usually be felt directly but the pulse can easily be felt over the femoral artery about a third of the way down on the inside of the thigh. The same location is satisfactory for young, thin pigs, but in most pigs the fat thickness precludes palpation of an arterial pulse. Practice taking the pulse on several normal animals until you can do so readily and with confidence if the need arises.

Check Respiration

Increased rate of respiration with fever and coughing is frequently indicative of pneumonia. Without fever it reflects anemia or impaired lung function such as pulmonary edema due to allergy, organophosphate poisoning, or circulatory collapse.

These three measurements — temperature, pulse, and respiration — provide easily obtainable information that helps to narrow the possible causes of illness. They even give some indication of what the final outcome may be.

Check the Rumen, Too

For ruminant animals, cows, sheep, and goats, a fourth measurement can be added, and that is **rate of rumen contraction.** The rumen can be likened to a mixing vat that churns periodically to stir up the ingested feed. In the normal animal, rumen contractions occur two to four times a minute. By pressing firmly on the left flank one can feel this movement when it occurs. Contractions will be slower than normal or absent with some types of indigestion, in the cow with traumatic gastritis or displaced abomasum, during milk fever, as a result of dehydration, and in conditions affecting the vagus nerve. Contractions will be faster than normal in the animal which has or is about to have diarrhea from any cause.

The examination so far permits some tentative conclusions whether the illness is due to infectious or noninfectious causes, and this helps to narrow the possibilities considerably. A preliminary judgment can even be made whether to call a veterinarian at this point. If you decide to call, tell your veterinarian what you have observed. He will appreciate it because what you describe will help him to decide whether he should drop everything else and come right out (often at added cost to you) or whether it is safe to wait until later when he will be in the area anyhow. As he develops confidence in your ability at preliminary evaluation you may find that he takes less time to make a final diagnosis. Since the veterinarian's time is worth money (yours), you ultimately save.

Further Examination

Ailments Causing High Fever

If you are still undecided what to do at this point, start methodically examining the accessible organ systems. If there is high fever, the odds favor disease involving the respiratory tract, the reproductive organs including the mammary gland, or the urinary tract.

For the respiratory tract look for nasal discharge, coughing, labored breathing, and in extreme cases, flaring of the nostrils during inspiration. In his examination, your veterinarian would also add careful auscultation of (listening to) the lungs with a stethoscope and percussion. In the case of such diseases as infectious bovine rhinotracheitis or influenza, samples may also have to be taken for virus isolation or serological work in the laboratory before a final diagnosis can be made.

But if nothing is obviously wrong with the respiratory tract the next good possibility is the mammary gland. Acute mastitis with fever is common in dairy cattle. While it is less common in beef cattle and other species, it should not be overlooked in any of them as a possible site of infection. The infected udder with acute mastitis will feel hot and swollen to the touch and will usually be very sore. The color and consistency of the milk will be abnormal. It may be watery and have clots, flakes, or pus in it. These abnormalities can best be detected by squirting some milk on a black plate strip pan. The type of strip cup employing a fine mesh screen will reveal clots and flakes but will not identify milk that is off color or watery. Most farm supply stores stock some satisfactory type of black strip plate. Acute mastitis is a serious disease that requires prompt and appropriate treatment locally and systemically.

Urinary tract infections such as leptospirosis and pyelonephritis may be difficult to diagnose based on physical signs alone. This is a job for the veterinarian unless you happen to see coffee-colored urine typical of leptospirosis.

Obviously there are many more diseases causing fever in domestic animals but the foregoing illustrates the steps to be taken in arriving at a diagnosis.

Disease Without Fever

Disease conditions not associated with fever are many and varied. Some are accompanied by loss of appetite but others are not. If appetite is lacking, think first of indigestion. Is there history of recent diet change which is a common cause? Is rumination slow and are feces scanty? Is there evidence of

A horse with colic will often stand in a stretched-out position and look anxiously at his belly.

abdominal cramps and pain such as restlessness, kicking at the belly, stretching and standing in a stretched-out, "saw-horse" attitude? All are indications of indigestion. Indigestion is a common cause of colic in the horse accompanied by rapid pulse, sweating, marked pain, and sometimes injection of the sclera. The latter is merely dilation of the blood vessels supplying the white part of the eye.

If there is no fever and no evidence of indigestion yet the animal refuses feed and water, look in the mouth for swellings, ulcers, and, in the horse, sharp teeth. One word of caution — if you live in an area where rabies is endemic, don't put your bare hands in the mouth of an animal that is not eating for an obscure reason. Wear leather or rubber gloves.

Sharp teeth or malocclusion may be a cause of failure to eat. The inside edge of the lower molars and the outside of the upper molars of the horse become very sharp and sometimes abrade the cheek and tongue. The resulting soreness leads to inadequate chewing which contributes to indigestion. Check, too, for tongue paralysis, a principal sign of botulism and a common finding with listeriosis in cattle, sheep, and goats. The latter disease also usually causes a unilateral facial paralysis and an inclination to walk in circles.

Lameness

Other non-febrile disease conditions will usually be obvious at least insofar as the affected area is concerned. One that commonly causes confusion is lameness. Lameness is common in all species and most of the time the trouble is in the foot itself. Every careful physical examination where lameness is a factor includes picking up the foot and examining it carefully. With a hoof pick, clean away all dirt and debris and with a hoof knife pare away all dead-appearing tissue. Cleaning frequently reveals puncture wounds, imbedded nails and stones, stone bruises, and infections. Sometimes trimming a badly overgrown foot is all that is required. **Foot rot** is a specific disease in cattle, sheep, and goats that is recognizable by the swelling, exudate, and the characteristic foul odor it produces.

Aside from fractures, **joint lesions** are the next most common cause of lameness in species other than the horse. Except where there is obvious swelling, diagnosis of these is best left to the veterinarian. Years ago a common cause of lameness in cattle was rubber canning jar gaskets encircling a single claw or the entire foot. When these were carelessly discarded, cattle would step on them and they would work up higher on the foot. The pressure they exert causes impaired circulation, and they cut into the skin, causing swelling and infection. As home canning became less popular, this type of injury almost disappeared, but with the resurgence of interest in home canning, it may become a consideration again.

Lameness in the horse has a variety of causes other than injuries to the foot. These are so varied and four sound legs are so important to the horse that diagnosis and treatment should be left to the veterinarian.

Consider Other Factors

When attempting to arrive at a diagnosis, consider extraneous factors as well as the clinical signs observed. Environmental factors influence the prevalence of some diseases. Pneumonia, for example, is relatively rare in the summer but common in the winter from October through March when rapid weather shifts occur. Conversely, labored breathing due to pulmonary edema is more common when animals are exposed to allergenic grasses at pasture. Internal parasitism with stomach worms in sheep, goats, and cattle is rarely a problem in the winter but is serious on some farms during the pasture season. The onset of acute haemonchosis in sheep can be dramatic a few days after a rain that follows a prolonged dry period because the moisture fosters maturation to the infective stage of the worm ova which have accumulated. Pregnancy disease or ketosis in the ewe as well as ketosis and milk fever in the cow are always associated with parturition. Similarly, metritis does not occur when the animal is pregnant but appears after parturition.

Regional Diseases

Some diseases occur only in certain regions. For example, winter dysentery in cattle occurs primarily in the Northeast. Piroplasmosis in horses is limited mostly to the Gulf Coast states because that's where the tick which transmits it lives. The strains of virus causing equine encephalomyelitis tend to be regionally specific and are identified as Eastern, Western, Venezuelan, and so on.

As you learn more about the pathogenesis of disease and take all factors into account, the problem of diagnosis — at least of the common diseases — becomes somewhat easier.

The foregoing by no means covers all the misfortunes that can befall animals and it will not make you an accomplished diagnostician. It does outline a procedure for preliminary examination which, when coupled with the specific disease information to follow, should allow you to distinguish between those things you can handle and those for which a veterinarian should be called.

Once the physical examination has been completed and the animal has been evaluated, the following tables may help to suggest some possible causes for the illness. These include most but certainly not all of the specific disease entities afflicting animals. This is essentially the procedure every veterinarian goes through in reading a diagnosis — complete history, careful physical examination, evaluation of clinical findings, differential, and final diagnosis. The veterinarian, of course, by virtue of training and experience will have a much greater depth of knowledge about the physiological and pathological processes involved, as well as the advantage of a battery of diagnostic tests when necessary.

Except in the most obvious conditions, it will always be to your advantage to have the diagnosis and therapeutic recommendations made by your veterinarian. I am always amazed at how many people who wouldn't think of attempting to repair the TV set themselves don't hesitate to use a variety of potions and remedies on a valuable sick animal before they call a veterinarian as a last resort.

Don't forget that nothing is absolute in medicine and there are many variables.

Although we may list and classify diseases and symptoms in a convenient manner, in reality medicine is not this orderly. Not all diseases produce all the clinical signs listed all the time and there are varying degrees of severity. Nothing precludes the possibility of more than one disease affecting the animal at the same time. In fact, malnutrition and some types of internal parasitism frequently coincide. A good example of disease interaction is the MMA syndrome in sows. Predisposing factors for this condition are lack of dietary roughage, lack of exercise, unsanitary surroundings, and constipation. The clinical signs include uterine infection (metritis), mastitis, and agalactiae, hence the acronym MMA. The implications for the sow are serious, but they are even worse for the piglets, which, because there is no milk, die of hypoglycemia or starvation.

The moral, if there is one, is that it is always better to prevent disease than to treat it, no matter how prompt the diagnosis and therapy. A better understanding of animal disease and its diagnosis will assist in development of programs for disease prevention.

TABLE 6-2

Common Livestock Diseases Characterized by Fever

Disease	Species	Primary Site	Remarks
Anaplasmosis	cattle, sheep, goats	red blood cells	insect borne, anemia, southern states
Anthrax	cattle, sheep, goats, horses, pigs	generalized	high mortality limited distribution
Babesiasis (Piroplasmosis)	horses	liver, spleen	insect borne, anemia, southern states
Bacillary hemoglobinuria	cattle	liver	western and southern USA
Blackleg	cattle, sheep, goats	muscle	young cattle, 6–12 months, usually acute
Bluetongue	sheep, cattle, goats	generalized	western states
Bovine virus diarrhea (BVD, Mucosal Disease)	cattle	alimentary tract	yearlings
Calf diphtheria	cattle	pharynx, larynx	2–6 months of age
Contagious ecthyma (sore mouth)	sheep, goats	lips, udder	contact transmission
Enzootic Pneumonia (Virus pig pneumonia, V.P.P.)	pigs	lung	3 weeks and older
Eperythrozoonosis	pigs, sheep, cattle	red blood cells	southern and midwestern states
Equine encephalomyelitis	horses	brain	several viral strains
Equine infectious anemia (EIA)	horses	generalized	acute, chronic, inapparent
Equine influenza	horses	upper respiratory tract	clinical signs during inclement weather
Equine rhinopneumonitis (Virus abortion)	horses	upper respiratory tract	abortion follows
Erysipelas	pigs	generalized	
Heat stroke	pigs, horses	generalized	weather influence
Hog cholera	pigs	generalized	high mortality
Infectious bovine rhinotracheitis (IBR, Rednose)	cattle	upper respiratory tract	all ages, highly contagious, low mortality
Infectious polyarthritis (Glassers Disease)	pigs	generalized	2–4 months of age
Leptospirosis	cattle, pigs, sheep, goats	kidney	any age
Listeriosis	cattle, sheep, goats	brain	silage thought to predispose
Lyme disease	horses, cattle	lameness	northwest, north central states

Table 6-2

Common Livestock Diseases Characterized by Fever

Disease	Species	Primary Site	Remarks
Malignant catarrhal fever	cattle	mouth, pharynx, generalized	sporadic
Malignant edema	cattle, sheep, goats, swine	local, generalized	wound infection, acute
Navel infection (Navel ill)	horses, cattle, sheep, goats, pigs	navel, joints	1–3 weeks of age
Necrobacillosis	cattle, sheep	liver	feedlots
Parainfluenza	all species	lungs	low mortality
Pasteurellosis	sheep, pigs, goats	lungs, generalized in swine	
Pasteurellosis (shipping fever)	cattle	lungs	all ages, highly contagious
Polyarthritis	sheep	joints	feedlot lambs
Potomac fever (Ehrlichiosis)	horse	large intestine	acute diarrhea equine
Pseudorabies	pigs, cattle	brain, nerves	severe pruritis
Pyelonephritis	cattle	kidney	sporadic
Salmonellosis	cattle, sheep, pigs, goats, horses	intestine	young more severely affected
Shigellosis (Sleepy foal disease)	horses	generalized	1–3 days of age
Strangles (Distemper)	horses	pharynx	young horses
Swine dysentery (Vibrionic dysentery)	pigs	intestine	8–12 weeks of age
Swine influenza	pigs	upper respiratory tract	clinical signs during inclement weather
Tetanus	horses, sheep, goats, pigs, cattle	nerves, brain	wound infection
Thromboembolic meningoencephalitis (TEM)	cattle	brain	feedlot cattle
Toxoplasmosis	sheep, goats, cattle	generalized	
Transmissible gastroenteritis (TGE)	pigs	intestine	1–4 weeks of age
Tularemia	sheep, pigs, horses	generalized	northwest U.S.
Vesicular stomatitis	cattle, horses, pigs	mouth	
Viral arteritis	horses	generalized	easily confused with rhinopneumonitis and influenza
Viral encephalitis (Teschen disease)	pigs	brain	1–2 weeks of age

TABLE 6-3

Common Livestock Diseases Not Characterized by Fever

Disease	Species	Primary Site	Remarks
Acetonemia (Ketosis)	cattle	liver, generalized	1–4 weeks after calving
Actinobacillosis	cattle	soft tissue, tongue	sudden onset
Actinomycosis	cattle	bone, jaw	chronic
Allergy	cattle, horses	skin, lungs	weeds, drugs, sprays
Anaphylaxis	cattle, horses, sheep, goats, pigs	lungs, general	vaccine injection
Anemia	all	red blood cells	variable causes
Aneurysm	horses	Mesenteric artery	follows trongyle infestation
Bloat	cattle, sheep, goats	rumen	lush wet legume pasture, chronic in some individuals
Botulism	cattle, horses, sheep, goats	nerve endings	paralysis
Brisket disease	cattle	heart	high altitudes
Brucellosis	cattle, pigs, goats, sheep	genital tract	abortion, infertility
Cardiac anomalies	all	heart	congenital, young animals
Caseous lymphadenitis	goats, sheep	lymph glands	chronic abscesses
Coccidiosis	cattle, sheep, goats, pigs, horses	intestine	bloody diarrhea
Colibacillosis	cattle, pigs, sheep, goats, horses	intestine, generalized	young animals, sudden onset
Contagious equine metritus (CEM)	cattle	lymph nodes	chronic
Displaced abomasum	cattle	abomasum	mature cows; easily confused with ketosis
Enterotoxemia	sheep, cattle, goats, pigs, horses	depending on type	young well-fed animals
Grass tetany (hypomagnesemia)	cattle	generalized, neurological signs	lush, grass pasture
Greasy pig disease	pigs	skin	easily confused with parakeratosis
Gut edema	pigs	intestine, generalized	thrifty feeder pigs
Indigestion	horses, cattle, sheep, goats, pigs	stomach	feed change, over-eating
Infectious keratitis (pink-eye)	cattle	eye	
Internal parasitism	sheep, horses, cattle, goats, pigs	variable depending on parasite	variable causes
Interstitial pneumonia (Lungers, fog fever)	cattle	lungs	variable causes

TABLE 6-3

Common Livestock Diseases
Not Characterized by Fever

Disease	Species	Primary Site	Remarks
Iron deficiency anemia (Thumps)	pigs	blood	1–4 weeks of age
Isoimmune hemolytic anemia	horses	blood	foals after nursing
Jowl abscess	pigs	throat	6 weeks and older
Laminitis (founder)	horses, cattle, sheep, goats	foot	sequel to overfeeding on grain or other disease
Lead poisoning	cattle, sheep, goats, pigs	generalized	paint, old motor oil, sprays, etc.
Lymphomatosis	cattle	lymph nodes	chronic
Mammillitis	cattle	teats, udder, skin	more severe than pseudocowpox
Myoclonia congenita (shaky pig disease)	pigs	brain	baby pigs, congenital
Necrotic pododermatitis (foot rot)	cattle, sheep, goats	foot	sporadic in cattle, contagious in sheep
Neoplasms	all	variable	slow onset
Nitrate poisoning	cattle, sheep, goats	blood	high nitrate forage
Nutritional deficiencies	all	variable	develop slowly
Osteodystrophic fibrosis (Big head)	horses, pigs	bone	adults
Osteomalacia	cattle, sheep	bone	adults
Papillomatosis (Warts)	cattle, goats, horses, pigs	skin	
Parakeratosis (Zn deficiency)	pigs, cattle, goats	skin	
Paratuberculosis (Johne's Disease)	cattle, goats, sheep	intestine	chronic
Parturient paresis (Milk fever)	cattle, goats	metabolic, generalized	associated with calving
Polioencephalo-malacia	cattle, sheep, goats	brain	6–24 months of age
Porcine parvovirus	pigs	embryo, fetus	reproductive failure
Pregnancy disease (Ketosis)	sheep	liver, generalized	occurs at lambing
Pseudocowpox	cattle	teats, udder	
Pulmonary emphysema (heaves)	horses, cattle	lungs	chronic
Purpura hemorrhagica	horses	blood	sequel to other illness sporadic
Rabies	cattle, horses, goats, sheep, pigs	nerves, brain	endemic areas, human health hazard
Ringworm	cattle, pigs, horses, goats, sheep	skin	human health hazard

TABLE 6-3

Common Livestock Diseases
Not Characterized by Fever

Disease	Species	Primary Site	Remarks
Salt poisoning	cattle, pigs	brain	high salt and low water intake
Spastic syndrome	cattle	rear leg muscles	adults, hereditary
Sporotrichosis	horses	skin	wound infection
Streptothricosis (Mycotic dermatitis)	cattle, sheep, goats, horses, pigs	skin	chronic
Swine pox	pigs	belly, snout	
Tuberculosis	cattle, pigs, goats	generalized	human health hazard
Urea poisoning	cattle, sheep, goats	generalized	acute, excess urea or inadequate mixing in feeds
Urethral calculi	sheep, cattle, goats	urethra	more common in castrated males
White muscle disease (stiff lamb disease)	sheep, cattle	muscle	young thrifty animals exercise accentuates
Winter dysentery	cattle	intestine	northeastern U.S. highly contagious

TABLE 6-4

Common Livestock Diseases
Characterized by Diarrhea

Disease	Species
Bovine virus diarrhea	cattle
Coccidiosis	cattle, sheep, goats, pigs, horses
Colibacillosis	cattle, pigs, sheep, goats
Indigestion	all
Internal parasitism (some types)	all
Malignant catarrhal fever	cattle
Paratuberculosis	cattle, goats, sheep
Salmonellosis	all
Swine dysentery	pigs
Transmissible gastroenteritis	pigs
Winter dysentery	cattle

TABLE 6-5

Common Livestock Diseases Characterized by Neurological Signs

Disease	Species
Acetonemia (occasionally)	cattle
Botulism	cattle, horses, sheep, goats
Equine encephalomyelitis	horses
Grass tetany	cattle
Lead poisoning	cattle, sheep, goats, pigs
Listeriosis	cattle, sheep, goats
Myoclonia congenita	pigs
Polioencephalomalacia	cattle, sheep, goats
Pseudorabies	pigs, cattle
Rabies	cattle, horses, goats, sheep, pigs
Salt poisoning	cattle, pigs
Teschen disease	pigs
Thromboembolic meningoencephalitis (TEM)	cattle
Urea poisoning	cattle, sheep, goats

TABLE 6-6

Common Livestock Diseases Characterized by Respiratory Distress

Disease	Species
Anaphylaxis	all
Brisket disease	cattle
Calf diphtheria (advanced)	cattle
Equine influenza	horses
Heat stroke	pigs, horses
Infectious bovine rhinotracheitis	cattle
Iron deficiency anemia	pigs
Malignant catarrhal fever	cattle
Nitrate poisoning	cattle, sheep, goats
Parainfluenza	all
Pneumonia (all types)	all
Pulmonary emphysema	horses, cattle
Strangles (advanced)	horses
Urea poisoning	Cattle, sheep, goats

ANIMAL DISEASES

Part Two of this book is devoted to a brief discussion of the diseases affecting livestock with suggestions for their prevention. Not every possible disease is covered, and the reader should keep in mind that two or more diseases can affect the same animal concurrently.

Familiarity with this section will not make the reader an accomplished diagnostician; that comes only with training and experience. It *will* help to promote understanding of the many ills that can befall livestock and should help the livestock owner to better understand the diagnosis and recommendations made when veterinary service becomes necessary.

Although most of the major disease entities affecting livestock in the U.S. are described in this section, little is said about treatment for several reasons. Effective treatment is contingent upon accurate diagnosis and selection of the most effective drugs available. Drugs for use on livestock are widely advertised but, unfortunately, the best advertisement and the best drug don't always coincide so, for the novice, making the appropriate choice is difficult. Secondly, where food-producing animals are concerned, government regulation is a factor. Effective drugs that were once on the market have been removed from the market by law because of prolonged residue problems. Drug residues in meat or milk are considered adulteration, and adulterated food products are illegal. To prevent adulteration, there are legally specified withdrawal times (the interval between administration of the drug and the time of slaughter for meat, or sale of the milk) for all the drugs available for food animals. This time varies for different drugs and sometimes even for the same active ingredient in different vehicles. Lastly, what might be recommended for treatment today could become obsolete tomorrow. For all these reasons, definitive diagnosis and treatment recommendations for major problems are best left to your veterinarian. Indiscriminate use of drugs may only confuse the diagnosis and may create violative residues leading to fines for you and bad publicity for your industry.

In keeping with the book's focus, although specific treatments for diseases are de-emphasized, general recommendations for disease prevention through management and immunization appear throughout.

Diseases Caused by Bacteria

MASTITIS

Without doubt, mastitis is the most prevalent disease afflicting dairy cattle, but its prevalence is not limited to them alone. It is a common problem in sows and dairy goats, occurs sporadically in beef cattle, sheep, and, rarely, in the mare. It may occur as a chronic, even inapparent infection, or as an acute febrile disease causing generalized illness in addition to local pain and swelling. The acute form especially in sheep and goats may be complicated by secondary infection with *Clostridium perfringens,* which causes gangrene. This sequel, commonly called "blue-bag," is life-threatening, and at the very least usually results in sloughing (falling off) of the infected gland.

There are a number of bacteria that have the potential to cause mastitis, including *Streptococcus agalactiae, Streptococcus dysgalactiae, Streptococcus uberis, Escherichia coli,* and several species of *Staphylococci.* Infections due to *Pseudomonas aeruginosa, Corynebacterium pyogenes, Aerobacter aerogenes, Klebsiella spp.,* and a group of organisms called *Mycoplasma* are less common. The latter share some of the characteristics of bacteria and viruses and although *Mycoplasma* mastitis is not common, it produces a severe udder reaction with the quarters becoming rock-hard and generally not producing any milk until the next lactation.

There are regional and species differences in the prevalence of these organisms as udder pathogens. *Str. agalactiae* is the most prevalent in cattle except on the West Coast where *E. coli, Staph.* and other *Streptococci* seem to predominate. *E. coli* is the predominant cause of mastitis in the sow and is often incriminated as a part of the MMA syndrome. *Staph, Strep and E. coli* are the most common causes in thc cwc, doc, and mare.

143

Udder abscess, the result of mastitis.   *Hard intramammary nodules caused by C. pyogenes infection.*

Signs of Mastitis

Clinical signs of acute mastitis include abnormal milk; a hot, swollen udder that is often painful; fever; lack of appetite; and greatly reduced milk flow. The latter has serious implications for the offspring of animals that are nursing their young and agalactia (lack of milk flow) in sows is a prominent cause of death loss of piglets due to starvation. Diagnosis of acute mastitis is not difficult.

Acute mastitis, as a result of treatment and occasionally spontaneously, may subside into a chronic form with a latent infection that subsequently flares up again, particularly when udder resistance is lowered. Localized abscesses are not uncommon as a sequel, nor is scar tissue, which develops from tissue destruction during the acute phase. This results in unbalanced udders with "slack" quarters. Abscesses and lumpy scar tissue are palpable if not actually visible and animals with such evidence of past severe infection are not good prospects for herd replacements.

Testing for Chronic Mastitis

Chronic mastitis is not as easy to diagnose. Characteristically, *Str. agalactiae* produces a low grade chronic infection that causes a gradual attrition of secretory tissue and loss of production. This unobserved infection accounts for production losses as high as 20 percent in some dairy herds, and lost production is the most costly part of chronic mastitis.

Daily use of the black plate strip pan will help to identify cows with chronic mastitis. A few squirts of milk on the plate prior to milking will reveal milk that is watery or contains clots and flakes. As a matter of routine it only takes a few seconds and as a fringe benefit helps to stimulate letdown, thereby facilitating milking.

An indirect but more sensitive and objective method of detecting abnormal milk is the use of a leucocyte screening test such as the California Mastitis Test (CMT), Wisconsin Mastitis Test (WMT), or Modified Whiteside Test (MWT). Of these, the CMT is the easiest to do at the side of the cow. These tests provide an estimate of numbers of somatic cells in milk. Since the leading cause of high numbers of cells in milk is mastitis, it follows that test results will give a reasonably good indication of udder health.

CMT test kits are available from most dairy farm supply dealers. The kit consists of a four-compartment plastic paddle and a bottle of reagent. The reagent is a liquid detergent to which has been added a pH sensitive dye, usually brom-cresol purple. Milk from each quarter is squirted into separate compartments of the paddle and an equal amount of reagent is added. The mixture is then gently swirled for ten to fifteen seconds and the reaction noted. An increase in viscosity and depth of color indicates the presence of somatic cells. The more cells present the greater the viscosity will be and results are recorded as negative, 1, 2, and 3, with 3 being indicative of the most cells. Quarters indicating 2 or 3 almost certainly have serious levels of infection.

Treatment of mastitis, however, should not be based solely on CMT results because cows recently fresh and those drying off will give high test results in the absence of any infection. Udder injury from improper milking machine operation will also raise cell counts but such injury also leads to mastitis very quickly.

The U.S. Public Health Service has adopted the somatic cell count as a measure of milk quality and all milk from commercial dairy herds is periodically screened. The federal standard is set at 750,000 cells/ml of Grade A milk, although many states and milkshed districts have adopted stricter standards. Since the screening is done on a pooled sample representing all cows in the herd, the dairy farmer who consistently meets the federal standard should not feel complacent about the mastitis status of his herd. When the somatic cell count of a pooled sample exceeds 500,000/cc it is virtually certain there are cows with subclinical mastitis in the herd. The higher the count, the more mastitic cows there are.

Neither should the farmer be lulled into complacency by few observed acute or clinical cases. A British study in 1971 of 1,344 cows in 31 herds demonstrated that for every quarter showing evidence of clinical infection there are 32 subclinically infected quarters. Similar results have been obtained in other studies in this country. While obvious clinical cases are bad enough, it's the unobserved subclinical cases that cause the serious production loss due to this disease.

Most of the staggering loss from mastitis can be prevented by application of inexpensive control methods if one understands the pathogenesis (origin and development) of the disease. First, a distinction must be made between udder infection and mastitis. It is possible, even common, for many potential pathogens to infect the mammary gland and not cause disease. Mastitis results when these are present in overwhelming numbers and when resistance of the udder tissue is lowered due to injury. In the dairy cow, an improperly functioning or misused milking machine is a constant source of udder injury leading to a high incidence of clinical mastitis.

Infection of the gland in all species occurs when pathogens enter the teat canal. For practical purposes, this is the only route of infection. It follows, then, that if pathogens are kept away from the teat end, infection will not result. The closer you can come to keeping the teat end sterile, the less the risk will be. Obviously it's impossible under farm conditions to keep teat ends sterile but many simple procedures will help. The first is to keep the animal in as clean and sanitary surroundings as possible to keep environmental pathogens down to a reasonable level. The animal who has no alternative but to lie down in mud and manure is more likely to get an infected udder than one lying on clean dry ground or a well-bedded stall.

An exception should be noted. Although not common, mastitis in cows due to *Klebsiella spp.* is a serious disease that has been linked to use of contaminated sawdust, wood chips, or shavings as bedding. *Klebsiella spp.* is a common saprophyte on tree bark, therefore the use of green sawdust is not recommended. Sawdust or shavings from kiln-dried lumber would be less hazardous.

There are other simple methods of reducing exposure. Milk known infected cows last so that infection will not be carried to others on your hands or the milking machine. Avoid the bad habit of stripping a little milk on the floor before attaching the milking machine. The highest concentration of bacteria is usually in the foremilk and stripping the milk on the floor only increases the level of environmental contamination. Keep animals out of situations likely to lead to high infection rates. For example, serious outbreaks of coliform mastitis have resulted when cows were allowed to wade in contaminated ponds.

Use of Germicide

The single most effective procedure for preventing new infections has proven to be dipping the teat ends in a residual germicide immediately after each milking. A number of teat dip products are available for the purpose, some of which are excellent and others not so good. In the three-year field trial conducted by Cornell University that confirmed the original work on teat dipping as a control procedure done in England, the germicide used was sodium hypochlorite in the form of the common household bleach, Clorox. Diluted at the rate of four parts water to one part of Clorox, this solution gave a residual germicidal effect lasting six hours or more. Commercially available teat dips, although more expensive, are equally good and less objectionable to use.

The teat is most vulnerable to bacterial invasion immediately after milking. The teat sphincter muscle is then relaxed and it's not unusual to find a drop of milk on the teat end when milking is completed. This is an excellent medium for bacterial growth and subsequent invasion of the teat canal itself. Dipping the entire teat in a sanitizer prevents this from happening.

Use of Antibiotics

As a control procedure, it has also been proven advantageous to infuse (inject via the teat canal) long-acting antibiotics into each quarter following the last milking prior to the dry period. This is the most practical time to treat the chronically infected cow because milk doesn't have to be discarded and the antibiotic has a longer time to work. Over a period of time, by following good sanitary practices, dipping teats after each milking, and treating all quarters of all dry cows, a number of herds have become free of infection with *Str. agalactiae* and some have even become free of *Staphylococci*. Once *Str. agalactiae* is eradicated from a herd it will not reappear unless the infection is introduced via an infected cow added to the herd, since, for all practical purposes, the organism lives only in the udder. In the badly infected herd, eradication of *Str. agalactiae* can increase milk production by 20 percent or more.

While an assiduously followed program of teat dipping and dry cow treatment will greatly reduce udder infection as all the herd goes through the treatment cycle, it may sometimes be desirable to reduce the infection level much faster. With the aid of your veterinarian and a diagnostic laboratory, this can be done by collecting milk samples from each quarter and culturing them to identify the bacteria present. Once they are identified and particularly if the organisms are checked for antibiotic sensitivity, the most effective antibiotic can be used to treat the infected quarters. This procedure is most effective for *Str. agalactiae* eradication, since this organism is an obligate udder parasite. The procedure usually has to be repeated several times to eliminate the last vestiges of infection. Although the level of infection with other pathogens can be reduced in this manner, total eradication is difficult because reinfection occurs through environmental contamination. That's why sanitation and avoidance of teat and udder injury is so important in control of mastitis. Treatment alone will never do the job!

Check Milking Machines

The leading cause of teat and udder injury for the dairy cow is improperly used or malfunctioning milking machines. While a detailed discussion of machine function is beyond the scope of this book, a few suggestions may be helpful. First, a great deal of research has gone into milking machine development and it's safe to say that all new milking equipment, properly installed and maintained, will do an adequate job. Trouble arises when dairy farmers forget that the milking machine operates more hours than any other machine on the farm and therefore requires periodic maintenance. All too often it is forgotten until it quits.

The milking system should be checked by a factory trained serviceman every six months. He will check such things as air flow, vacuum level at the pump, stall cock and teat end as well as pulsation rate and interval. On some types the pulsators must be dismantled and cleaned, and worn parts replaced. The rubber teat cup liners must be properly cared for and replaced frequently. Impregnation with butterfat causes them to swell and lose elasticity, thereby reducing their effectiveness. The life of liners can be prolonged by using two sets and rotating them weekly. The used set can be boiled in lye solution to remove accumulated fat and then rested until the next week. Liners used in this manner will last more than twice as long as a single set. The alternative is simply to buy new ones more often. The vacuum pipeline should be flushed monthly to remove accumulated debris that restricts air flow. If you don't know how to do this, your serviceman can show you.

Milking machine problems seem to be more frequent in the small expanding herd. Too many people, as they add more cows, simply add more milker units until they unwittingly exceed the capacity of the vacuum pump and line. The effect is insidious because although the pump may be overloaded, the machines will usually still pulsate and milk cows. But, because of inadequate vacuum, milking time will be increased which means greater irritation for the udder. Be sure you don't exceed the rated capacity of your equipment.

Milking Procedures

Even a properly functioning machine can cause udder irritation if it is not properly used. The longer the machine is attached to the cow the greater the opportunity for irritation and subsequent infection. The vast majority of properly prepared cows will milk out in five minutes or less and the machine should be removed as soon as milking is complete. Some of the new machines are designed to detach automatically when milk flow stops.

To reduce machine on-time, let down of milk must first be stimulated. Milk secretion occurs as a result of hormonal influence. The udder is not a bagful of loose milk, as some people think. It is a gland whose cells secrete milk in response to oxytocin (a hormone) released by the pituitary gland under certain stimuli. One stimulus is washing the udder with warm water, which has the added benefit of removing any accumulated dirt. Individual paper towels are recommended for this purpose to avoid spreading infection from one cow to another, and to wipe excess water from the teats and udder.

In the milking parlor, a warm water spray accomplishes the same thing with less risk of contamination. After washing the udder and wiping it dry, use the strip pan as explained earlier and then attach the machine. The stimulative effect of udder massage is lost in a few minutes if the machine is not promptly attached. Addition of a sanitizer to the wash water has some germicidal effect but only if the water is changed frequently because most sanitizers are rapidly inactivated by organic debris.

Proper milking requires undivided attention and it's a rare individual who can do a good job in a stanchion barn handling more than two milker units. As soon as milking is complete, turn the unit off, break the vacuum by pressing the base of one teat against the side of the teat cup to admit air and remove it. Remember that the teat cups are held on by vacuum and that remains for a time after the unit is shut off. Pulling the teat cups off without first breaking the vacuum contributes to everted teat ends, which provide better avenues for infection.

Handling "Slow" Milkers

Some cows congenitally or as a result of injury have unusually tight teat sphincters and as a result are "slow" or "hard" milkers. The condition can usually be corrected surgically but hard milkers should be milked last so they don't impede progress in milking the rest of the herd. The use of teat dilators is a necessary evil in management of some cases of teat injury but they should not be used routinely for hard-milking cows. Anything introduced into the teat end carries with it a risk of introducing infection despite the most sanitary technique including wiping the teat end with 70 percent alcohol first. Routine use of teat dilators sooner or later results in mastitis.

Although considerable research is in progress, results thus far in attempts to find a vaccine capable of preventing mastitis have been disappointing. Staphylococcus bacterins and toxoids are commercially available but reported results from their use are inconsistent. Many different strains of *Staphylococcus spp.*, each antigenically a little different, are capable of producing mastitis. If the mastitis in your herd is due to a strain incorporated in these products they may be helpful. If not, they will be useless. The same may be said of *E. coli* bacterins/toxoids for the control of mastitis due to this organism. In herds with severe problems due to *Staphylococcus spp.* or *E. coli* some relief may be obtained by using an autogenous bacterin prepared from organisms isolated from the herd. Your veterinarian can advise you in this regard.

Minimizing Problems

Ways have been suggested to minimize problems with mastitis. *Str. agalactiae*, the most prevalent and insidious pathogen, can and should be eradicated from every dairy herd for economic reasons if nothing else. But despite your best efforts there will be occasional cases of mastitis in all species and these will generally be acute in nature, recognizable by heat, swelling, and abnormal milk. If the problem is limited to the udder these may usually be handled by infusion of antibiotics into the affected gland in the cow, doe, ewe, or mare.

The mammary glands of the sow are anatomically quite different and parenteral medication routes must be used. Your veterinarian may ask you to infuse follow-up medication using commercial preparations he provides or prescribes. You may even feel confident in doing this without veterinary advice. In any case, strip out all the milk you can and then wipe the teat end carefully using a cotton swab and 70 percent rubbing alcohol. If this precaution is not observed, when introducing the tube or syringe cannula you may push bacteria into the teat, making the problem worse. Simply because the gland is already infected doesn't mean it can't be infected concurrently with other organisms. Many serious yeast and mold infections occur this way. Use reliable products from reputable manufacturers and don't buy on the basis of price alone. When an expensive animal is at stake, a few cents on a drug is a poor place to economize. Your veterinarian can advise you what to use when the need arises.

Complications

Acute mastitis is often complicated by generalized, septicemic infection in all species. In addition to the clinical signs involving the udder, there will be high fever, lack of appetite and often, dehydration. The animal will appear dull and depressed. Milk flow may cease entirely especially in the sow and the onset is usually rather sudden. The first observed sign in the ewe may be an unusual rear leg gait because of udder soreness. Pulse and respiratory rate are usually high early in the disease declining as the temperature falls prior to death. Acute septic mastitis is a serious disease calling for prompt vigorous treatment to save the animal's life.

Although *E. coli* and *Staph aureus* are common causes of septicemic mastitis, it is not possible to determine the causative organism with any degree of accuracy on the basis of clinical signs alone. A number of organisms identifiable only by culture can cause similar signs. Although culture results are useful as a guide for management of similar future cases in the herd, treatment must be initiated on the basis of clinical signs and good judgment without waiting for a laboratory report.

Before the Veterinarian Arrives

Treatment of these cases is a job for the veterinarian but pending his arrival there are some things you can do to help insure a successful outcome. First, in the case of *E. coli* infection, endotoxin, a poisonous substance produced by the organism, causes a shock-like syndrome that accounts for most of the acute signs. The level of toxin and toxin-producing organisms in the udder can be reduced by stripping out all the secretion at least every hour. This of course is not so easy in the sow although it can readily be done in the other livestock species.

Second, the rate of swelling, tissue destruction, and absorption of toxic products can be slowed by packing the udder in ice. The mare, cow, ewe, and doe will usually tolerate an udder support improvised with a feedbag and bale twine. Once in place this can be packed with ice or snow. For the sow and other animals that won't tolerate it, cold showers from a garden hose will help.

Treatment of septic mastitis generally includes broad-spectrum antibiotics via the intramammary and intravenous or intramuscular routes as well as supportive therapy in the form of electrolyte solutions given intravenously, and sometimes aspirin to reduce the fever. Pituitrin or oxytocin helps to evacuate the udder prior to treatment. Each case must be evaluated on the basis of signs presented, and treated accordingly. This is a job for the veterinarian.

Antibiotic Withdrawal Time

Before leaving the subject of mastitis, a precaution for those selling milk should be mentioned. Antibiotics given via any route for any purpose will appear at some level in milk. Concentration will be much higher when the antibiotic is infused into the udder. Every antibiotic approved for use in lactating animals has a milk withdrawal time on the label and the time varies with the product. Withdrawal time is the interval that must elapse between last treatment and sale of the milk. Typically it will be 72–96 hours. A withdrawal time is also given for use of meat from a treated animal. **Read the label and observe the withdrawal time.** Residues of antibiotics in animal products may result in penalties for the producers. Worse in the long run, repeated violation will result in even greater restriction of the drugs that may be used in food producing animals.

Udder Edema

Udder edema may be associated with mastitis but more often it is not; nevertheless, it is appropriate to discuss it here. Edema is an excessive accumulation of body fluid outside the body cells and vascular pathways. Swelling is a form of edema in response to infection or injury. A physiological edema in the absence of udder infection is rather common, particularly in animals lactating for the first time. It generally disappears a few days after parturition and causes no problem. But a few dairy heifers develop a severe and persistent edema that requires some care.

Testing for Edema

Physiological edema can readily be distinguished from the swelling caused by acute mastitis. Edema, on one hand, is usually symmetrical (equal on both sides), involving the lower third of the entire udder and extending forward sometimes to the belly wall. Mastitis, on the other hand, usually affects only one quarter or half of the gland. Furthermore, edema does not produce heat as infection does. As a further test, press a finger into the swollen area. If it is edema, this will force extracellular fluid out of the compressed area, leaving a pit which will last for several minutes. This is a good diagnostic test for edema.

The causes of udder edema are probably multiple although there is some hereditary predisposition. Lack of exercise prior to parturition is certainly a factor and there is some evidence that high protein diets during the weeks preceding parturition contribute to the problem.

Generally the swelling will gradually subside following parturition and milking or nursing and no special care is necessary. But in a few animals it may be severe enough to interfere with milking and even walking. The objective is to get the excess fluid absorbed back into the general circulation, and anything that stimulates blood circulation will help. Exercise and massage are particularly helpful. Frequent application of alternate hot and cold packs will also help as will massage with a mild liniment. If these measures don't help, your veterinarian can give oral or intravenous diuretics which will. In a few individual cows slight edema will persist for several weeks or months, particularly on the lower and posterior aspects of the rear quarters. It will appear quite firm to the touch and will resist most efforts to remove but, fortunately, it does not harm and has little significance.

Pneumonia

Although the symptoms are rather clear cut, pneumonia is a very complex disease with several different predisposing or contributing factors. Because of its complexity, pneumonia is often described by various terms. For example, the pathologists will speak of **bronchopneumonia,** that in which the infection involves primarily the bronchi and bronchioles and the alveolar tissue, or pneumonia may be described as **interstitial,** in which the lung connective tissue is the primary site of infection. We also speak of **inhalation pneumonia,** which results from inhalation of liquids usually because of improperly administered medications, or

verminous pneumonia, in which the underlying cause is parasites, particularly lungworms.

Several viruses can cause pneumonia, particularly in swine and calves. The myxorivus, *Parainfluenza-3*, SF$_4$, or *bovine respiratory syncytial* virus working in concert with *Pasteurella multocida* causes a very serious form of pneumonia in cattle and sometimes in sheep. *Corynebacterium equi*, which produces serious generalized disease in foals on some farms, commonly causes pneumonia as one of its principal signs. A very serious disease when pigs are brought together in large numbers, formerly called virus pig pneumonia, now is known to be due primarily to *Mycoplasma hyopneumoniae*. This disease and shipping fever or pasteurellosis in cattle are highly contagious and devastating when they appear in a herd. Regardless of the cause, the most serious effects of pneumonia are generally caused by bacteria either as primary or as secondary invaders.

How it begins. Management plays an important role in the onset of pneumonia. Most of the organisms that cause the disease can be found in apparently normal and healthy animals. Only under adverse conditions when the animals' resistance is lowered does the disease appear. Unsanitary conditions, overcrowding, poor ventilation, drafts, and other stress are known to be predisposing factors. Pneumonia can occur in all species but is most commonly seen in cattle and pigs, perhaps because these are the species more likely to be kept under crowded circumstances.

Symptoms. The clinical signs of pneumonia are generally not difficult to recognize. There is fever, coughing which is more pronounced on exercise, and labored breathing to varying degrees. Usually the respiratory rate will be fast but the depth of respiration may be shallow, probably because of pain. In most cases of pneumonia, there is some inflammatory involvement of the pleura, the membrane lining of the chest cavity and covering the lungs, which causes considerable dis-

Open mouth breathing typical of advanced severe pneumonia. Note the sunken eye indicating prolonged illness and dehydration.

comfort when the chest is expanded during inspiration.

Pneumonia is an inflammation of the lungs and with the inflammation there is an accumulation of mucus and debris in the smaller air passages as well as some swelling of the lung tissue itself. This results in an interference with air flow and absorption of oxygen which is necessary to convert carboxyhemoglobin in red blood cells back to hemoglobin.

When the inflammation is severe, there will be an oxygen deficiency resulting in varying degrees of cyanosis (bluish discoloration of mucous membranes) with very labored breathing to the point where the head and neck are outstretched and the tongue is protruding. Needless to say, this is a very grave sign, and points out the need for early effective treatment. In human medicine, administration of oxygen helps alleviate the condition. But oxygen is difficult to administer to animals because of the restraint problem. The exudate (fluid) in the lungs when air passes through or around it will give rather typical abnormal lung sounds if one listens over the chest cavity with a stethoscope. If a portion of the lung becomes so congested that no air passes through, no sounds will be heard, which is just as significant if not more so than the abnormal sound.

SHIPPING FEVER

The respiratory disease complex is probably the most important faced by the cattle feedlot operator and is the greatest source of economic loss in feedlot cattle, not only because of significant mortality but because of unthriftiness and decreased rate of gain. There are several factors known to make up the respiratory disease complex and some that are probably unknown as well. But one of the most significant is the disease called **shipping fever** or **pasteurellosis.** It is caused by a bacterium, *Pasteurella multocida,* and a virus, *Parainfluenza-3* (PI-3), working together at a time of stress. Recent work has incriminated bovine respiratory syncytial virus (BRSV) as an additional factor. Although each of these viruses may cause infection by themselves with mild clinical signs it is when *P. multocida* appears as a secondary invader that serious disease results. The more common stress is that of moving animals from one location to another, sometimes over great distances, hence the name shipping fever. It is not limited to feeder cattle and can be equally disastrous in the dairy herd. Shipping fever differs somewhat from a simple pneumonia in that it tends to be quite contagious. These organisms apparently increase in virulence as the disease becomes active in animals under stress and their invasiveness increases so that even animals not under stress soon come down with the disease.

Shipping fever in cattle is basically a severe contagious bronchopneumonia. The earliest sign is a high fever ranging up to 106°F and occasionally higher with lack of appetite, coughing, nasal, and occasionally ocular discharge. As the disease progresses, respiration becomes rapid and shallow. As the disease progresses further, there is an accumulation not only of fluid in the smaller air passages, but cellular debris and occasionally outright pus, which restricts air flow. Consolidation of lung tissue will become so severe that cyanosis results from lack of oxygen.

Animals in this extreme condition will be reluctant to move and will stand with head and neck outstretched, sometimes with tongue protruding, literally gasping for air. Some outbreaks of pasteurellosis in cattle are characterized by diarrhea as well as the respiratory signs. Because of the respiratory distress the clinical signs are greatly aggravated by exertion. It's extremely important, therefore, that animals with pneumonia be handled quietly and gently. If you have to chase them around the pen to treat them, they may be better off untreated.

Treatment

Fortunately, *Pasteurella multocida* responds well to treatment that is initiated early. Treatment has no effect on the virus components of the complex. Several antibiotics, penicillin and its synthetic derivates, tetracycline, tylosin, erythromycin, and cephalosporin are all reasonably effective. The key is to start treatment early before too much damage is done to the lungs and to continue it long enough so the last vestiges of infection are removed. The longer treatment is delayed, the less likely a successful outcome will be.

Advanced cases generally end up with impaired lung function and even walled off abscesses of the lung that make the animal unthrifty and unprofitable even if it survives. The latter is a common complication in the feedlot where hundreds of animals and sometimes even thousands are kept, making it difficult to observe them individually to detect early signs of pneumonia. Furthermore, treatment of animals under these conditions is difficult on an individual basis because of the time and labor factor involved. Medication of drinking water or feed with a broad spectrum antibiotic is helpful, but unfortunately, the really sick animals usually don't eat or drink as much as they should and the problem of regulating drug dosage is almost unsurmountable when administered in this manner.

Prevention

The key is to do everything possible to prevent this disease from occurring in the first place. It goes without saying that you should start with healthy cattle insofar as possible. The best way to do this when you are buying replacements is to buy directly from the farm where the animals have been raised, rather than through a commission sale. While the sales managers do the best they can to provide you with healthy cattle, it is not at all unusual for cattle going through commission sales to have been enroute from the farm of origin for two weeks or more, often traveling through several commission sales before they get to their final destination. This kind of stress almost insures that they are going to have disease problems of some kind.

Second, regardless of the source and whether you are dealing with dairy cattle or beef cattle, it's effort well spent to keep the animals separated from the main herd for at least two weeks when you get them home. In that way, if they do develop shipping fever or some other disease, they at least will not endanger your other animals.

If you are dealing with feeder calves, remember that these are usually right off the range and rather unaccustomed to being handled and equally unaccustomed to anything but grass to eat. Therefore, they should not only be segregated in clean surroundings, but should be left alone with hay and clean water to rest and become accustomed to their new environment. Similarly, avoid the temptation to put them on full feed immediately in hopes of getting a faster rate of gain. This is usually self-defeating because they aren't accustomed to grain and frequently will get a digestive upset, which is sufficient added stress to contribute to the onset of shipping fever.

With dairy cattle, the same general recommendation holds true. Buy them from the source least likely to contribute to disease and segregate them from the main herd for a minimum of two weeks.

The same precaution should be observed for your own animals that you may be bringing back from a fair or show. There is no way of knowing what diseases they have been exposed to when mixed in with other animals at a show and, therefore, they can be just as dangerous to bring directly back into the herd as entirely new replacements. These management procedures will do much to prevent shipping fever from appearing in the herd. In addition, vaccine given early enough can be helpful.

Vaccines

There are several vaccines available that will help to prevent shipping fever, but they are not 100 percent effective. The simplest of these is a bacterin for *Pasteurella multocida*. The more commonly used ones also incorporate antigens for other organisms such as *Corynebacterium pyogenes*. These bacterins are moderately effective for a short period of time but generally must be given every sixty days to provide any real value. Vaccines are available for protection against *Parainfluenza-3*, *Bovine respiratory syncytial virus*, *Pasteurella multocida*, *Pasteurella hemolytica*, and *Infectious bovine rhinotracheitis*, all organisms that contribute to the respiratory disease complex. These are available singly or in various combinations and, depending on formulation, are given subcutaneously, intramuscularly, or intranasally so the choice can be quite confusing. Your veterinarian can best advise you what vaccines should be used in your area under your conditions. But in any case, remember that although intranasal IBR/PI-3 vaccine produces local cellular immunity in the upper respiratory tract in forty-eight hours, it takes at least two weeks for solid immunity to develop following administration of vaccine. Vaccine given the day the animal was shipped or the day they arrive will be of very questionable value in preventing disease outbreaks.

If you are in the business of finishing beef cattle, whenever possible buy feeder calves that have been preconditioned. These will have been weaned, castrated if necessary, vaccinated, and accustomed to grain well before their shipping date. Experience has shown that they arrive in better condition with fewer problems than those taken directly off the range.

Related factors. Although as the name implies, pasteurellosis is commonly associated with shipping, this is not the only factor that can trigger an outbreak of the disease. Since many healthy cattle harbor the organisms responsible, it requires only a lowering of resistance from any cause to induce an outbreak. The stress of a radical change in diet if the animals don't eat well for a day or two has occasionally been incriminated as a factor. The disease is seen more commonly in the fall and winter months during or following periods of inclement weather, but cold does not seem to be an important factor provided the animals have at least a windbreak or some sort of minimal shelter. In fact, it occurs more frequently during the winter in herds that are stabled in enclosed barns where the ventilation is poor. The build-up of ammonia fumes from decomposing manure and high humidity provides sufficient stress. Also, of course, in an enclosed barn lacking frequent air change, the concentration of infective moisture droplets in the air will be considerably more than it would be outside.

Last, it appears possible, circumstantially at least, that shipping fever can be spread from farm to farm on boots and clothing, etc., because it is not unusual to find the disease appearing sequentially on adjacent farms where there has been traffic in and out.

PNEUMONIA OF PIGS

A contagious pneumonia of pigs, sometimes called *enzootic pneumonia* and formerly called "virus pig pneumonia," is probably the most important disease encountered in the swine industry from an economic standpoint. It is caused by an organism called *Mycoplasma hyopneumoniae* which, while not classified as a bacterium, causes a chronic disease that is made much more acute in the presence of a secondary bacterial invasion. The severity of the lung lesions that it causes is also increased in the presence of migrating ascarid larvae or lungworms.

The disease is more prevalent in swine herds where replacements are frequently added from random sources. It differs from the usual concept of pneumonia in that typically it does not produce a serious febrile (fever) reaction nor do the pigs go off feed. But, it does cause lung lesions and a chronic cough, a combination which leads to decreased rate of gain and therefore increased cost of pork production. It is widespread and its principal effect is economic. When complicated by secondary bacterial infection, the clinical signs more nearly approximate those of the types of pneumonia we have discussed thus far.

The disease is more prevalent and more persistent in younger swine beginning about the age of three weeks and older. Unlike bacterial pneumonia, mycoplasma pneumonia will appear at any time of the year with no increased prevalence noted during the fall and winter months. The organism persists for months in infected pigs and transmission to susceptible ones is by direct contact or aerosol inhalation.

Mortality Low

Generally, a high percentage of the younger pigs in the herd will be infected, but if the disease is not complicated by other factors, mortality will be rather low. Coughing aggravated by exercise and unthriftiness are the principal and often the only clinical signs. But, diagnosis can be confirmed by typical lesions found in the lungs (examination after death) or by serological tests. By special cultural techniques in the laboratory, the organism can be isolated from infected pigs, which confirms the diagnosis.

Attempts to control the disease or treatment have generally been unsuccessful. Antibiotics and sulfa drugs are ineffective against *M. hyopneumoniae,* but they do have value in controlling secondary bacterial infection which may occur, thereby reducing pig mortality. Control of ascarids and lungworms through the use of good sanitary practices and anthelmintics when indicated also helps to reduce losses from *mycoplasma pneumonia.*

Methods of Control

Control of the disease in some herds has been accomplished by rather radical changes in swine herd management. Where the infection rate is severe, perhaps the best solution is depopulation of the entire herd and replacement of breeding stock with pigs purchased directly from specific pathogen-free (SPF) herds. Once this step is taken, however, to maintain an infection-free herd, one must buy all subsequent herd replacements from herds of equal or better disease-free status. This may limit the options and choice of breeding stock and usually increases the cost of those replaced. However, the improved performance of the pigs in the herd may well justify the added cost.

A second moderately successful method used where physical facilities permit is to attempt to provide a degree of isolation within the herd between infected and noninfected pigs. With this method sows are farrowed in isolation to help insure that there is no cross-infection between litters. The litters are then observed for clinical signs of infection and those that appear to be free, at least upon observation or even necropsy (examination after death) of one of the piglets, can be grouped together and segregated from all other pigs on the farm. If the infected and noninfected groups can be kept separate, the infected group can be gradually eliminated, leaving only the non-infected breeding stock behind. While both of these methods present obvious problems, the economic effect of this disease is so great that any control attempt is worthwhile. *Mycoplasma hyopneumoniae* apparently stimulates some immunity, since older swine are less frequently found to be infected than the younger groups. Attempts thus far to produce an effective vaccine have not been successful.

With the exception of contagious pasteurellosis in cattle and mycoplasma pneumonia in swine, most cases of pneumonia in livestock, as in people, are isolated and sporadic. Each must be managed on the basis of clinical signs observed and treated accordingly.

COLIBACILLOSIS

Colibacillosis is a major disease of the young encountered primarily in calves, pigs, and lambs. It also affects foals and kids, although less frequently. The disease takes two primary forms, **enteric,** involving the intestinal tract to cause profuse diarrhea, and **septicemic** (in the blood stream), which may cause sudden death with no premonitory signs. Colibacillosis is the leading component of the neonatal diarrhea complex commonly called "scours."

The causative organism, *Escherichia coli*, is a common environmental contaminant found universally in manure. As a sidelight, the count of *E. coli* per cc is the standard for potability of public water supplies and a particular serotype has recently (1993) been incriminated in the death of several children who ate inadequately cooked meat. There are many different strains of the organism, some relatively innocuous and others highly pathogenic. A few of the highly pathogenic strains produce an endotoxin that accounts for their detrimental effect. Experimentally, minute quantities of *E. coli* endotoxin given intravenously have been shown to produce circulatory collapse and death in a matter of minutes. Lesser quantities perfused into an isolated loop of intestine will cause complete paralysis and dilatation of the loop. This effect is undoubtedly a factor complicating the enteric form of the disease. Colibacillosis is more frequent when large numbers of young animals are housed in close confinement.

The Enteric Form

The enteric form is most common in dairy calves, pigs, and lambs, probably as a reflection of intensified husbandry methods. The route of infection is primarily oral, making sanitation an important factor in control. Typically it appears within the first week after birth. Although there is usually a moderate fever at the outset, the first sign noted may be a pasty or watery yellowish diarrhea which has a foul odor. There is some abdominal pain and frequent defecation and straining. Affected animals refuse feed and because of tremendous fluid loss from the diarrhea, rapidly become dehydrated. Without treatment the disease usually terminates in coma and death within three to five days. In some dairy herds calf mortality from this disease may approach 100 percent. In piglets, perhaps because they are weaker at birth than calves, the disease is more acute. Although the symptoms are quite similar, onset in pigs is usually within twelve hours after birth and they will die a day later.

A specific enteric colibacillosis called **gut edema** occurs in pigs two to four months old and occasionally earlier. Evidence to date indicates that this disease is not due to the infection itself but is a reaction to endotoxins produced by several strains of *E. coli*. The condition occurs at any time of the year and on a given farm will appear only in pigs in the same age range. It is most likely to appear during the interval between weaning and establishment on full feed.

The Septicemic Form

The other major form of colibacillosis is septicemia with generalized infection. This is an acute disease of the very young that frequently causes death with no warning signs. Septicemic colibacillosis is the most common form of colibacillosis in lambs and foals. When the syndrome is less acute, meningitis commonly occurs, causing a variety of central nervous system disturbances. Animals that recover from the acute disease often develop an arthritis due to localization of the infection in the joints. A common route of infection for septicemia is via the navel.

The result of septicemic colibacillosis.

Prevention

Clearly, colibacillosis is a serious and complex disease that must be prevented by whatever means are possible. **The single most effective method is to ensure that all newborn animals receive colostrum as soon as possible after birth.** The majority of older animals, through prior exposure to pathogenic strains of *E. coli*, will develop protective antibody that is transferred in colostrum. To insure exposure, some hog farms make it a practice to feed some manure to the sows during the last month of gestation. While this may increase the sow's *E. coli* antibody level, it also may expose her to other pathogens such as enteroviruses that can cause abortion, so it isn't a good practice that can be universally recommended.

Overeating is a common predisposing factor for all types of gastrointestinal disease and is a frequent cause of nonspecific diarrhea in dairy calves. Restricting milk intake to 10 percent of body weight daily for the first seven to ten days will help to prevent trouble. And of course, sanitation is important. Animals born in a filthy environment are certain to be exposed to overwhelming numbers of *E. coli*.

There is a direct correlation between concentration of animals in the susceptible age range and the prevalence of colibacillosis. The rate of infection accelerates either when animals are all born in the same pen or area without adequate intervals for thorough cleaning or when they are all grouped together in the same pen after birth. Many dairy farmers have been able to almost eliminate the enteric form of the disease by rearing calves in isolated hutches, referred to in the section on housing. Dipping the navel in tincture of iodine is strongly recommended to prevent infection via that route.

Numerous attempts have been made to prevent colibacillosis through immunization of the dam or the offspring immediately after birth. None has been very successful because of the number of antigenically different strains of the organism involved. Autogenous bacterins incorporating strains found on the farm may be helpful when other methods fail. Genetically engineering vaccines that incorporate only specific antigenic components of the organism show considerable promise. Continuous low-level administration of antibiotics in the feed or drinking water may also be helpful. But, E. coli is not only widespread; it is also very adaptable and readily develops antibiotic resistance. Constant low-level feeding of the same antibiotic promotes resistance and is therefore self-defeating. Administration of antiserum or antibody concentrate to valuable newborn animals may be worthwhile if the pathogenic strains of organism present on the farm are present in the product.

Treatment

Treatment of the enteric disease in all but baby pigs is reasonably successful. Newborn pigs die so quickly and there are usually so many of them that treatment is not very satisfactory but nevertheless should be attempted. Use of antibiotics and antidiarrheal oral medications alone however may not do the job. The effects of endotoxin produced by some strains will linger after the bacteria have been destroyed. Furthermore, in many cases the enteric disease is compounded by the loss of tremendous volumes of fluid and electrolytes resulting in dehydration. For best results this loss must be replaced by equivalent quantities of electrolyte solution given intravenously and orally. Good results have been reported in calves when no milk at all is given for twenty-four hours. Instead, a simple homemade electrolyte formula (see box) is given.

HOMEMADE ELECTROLYTE FORMULA

Table salt — one heaping teaspoon
Baking soda — one heaping teaspoon
Water — one gallon

While commercially prepared electrolyte solutions are more complete and better balanced, this simple, readily available formula given instead of milk for twenty-four hours will help to relieve the diarrhea by reducing the number of organisms present, and at the same time counteract loss of sodium and chloride ions as well as correct the acidosis that occurs with dehydration. The calf with diarrhea but not yet severely dehydrated will need two quarts of this warmed solution every eight hours for the first day. After that, milk or milk replacer diluted with the same solution to fifty percent of normal concentration can be fed. Gradually increase the percentage of milk until it is back to normal at the end of the third day. This procedure alone will save many calves that would otherwise die.

If the dehydration is severe, regardless of species, electrolyte solutions will need to be given intravenously in addition to being given orally. Although it is time-consuming, for the animal that is seriously ill with either the septicemic or enteric forms of colibacillosis, nothing is better than a blood transfusion. This, however, is a job for the veterinarian.

Antibiotics in injectable or oral preparations are routinely given to control or treat "scours" in farm animals with variable results. Because of its acute onset, antibiotic therapy for septicemic colibacillosis is only moderately helpful, although for the animal that survives the acute phase, antibiotics help to prevent secondary complications. Treatment of the enteric form must include fluid replacement and good nursing care for satisfactory results.

Prevention

The really important thing is to prevent the disease from occurring in the first place. The following suggestions have all proven helpful:

- Keep the calving pen, farrowing house, lambing shed, and other facilities, as clean and sanitary as possible.
- Insofar as possible, isolate newborn animals from each other.
- Don't overfeed. Although it may seen heartless, keeping newborn animals on the hungry side for the first few days helps to ensure their survival.
- Thoroughly scrub and sanitize feeding equipment after each use.
- Provide supplemental heat especially for piglets and lambs.
- **Be certain** newborn animals get colostrum as soon as possible after birth. If there is doubt whether a newborn animal has nursed colostrum, then zinc sulfate turbidity test can be applied to a small amount of blood serum. This gives a rough estimation of the amount of globulin absorbed. Your veterinarian can do it for you. Colostrum can be frozen in plastic bags and kept almost indefinitely. It's a good idea to keep some on hand to feed the animal that becomes an orphan soon after birth.
- Routine oral use of a new **E. Coli monoclonal** antibody product may prove helpful.

PODODERMATITIS

Pododermatitis, commonly called **foot rot,** is a disease of cattle, sheep, and, to a lesser extent, goats. In cattle, the disease is caused by a soilborne organism, *Fusobacterium necrophorum,* that gains entry via minute cracks or abrasions. In sheep, *F. necrophorum* working in concert with another pathogen, *Fusiformis nodosus,* appears to be responsible. The latter organism seems capable of penetrating unbroken skin, causing severe foot lesions that may affect entire flocks, particularly during warm wet weather. Foot rot in cattle is more sporadic, rarely affecting more than 10 percent of the herd at one time.

The first clinical sign noted is generally lameness, which gets progressively worse. In cattle usually only one foot at a time is affected, whereas in sheep infection of all four feet is not uncommon. In cattle, the infection commonly starts at the bulb of the heel and extends up to the fetlock and into the interdigital space, causing swelling and tissue necrosis. This dead and dying tissue has a characteristic odor which gave the disease its early name of "fouls." As the disease progresses and swelling extends, cracks open that permit infection with a variety of secondary invaders. Left untreated, the infection may extend into the coffin joint, causing permanent lameness. The lameness and acute pain, of course, lead to rapid weight loss and in the dairy cow, decline in milk production. Foot rot is a troublesome and costly disease on some farms and any effort expended to control it is well worthwhile.

Although foot rot is common, relatively little research has been done on it. As a result there is confusion in terminology and even etiology. It may involve the sole, the heel, the interdigital space, or the skin on the posterior aspect of the pastern, and be named according to the anatomical site of the initial lesion. **Thrush,** which involves the frog of the horse's hoof, is a form of foot rot attributable to poor foot hygiene.

The organisms causing foot rot thrive best in a warm, moist anaerobic environment. Underrun soles and cracks in the feet provide an ideal environment for them. A good foot rot control program therefore includes regular periodic examination and trimming of the feet.

Regardless of the name or the multiple etiology, the measures outlined here will do much to control the disease.

Sagittal section through one claw of the bovine foot. Infection readily extends into the coffin joint to cause severe lameness.

Neglect of the feet and unsanitary conditions contribute to foot rot.

Early Treatment

Like all diseases, treatment is most effective if begun early. The first essential step is to examine the foot and carefully pare away all dead and underrun sole tissue. Foot rot is not the only cause of foot swelling and lameness. On more than one occasion I have seen cases that didn't respond to intramuscular injection of antibiotics because there was a nail in the foot or a stone lodged between the claws. Always examine the foot! When only a few animals are involved it's practical and advantageous to treat the infection locally and bandage the foot. This is more comfortable for the animal and promotes more rapid healing.

Once the infected area has been debrided and cleaned up several different medications can be used. Among these are 20 percent icthammol ointment, copper napthenate solution, 5 percent formalin solution, and sulfanilamide powder to which has been added copper sulfate powder at the rate of 5 percent. Any of these will be beneficial when coupled with parenteral administration of penicillin and streptomycin or one of the sulfonamides such as sulfapyridine, sulfamerazine, or sulfamethazine. Some other antibiotics and sulfa drugs work equally well; the choice is largely one of preference and economics and, in the case of food producing animals, legality. Aside from helping the animal, bandaging the foot has value as a control procedure as well. An open, discharging foot rot lesion sheds millions of organisms onto the ground to serve as a source of new infections. For this reason, infected animals should be segregated from the rest of the herd or flock.

Foot Bath

When too many animals are involved to make bandaging practical, and as a general control procedure, a foot bath of 5 percent copper sulfate through which the animals must walk at least daily is helpful. The trough containing the solution should be about four inches deep and wide enough so the animals can't jump over it. In freezing weather or when solutions are objectionable, the same thing can be accomplished with a shallow box filled with a mixture of 5 pounds of copper sulfate powder to 100 pounds of hydrated lime. This of course, must be placed in an area protected from rain or snow. The use of EDDI as a feed additive or in salt blocks has been recommended as a control procedure, but results have been inconsistent.

Fusobacterium necrophorum can survive in the soil for long periods, so that once infection appears in a cattle herd new cases will appear sporadically thereafter. Rotating pastures and reducing the concentration of cattle in the pasture lessens the rate of ground contamination but won't prevent it entirely. Prevalence is greatly reduced when cattle are kept in a paved drylot that is regularly cleaned.

Sheep

Fusiformis nodosus, a component of the disease in sheep, is an obligate parasite that probably doesn't survive outside the sheep for more than a week. This makes it possible to eradicate the disease and many flock owners have done so. Eradication requires some effort but is worth doing. It requires examination of the feet of each individual sheep and separation of infected and non-infected. The non-infected are then given a dose of antibiotic, usually penicillin and streptomycin, and put into a pasture that has not held any sheep for at least two weeks. It also helps to walk them through a foot bath as described above as they enter the clean

Methods of supporting front and rear legs for examination and foot trimming.

Example of a neglected foot. The sole of the left claw has been trimmed for comparison.

pasture. As individuals in the infected group recover, they are given additional antibiotic and added to the clean flock in the same manner. The clean flock should be carefully observed every day for a week or two for any sign of lameness. Lame ones should immediately be put back with the infected flock. Once the entire flock is free of infection, special measures must be taken to keep it that way.

If possible, replacement sheep should be purchased directly from flocks known to be free of infection. Where the history is unknown, they, and your own animals returning from a show, should be considered infected, treated with antibiotics on arrival, and kept separate from the main flock for two weeks. At the end of that time, if no problems develop, they can join the clean group.

A word of caution should be added. Don't forget that you can carry *F. nodosus* on your shoes or boots from the infected to the clean flocks. Always disinfect your boots when moving from one flock to the other as long as any vestige of infection remains.

A vaccine for prevention of foot rot in sheep appears to be a useful aid but does not supplant the need for the control measures outlined above.

Poll evil.

BRUCELLOSIS

Brucellosis is a disease of great economic significance that occurs principally in cattle, swine, and goats. Three distinct species of *Brucella* are responsible. *Br. abortus* (cattle), *Br. suis* (swine), and *Br. melitensis* (goats) tend to be host-specific. The principal and usually only clinical sign they produce is abortion, typically during the last third of gestation.

All three cause a serious, generalized febrile disease in man called **undulant fever.** In animals, however, the infection is concentrated in the reproductive organs where it localizes in the uterus, udder, and placenta of the female and the testicles of the male. A fourth species, *Br. ovis*, causes ram epididymitis although ewes tend to be resistant so that ram infertility, not abortion, is the principal sign. Infected cattle and goats shed the organism in milk, and drinking raw milk from infected animals is a public health hazard. The organism is readily killed by pasteurization. *Br. abortus* was the cause of the suppurative diseases, poll evil and fistulous withers, in horses when draft horses were kept in close association with infected cows. With the decline in draft horses and the much lower infection rate in cattle, these diseases are now rare.

Treatment of brucellosis in animals is generally unsatisfactory because of inconsistent results and cost. Ram epididymitis has been successfully treated with high levels of antibiotics over a long period of time. But the total cost of drugs usually exceeds the value of the ordinary commercial ram.

Eradication Program

Because of the economic and public health significance of brucellosis and because treatment is of little value, the state and federal governments many years ago adopted a policy aimed at total eradication. Basically this involves identification and slaughter of infected animals with indemnity paid to owners to offset the difference between meat price and appraised value. Meat from infected animals is not a health hazard.

During the early stages of the eradication campaign in cattle, when infection rates ranged up to 25 percent or more, vaccination of calves was a useful adjunct. The vaccine used is a live modification of *Br. abortus* designated Strain 19 which reduces the rate of spread and number of abortions but it does not provide complete protection. Two other vaccines used in Europe, 45/20 and H38, are currently being evaluated in this country. Vaccines for *Br. suis* and *Br. melitensis* are not available, but a vaccine is being used to control ram epididymitis.

Diagnosis

Brucellosis is readily identifiable by several serological tests as well as by the milk ring test, applicable for dairy cattle and goats. Diagnosis is sometimes handicapped, however, by a long interval between exposure and having the infection show up in the test. This may take up to sixty days. Therefore, a negative test on a recently exposed animal may be misleading. The significance of this delay will become apparent when we discuss ways of preventing infection.

In species other than sheep, spread of infection is primarily oral. Infection of rams occurs primarily during mating, particularly when the ewe has recently been bred by an infected ram. The vaginal discharges of infected animals and especially aborted fetuses are literally teeming with the organism. Although *Br. abortus* has

Aborted fetus due to brucellosis. These curious cows are certain to become infected.

the capacity to penetrate the unbroken skin and infection caused by a droplet of infective material in the eye has been recorded, it's probable that most infections occur via the oral route because of the propensity of animals to sniff each other's genital areas.

Abortion is the primary evidence of infection with brucellosis, and infection apparently produces some degree of immunity because typically animals that abort will conceive again after a time and carry subsequent fetuses to term. Nevertheless, the infection persists in a latent form and these infected animals remain a source of infection for others.

Vaccination vs. Eradication

Because of its economic importance and the test and slaughter eradication program in effect for cattle, brucellosis often becomes a very emotional issue. The question most often asked is, "Won't my herd be protected if I vaccinate every calf?" The answer is no. The Strain 19 vaccine used will immunize only about 65 percent of those calves to which it is given and the immunity produced only lasts a few years. So, despite an intensive vaccination program, new infections will continue to occur. Experience has shown that in the long run the cheapest way to control a disease like this is to eradicate it. There is ample evidence to indicate that this can be done. Vaccination has value only in areas where the infection rate is so high as to make a test and slaughter program prohibitively expensive. Nevertheless, legislatures of a few states, responding to strong political pressure based on misunderstanding of the disease have mandated compulsory calfhood vaccination.

To avoid residual antibody titers which interfere with diagnostic tests, any calfhood vaccination should be done close to the minimum legal age of two months. In special circumstances where the herd infection rates are very high and husbandry methods preclude eradication, cows may be vaccinated to reduce abortions. This however, requires special permission from state and federal authorities and permanent quarantine of the herd.

Eradication of brucellosis depends on identification and slaughter of infected animals, quarantine of infected herds, and restriction on movement of animals. It also requires accurate identification of animals and good records of acquisition and disposition, so that when a reactor is found she can be traced back to the point of origin and all contact animals individually tested to detect any spread of infection. Perhaps most important, it requires understanding and cooperation on the part of livestock owners, veterinarians, and regulatory program officials. At the end of 1993 there were only 283 cattle herds under quarantine for brucellosis in the U.S., with thirty-two states rated free of the disease. It seems to me that we have reached a point in the eradication program where it would be advisable and most economical to depopulate the few remaining infected herds and to cease vaccination. At the same time, we need to intensify the surveillance program to detect new infections before they spread through market cattle testing and the milk ring test. This is a decision in which producers and veterinarians as well as regulatory officials should be involved.

How to Prevent Infection

There is much that the livestock owner can do to ensure that his herd does not become infected. In fact, he can do more than anyone else — by following these recommendations.

- If an animal aborts, don't ignore it and write it off as bad luck. Have your veterinarian examine the fetus and collect samples from fetus and dam for laboratory analysis. Brucellosis is readily identifiable at the time of abortion. Then segregate the dam from all other animals in the herd until the cause is determined and thoroughly disinfect the area where the abortion occurred.
- Remember that brucellosis does not appear in a herd by spontaneous generation. Almost without exception when the disease appears in a previously clean herd it was bought along with replacement animals. Be selective in your source of replacements, buying only from known clean herds whenever possible. If there is any doubt about the status of the animal, insist that it have a negative blood test within thirty days of the time you bring it home. And, for added insurance, keep the animal separated from the main herd for at least thirty days until it is tested again and found negative.
- As a general disease control procedure, ask visitors to stay out of the stable area. Keep buyers, trucks, or trailers away from areas that are accessible to your herd.

Following these few simple rules will do more — at less cost — to keep brucellosis out of your herd than a vaccination program.

Brucellosis in Swine

Brucellosis in swine more closely resembles undulant fever in humans, in that it frequently causes a systemic infection with bacteremia. Because, in the early stages, *Br. suis* can be found in all body tissues, infected swine present a special hazard to packing house workers. Transmission in swine as in cattle and goats occurs via the oral route and also during mating. Infected boars may have a swollen testicle and impaired fertility. Palpation of the testicles and examination of the semen coupled with serological testing will identify infected animals. In an infected herd, low fertility, abortions, stillbirths, and weak piglets are common. Neither vaccination nor treatment is effective in swine, and eradication through depopulation or a testing program with total segregation of positive and negative animals are the control methods used.

Brucellosis in Sheep

Ram epididymitis is unique in that ewes, although they may become infected and occasionally abort, tend to be resistant and recover spontaneously. It is primarily a disease of the ram detectable by palpation of the testicles and blood test. One or both testicles may be involved. The affected testicle, especially the epididymis (tubes at the back of the testicle), will feel swollen and even fibrous in the later stages. The first intimation of infection is usually a gradually reduced fertility. Susceptible rams become infected when they breed a ewe recently bred by an infected ram. The rate of spread therefore is greatest during the breeding season, particularly when young rams are put with a flock along with older rams that are more likely to be infected.

Control can be achieved through vaccination and by splitting the ewe flock into two or more groups. Only young rams are kept with one group and the older rams kept with the other. In this manner a clean and an infected, or suspect, flock can be maintained separately. Rams known to be infected should be slaughtered.

Brucellosis in Goats

The disease in goats closely parallels that found in cattle and control measures are basically the same. In fact, regardless of some species differences, the prevention recommendations listed for cattle are equally applicable for all species.

Brucellosis in Exotic Species

Unfortunately the disease is transmissible to other species such as bison and llamas. While the latter are sufficiently docile to be blood tested, feral bison present a different challenge. These animals provide a reservoir of infection that is of concern primarily to cattle ranchers on the borders of parks where bison roam.

LEPTOSPIROSIS

This disease is seen in all species but is most frequently reported in cows, pigs, goats, sheep, and horses in that order. It is also transmissable to man and human cases are not rare. It is caused by several species of *Leptospira* including *L. pomona, L. hardjo, L. grippotyphosa,* and *L. icterohemorrhagiae. L. canicola,* a species affecting dogs, rarely is found in livestock other than swine.

Clinical signs of the disease are very variable and diagnosis may be difficult. It tends to be much more acute in young animals, resulting in high fever, complete lack of appetite, hemoglobinuria (bloody urine), jaundice, anemia, and death. Calf mortality, for example, may range up to 15 percent. Although a few adult animals may show similar clinical signs, the infection is often inapparent. In milking cows or goats there may be a sharp drop in production and a few may produce thick, ropy, blood-tinged milk without evidence of udder inflammation. Abortions several weeks after the infection passed through the herd or flock may be the only evidence the infection was there. Serologic testing or identification of the organism from the stomach contents of an aborted fetus will confirm the diagnosis. There is strong evidence linking prior leptospirosis infection with recurrent iridocyclitis (periodic ophthalmia, moon-blindness) in horses.

Kidney Infected

The primary site of infection is the kidney. Many recovered animals will continue to shed the organism in their urine for considerable periods of time without themselves showing any clinical signs whatever. Such carrier animals are an obvious hazard to other susceptible animals in the herd. The organism survives well in water such as in ponds or potholes. Water from these sources, when contaminated by urine from infected animals, or the urine droplets themselves are the primary sources of infection. Although most infections are probably acquired orally, the organism is quite invasive and infective urine droplets splashing into the eye can result in infection. For this and other reasons, persons handling aborted fetuses should wear gloves and wash thoroughly afterward.

Leptospirosis occurs in wild as well as in domestic animals, and it is probable that many swine herds become infected through contamination of feed by carrier rodents. Similarly, the infection occurs in deer and it has been postulated but not proven that the initial infection in some cattle herds occurs when carrier deer and cattle share the same pasture.

Vaccination

When treated early, animals with the acute infection respond well to antibiotic therapy but since the most important economic effect is abortion following acute or inapparent infection, prevention is much more desirable. Several steps are effective. One is to insure that purchased replacements are negative to a blood test for leptospirosis done by a reliable laboratory. Protecting the feed supply from rodent contamination and fencing animals away from potentially contaminated water supplies are also helpful. But routine vaccination is by far the most effective.

Although *L. pomona* is the most common serotype affecting livestock there are farm and regional variations. Bacterins are available now which incorporate antigens to stimulate immunity against all the common types of the organism. Depending on the manufacturer, these are available in several combinations or as *L. pomona* bacterin alone. The latter is relatively inexpensive and will provide good protection for almost a year. All animals on the farm should be vaccinated annually, especially when the possibility of carriers from prior infections exists in the herd.

BLACKLEG

On some farms blackleg is the most common of a group of diseases caused by spore-forming soilborne organisms belonging to the genus *Clostridium*. It occurs most frequently in well-nourished cattle of the beef breeds in the age range of six to twenty-six months. It also occurs in sheep and goats but in these species the disease is more commonly associated with wound infection such as occurs in sheep following docking, castration, or shearing. The mechanism by which infection occurs in cattle is less clear.

The spore form of the organism persists in the soil for many years and is very resistant to environmental changes such as drying, high temperatures, or freezing. The organism can commonly be found in the digestive tract of normal cattle. Once contaminated, a pasture will remain that way for years and in floodplain areas, pastures downstream from the originally infected pasture will also become contaminated. The disease is primarily seasonal and is seen most frequently in the late spring and summer when animals are at pasture.

Blackleg in cattle is a dramatic disease. Dead animals will be the first indication that the disease is present. Typically, one or two animals will be found dead in the pasture without any evidence of their having died other than suddenly and quietly. In fact, the disease at first glance could easily be confused with lightning stroke. However, with blackleg, decomposition of body tissues occurs very rapidly and the dead animals will invariably be found lying on their sides, extremely bloated with the upper legs rigidly extended. Similar sporadic losses will continue if nothing is done about it.

Diagnosis

Although the mechanism by which infection occurs in cattle or why it occurs is not really known, it is apparent that the organisms in the digestive tract become vegetative (growing and multiplying) and migrate through the intestinal wall to the blood stream where they are carried to all parts of the body, resulting in a bacteremia. *Clostridium chauvoei* in infected cattle can readily be isolated from the blood and vascular organs such as the liver and spleen, but its most pronounced effect is in the heavy muscles. Toxin produced by the organism produces a severe muscle inflammation and death of muscle tissue with gas formation. Muscles in the hip area and loin are most commonly affected. Running your hand over the back and hips of the dead animal will often give a clue to the cause of death. If it is blackleg, gas produced during muscle necrosis gravitates upward under the skin to cause a palpable crepitation (crackling-feeling). At necropsy the affected muscles will be dark, hemorrhagic and visibly necrotic. Because the carcass will be teeming with the organism, to avoid further pasture contamination, dead animals should be deeply buried right on the spot.

Once the diagnosis of blackleg has been made, careful examination of other animals in the herd may reveal a few in the early stages of the disease. It causes a very high fever, complete lack of appetite, depression, and lameness. These signs are generally not observed in the initial cases because the disease will be fatal in twelve hours or less. Given very early in the course of the disease, large doses of penicillin may prevent death of the animal although, depending on the degree of muscle damage done, lameness may persist if the animal survives.

Prevention

Blackleg is readily preventable by immunization with bacterin. Because mixed infection is a common occurrence, the bacterin usually used contains *Clostridium chauvoei* and *Clostridium septicum* antigen. A single dose provides reasonably good protection, but a second dose a month later is even better.

On farms where the infection is known to exist, this should be done with calves beginning at about six months of age and they should have another dose a year later. In the face of an outbreak, further losses can be minimized by vaccinating all animals in the susceptible age range immediately, giving them a large dose of penicillin to provide some protection in the interval required for immunity to develop, and putting them in another pasture. Most people experienced with blackleg routinely immunize susceptible animals every year in the early spring.

Blackleg in Sheep

The disease in sheep is somewhat different from that in cattle, although the end result, death, is usually the same. In sheep it is almost invariably a wound infection, either through a mechanical procedure such as docking, castration, or shearing or via vulvar lacerations incurred during lambing. If the lesion is in the leg muscles the animal will walk with a stiff gait if it walks at all. But the extreme swelling and gaseous crepitation found in the lesions in cattle are not nearly as apparent in sheep. The early stages of the disease are always associated with high fever, complete lack of appetite, and depression.

In sheep, as in cattle, the disease is readily preventable by vaccination, although sheep vaccinated under one year of age do not develop as solid an immunity as those vaccinated later. Vaccination of ewes three to four weeks prior to lambing will not only provide protection to the ewe but, because of colostral antibody, will afford some protection to the newborn lamb. In areas where the disease is prevalent, injection of penicillin following surgical procedures or difficult lambing may prevent infection from occurring.

Although the diagnosis of blackleg on the basis of history and necropsy alone is generally not difficult, it can be confirmed by isolation of the organism from infected tissues or fluorescent antibody test in the laboratory.

MALIGNANT EDEMA

This is an acute commonly fatal disease of cattle, horses, sheep, goats, and swine, that in some respects resembles blackleg. It is caused by *Clostridium septicum* and in cattle and sheep mixed infection with *Clostridium chauvoei* is not rare. Like the other *Clostridia*, *Cl. septicum* is a soilborne spore-forming organism that can survive for long periods of time under favorable conditions. Infection when it occurs is usually through contamination of wounds particularly bruising type injuries where there is considerable damage to tissue. The organism is anaerobic, and deep puncture wounds provide a very favorable site for its rapid multiplication. Although *Cl. septicum* is the principal organism causing malignant edema, other species of *Clostridia* can be involved. For example, the swelled-head condition sometimes seen in rams as a result of post-fighting infection is usually due to *Clostridium novyi*.

Cl. septicum is a potent toxin producer that causes profound rapidly fatal clinical signs. The first indication of its presence is generally soft swelling in the area of the wound that extends very rapidly because of exudation and infiltration of the surrounding areas. The adjacent muscle will become dark brown to black in color but without the gas production and subcutaneous crepitation commonly seen with blackleg. There is always high fever, and affected animals are depressed, weak, and may show muscle tremors and lameness before they die. Death may occur in twenty-four hours or less.

At necropsy there is usually gangrene of the skin overlying the infected area and the subcutaneous and intramuscular connective tissue around the site will be very edematous (filled with fluid). Small hemorrhages and blood-tinged edema fluid will be found in all of the body cavities.

Because of the similarity of malignant edema to blackleg and especially to anthrax, diagnosis based upon post-mortem examination alone is sometimes difficult. A fluorescent antibody test in the laboratory is helpful in distinguishing between these clostridial infections and anthrax.

Malignant edema is preventable by vaccination as outlined for blackleg but because of its acute nature and rapid progression, treatment of infected animals is generally not very satisfactory. The organism is susceptible to penicillin and broad spectrum antibiotics if they are given early enough. Antitoxin used to treat the toxemia caused by the disease in man is too expensive to be of practical value for use in animals.

Other clostridial infections, such as *Cl. sordelli* on the West Coast, have been incriminated as a cause of sudden death in feedlot animals. Those are controllable by use of specific bacterin.

ENTEROTOXEMIA

This is an acute, highly fatal disease most commonly encountered in lambs and calves, although it is occasionally seen in kids, piglets, and foals. It is the result of toxins produced by *Clostridium perfringens* and several different toxins are recognized, each producing a slightly different but overlapping clinical pattern. Types B, C, and D are the most frequently seen in the United States although Type A has been reported in California lambs. Enterotoxemia is most frequent in young animals but it can cause sudden death in adults as well.

Regardless of toxin type, onset is sudden and mortality is high. Type A in lambs causes severe depression, pallor, jaundice, hemoglobinuria (hemoglobin in urine), and rapid breathing. It is a hemolytic (causing blood breakdown) disease that in some respects resembles leptospirosis in calves. Type B enterotoxemia is responsible for the severe enteric disease often called lamb dysentery. It usually occurs in lambs less than two weeks old and may cause death without any premonitory signs. Less acute cases will demonstrate severe abdominal pain, failure to nurse, and profuse, often bloody, diarrhea. The disease rapidly progresses to coma and death in twenty-four hours or less.

Type B generally affects calves seven to ten days old but occasionally older calves will be affected. The symptoms in calves are similar to those in lambs, but calves that don't succumb in a few hours may develop central nervous system signs as well. The disease in piglets, foals, and kids is essentially the same as that seen in lambs. Because of its very acute nature, diagnosis of enterotoxemia is generally based on post mortem lesions. Hemorrhagic enteritis with ulcers and peritonitis is a common finding. Laboratory examination of a portion of intestine and intestinal contents will confirm the diagnosis.

Type C causes similar lesions and typing of *Cl. perfringens* exotoxin in the laboratory gives a definitive diagnosis. Type C is responsible for the disease known as "struck" in adult sheep in Great Britain and occasionally seen in this country.

Type D enterotoxemia is a major problem in feedlot lambs although it can affect those under two weeks of age. Characteristically, those in the best nutritional state will be the first of the group affected. Because the disease is usually seen in well-fed animals it is commonly referred to as "overeating disease." Sudden death may be the only sign. Those that live a little longer may exhibit excitement, incoordination, and convulsions. Depending on how soon the animal dies, post mortem lesions may range from almost none to hemorrhages of heart muscle, abdominal muscles, and the surface of the intestines. Rapid post-mortem decomposition of the kidneys is the basis for its other common name of "pulpy kidney disease."

Control Methods

Regardless of type, enterotoxemia shares some common characteristics and control methods. *Cl. perfringens* is a common soilborne inhabitant of the intestinal tract of animals. Although the exact mechanism is obscure, it's apparent that under some conditions the organism produces exotoxin, a poison, in excess of the animal's capacity to cope with it. Excessive consumption of milk or grain is a known predisposing factor. As evidence of this, the fattest animals are usually the first affected and the disease is rarely seen in nursing twin lambs because they simply don't have that much milk available. Similarly, in the feedlots, outbreaks are most common a few days after the animals are put on full feed.

Regardless of type a standard recommendation for control of enterotoxemia is to reduce feed intake whether it be milk for the very young or grain for the older groups. Unfortunately, in the feedlot, reduced grain feeding is inconsistent with rapid rate of gain. Some feedlot operators have successfully reduced the incidence through continuous low-level feeding of broad-spectrum antibiotics such as tetracycline to reduce the bacterial population.

These antibiotics and immunization are the most effective means of controlling the disease. Several types of biological products are available including toxoid, antitoxin, antiserum, and bacterins. Each is type-specific, although polyvalent products are available and recommended, even though more expensive, unless the specific type of toxin causing the problem has been identified. The choice of product to use depends on circumstances, and advice of a veterinarian is highly recommended.

Generally speaking, antitoxin and antiserum are used to provide immediate protection such as when animals are first put in the feedlot or during an outbreak. If antiserum is used, animals should be carefully watched for a few hours afterward for signs of anaphylactic shock. Some protection can be provided to the newborn through colostral antibody when the dams have been actively immunized with bacterin or toxoid. When using these products, be sure to follow the manufacturer's recommendations for dose, site, and route of inoculation because tissue reactions from these products are not unusual.

Lamb with tetanus.

TETANUS

Humans, horses, and sheep are the most susceptible to tetanus or "lockjaw" but the disease occasionally occurs in cattle, goats, and pigs as well. The clinical signs are caused by a neurotoxin produced by *Clostridium tetani*. Tetanus is a wound infection disease most common with deep penetrating wounds when tissue damage is extensive. The organism requires anaerobic (without oxygen) conditions for growth and will not thrive in a surface laceration where the blood supply is good. The interval between infection and clinical signs may range from four days to several weeks and it's not unusual for a puncture wound of the foot to be completely healed on the surface when symptoms of tetanus develop. The disease is usually individual and sporadic, although serious outbreaks have been reported following castration, shearing, and docking of pigs and lambs. The use of elastic bands for castration and docking is conducive to conditions favoring growth of *Cl. tetani*.

As infection proceeds, neurotoxin travels along nerve pathways increasing irritability of the motor nerve end plates so the effect is an overreaction to external stimuli. This may be seen first as muscle stiffness, particularly in the legs, muscles of the jaw, and around the wound itself. This progresses rapidly to a point where muscle rigidity increases. Difficulty in chewing or swallowing gives the disease the name "lockjaw." One of the early diagnostic signs in the horse is a "flash" of the third eyelid in response to a loud noise or sudden movement. Temperature is usually normal at the outset but the exertion of constant muscle contraction may cause sweating and temperature rise a few hours before death. Affected animals move with great difficulty if at all. Extensive rigidity of leg muscles may cause a "saw horse" stance and if the horse should happen to fall, fractures are a distinct possibility.

Prevention

Prevention of tetanus is far more rewarding than treatment. Mortality is very high in horses and sheep and less so in other species. Treatment with massive doses of penicillin and antitoxin is helpful, but the excitement of treatment itself may stimulate a fatal spasm. Use of sedatives, tranquilizers, and anesthetics may be helpful. Good nursing care is essential.

Prevention is far more satisfactory. Proper sterilization of surgical instruments between animals when castrating or docking will help to prevent infection as will careful cleaning and debridement of wounds. *Cl. tetani* spores are commonly found in soil and in the digestive tracts of animals, especially horses. It's safest to assume that any penetrating wound is contaminated and give tetanus antitoxin along with the usual wound treatment. Horses can be permanently immunized with two doses of tetanus toxoid given a month apart followed by an annual booster dose.

BOTULISM

This is not a common disease in farm animals but it must be considered when signs of progressive paralysis of unknown origin are seen. It is not an infection but is a toxemia caused by ingestion of the neurotoxin produced by *Clostridium botulinum*. Spores of the organism are widespread in nature and under favorable conditions of warmth, moisture, pH and low oxygen tension multiply rapidly in decomposing animal and plant material. Several types of toxin are recognized and all are quite stable, persisting for long periods of time even when the organism is no longer present.

Causes and Diagnosis

The clinical signs are those of progressive paralysis with the muscles of the tongue and throat being affected first. Tongue paralysis is considered one of the early specific signs. Death usually occurs in a few days due to respiratory paralysis.

The disease is common in wild waterfowl and is often called "limber neck" because of the neck muscle paralysis. It has been reported in horses, cattle, sheep, and goats but less frequently in swine. In range animals it is more likely to occur during periods of drought or when, as a result of phosphorus deficiency, animals are more likely to chew on carrion.

These are not the only circumstances, however. Improperly stored and cured silage can be a factor. I recall one instance where a dairyman had put oat silage on top of corn in a conventional wood silo. Several months later as he was feeding from the interface of the corn and oats, cows began to die from botulism. Apparently there was sufficient spoilage at the interface for *Cl. botulinum* to proliferate. After he removed and dumped about three feet of stored silage at that point, no further cases occurred. Silage stored in airtight silos has also been incriminated in at least two outbreaks of botulism in dairy cattle.

Botulism from spoiled canned food is hazardous to man and spoiled food should not be fed to animals because it's equally hazardous to them.

Antitoxin is the only specific treatment for botulism and the amounts required for animals are usually too costly to be of practical value. With good nursing care, some animals recover if the dose of toxin consumed is small.

Infectious Necrotic Hepatitis

This is a highly fatal disease of sheep, and occasionally seen in cattle and pigs, caused by *Clostridium novyi*. It occurs, like bacillary hemoglobinuria, when liver damage from any cause creates an environment in which the organism already present can proliferate. The toxin it produces causes extensive tissue destruction, disrupting capillaries and causing hemorrhagic areas in many body organs. Small subcutaneous hemorrhages give the underside of the skin a black appearance when observed at necropsy, hence the common name, "black disease."

Normal animals harbor the organism in areas where it is found and fecal matter from them further contaminates pastures. In sheep, the primary triggering factor is migration of immature flukes through the liver. They provide sufficient liver injury for *Cl. novyi* to multiply, which in turn causes more liver destruction, making conditions even more favorable. Flukes can be a factor in cattle, too, although other liver disease may be more significant. Liver abscesses commonly encountered in feedlot cattle and pigs on high-concentrate diets may account for the greater frequency of the disease in these species in feedlots. In sheep the disease is more prevalent from midsummer until early fall when the snail population (the intermediate host for liver flukes) is at its peak. High moisture conditions that favor snail growth make the disease more prevalent on irrigated pastures. Adult sheep are most commonly affected, and with few exceptions those affected will go from an apparently well-nourished, healthy state to death in a few hours. Mortality is 100 percent and anywhere from 5 to 30 percent of the flock may be affected.

Diagnosis

At necropsy the dark areas under the skin coupled with necrotic areas in the liver and accumulation of blood-tinged fluid in body cavities helps to distinguish this from other diseases causing sudden death. The fluorescent antibody (FA) test applied to liver tissue in the laboratory confirms the diagnosis.

Control Methods

While immunization with toxoid will control the disease even during an outbreak, control of the fluke population should be attempted as well either by fencing sheep out of wet areas or using a molluscicide where this is legally permissible because heavy fluke infestations can cause serious primary disease without bacterial complications. Feeding some hay in addition to concentrates to feedlot cattle helps to reduce the incidence of liver abscesses that predispose the animals to black disease.

Bacillary Hemoglobinuria

This disease of cattle and sheep, sometimes called "redwater," is caused by *Clostridium hemolyticum* and occurs primarily in the Western States in animals on irrigated pasture. The organism appears to produce two toxins, one causing tissue destruction similar to other *Clostridia spp.* and the other causing destruction of red blood cells. The result is severe anemia and loss of hemoglobin from red blood cells through the kidney to give the urine a dark red color, from which the disease gets its common name.

The organism is a soilborne spore-former and where the disease is prevalent spores are commonly found in the livers of normal cattle and occasionally sheep and goats. Liver damage, as from flukes, is apparently necessary before the spores become vegetative and start producing toxin. Initial infection occurs orally in animals grazing contaminated pasture or forage. Losses may begin seven to ten days after susceptible animals are put into the pasture. Sudden death may be the only clinical sign but more often there is evidence of acute abdominal pain, fever, rapid respiration, and reluctance to move. Profound anemia with hemoglobinuria and edema (swelling) of the brisket is a common finding. Anoxia (lack of oxygen) attributable to the anemia occurs late in the disease which is frequently fatal in anywhere from less than one to four days.

Diagnosis is based on history, symptoms, post-mortem examination and serologic testing. The blood test however is not completely specific, and blood or tissue cultures are more positive.

Treatment

Early treatment with penicillin or broad-spectrum antibiotics coupled with blood transfusion, good nursing care, and antiserum, if available, will save some animals. Annual subcutaneous vaccination with *Cl. hemolyticum* bacterin provides a fair degree of control although in high risk areas a second dose during the pasture season may be necessary.

Anthrax

This disease affects all species including man and in its most common form is a highly fatal septicemia, or blood poisoning. It is caused by *Bacillus anthracis*, the spores of which are resistant to heat, cold, drying, and most disinfectants and persist in the soil for years. Anthrax spores on hides and wool have been responsible for many cases of the disease in man. Similarly, contaminated feedstuffs, especially bone meal, have been the source of outbreaks in animals. There are areas of known soil contamination in some of the Central and Western States, and a few other states as well, where vaccination must be done regularly to prevent death losses. Outbreaks are more common in hot weather in animals grazing on alkaline soils. Outside those areas infection is rare, resulting only from contaminated feed or materials brought in.

The peracute (more acute) form of anthrax generally seen early in new outbreaks may cause death of cattle, sheep, and goats in as little as two hours. Swine and horses tend to be more resistant, generally showing clinical signs over a period of one to two days. In fact, in swine the infection may be limited to the throat area, and some may survive. In animals that live long enough for clinical signs to be observed, there will be high fever, muscle tremors, abdominal pain, respiratory distress, staggering, and convulsions prior to death. Blood discharges from all body openings just prior to death and after death are common. Recovered swine may develop chronic abscesses in the lymph nodes of the cervical region.

With such a rapid, violent, and fatal syndrome, it isn't hard to visualize why, historically, anthrax was such a feared disease. It still causes serious losses in many parts of the world but vaccination and quarantine procedures in this country have made it much less important than it once was.

Diagnosis

The initial cases of anthrax can easily be confused with other diseases causing sudden death such as blackleg, poisoning and lightning strike. There are, however, some distinguishing characteristics. Unlike blackleg it occurs in animals of all ages. The blood is very dark and does not clot, which is unique, and blood discharges from mouth, nose, and rectum are a fairly constant finding. These factors, plus the lack of rigor mortis and the disease's limitation almost entirely to known areas tends to clinch the diagnosis. It can be confirmed by microscopic examination of a stained blood smear, culture of the organism from body fluids, or injection of body fluid into guinea pigs in the laboratory.

Necropsy of suspected anthrax cases should be avoided for two reasons. First, all body tissues are loaded with the organism, and human infection can occur through minute scratches or abrasions, by inhalation, or by ingestion. Second, *B. anthracis* from the carcass that get onto the ground will sporulate, or become resistant spores, on exposure to the air in just a few hours. These spores will then contaminate the premises almost indefinitely. Anthrax is a serious, dangerous, reportable disease that when suspected should be brought immediately to the attention of your veterinarian.

Vaccination

Anthrax is preventable by vaccination but many states limit the use of vaccine to those areas where, through prior experience, anthrax is likely to occur. This precaution was made necessary by the type of vaccine in use for many years. It was, and is, an attenuated spore vaccine. Although the earlier vaccine produced a reasonable degree of immunity most of the time, individual and species differences in resistance caused some animals to develop the disease as a result of vaccination. More highly attenuated spore vaccines reduced this risk but did not provide as good an immunity. As a consequence, several vaccines with varying degrees of attenuation were marketed. These have been largely superseded by an avirulent attenuated vaccine developed by Stern, which is safer but nevertheless frequently causes fever, drop in milk production, and abortion in swine.

Treatment of anthrax usually isn't possible because of its acute nature but the organism is sensitive to penicillin, streptomycin, and the tetracyclines. Use of one or more of these on all animals in the herd when the disease is diagnosed may forestall additional cases. Given in large doses early in the disease, antibiotics will save some animals.

SALMONELLOSIS

This disease, affecting all species including man, is caused by species of the genus *Salmonella* and is sometimes called paratyphoid. Several hundred species and subspecies are widely distributed in nature, but fortunately only a few are highly pathogenic. *S. typhimurium* and *S. dublin* commonly affect livestock. *S. abortivoequina* was once commonly incriminated as a cause of abortion in horses but seems to have virtually disappeared from the United States. *S. cholerasuis* is limited primarily to pigs.

Forms

Three distinct forms of salmonellosis are recognized: peracute, acute, and chronic. The peracute form occurs primarily in young animals, especially those such as calves and pigs maintained under concentrated husbandry methods. It is a septicemic (generalized), rapidly fatal disease that in calves is indistinguishable from the septicemic forms of colibacillosis although it is inclined to occur sometimes in calves a week or so older. It causes high fever, dullness, depression and death in twenty-four to forty-eight hours. Foals, piglets, and lambs show similar signs. The peracute form generally occurs in animals under four months of age. Calves infected with *S. dublin* may also develop staggering and incoordination. In piglets where the infection is due to *S. cholerasuis*, a red to purple discoloration of the skin of the ears and abdomen occurs along with weakness, paralysis, and convulsions prior to death.

In adult animals and man, salmonellosis usually takes the form of an acute enteritis, or intestinal disorder. Onset is sudden with fever, abdominal cramps, and watery diarrhea. As the disease progresses the fever disappears but blood clots may appear in the feces. The diarrhea is accompanied by straining, and often mucus and mucous casts of the intestinal lining may appear. To the inexperienced, these mucous casts may look like the intestinal lining itself. Lack of appetite is usually complete and affected animals dehydrate rapidly and show extreme thirst. Horses will show violent colicky symptoms and pigs in addition to the above may show signs of central nervous system disturbance as well. Abortion is a common sequel in all species.

S. dublin is reported to cause abortion in cows and ewes without any other clinical signs. The acute form of the disease in the majority of animals terminates fatally in two to five days. Those that survive are debilitated for long periods of time. In horses, onset of acute enteric salmonellosis often follows the stress of transportation.

May Become Chronic

In pigs and sometimes in cattle following the initial acute attack, the disease will become chronic with persistent diarrhea, emaciation, and occasional episodes of fever and blood clots in the feces. Chronically infected animals should be culled from the herd.

Salmonellae are ubiquitous and many animals become infected without showing signs of disease. Development of clinical signs is dependent on the size of the infecting dose, pathogenicity of the particular organism, and resistance of the animal. The organism colonizes in the bile ducts and gall bladder and is intermittently shed in feces. Recovered and sub-clinically infected animals remain carriers, and fecal contamination from them is the primary source of infection. Under favorable conditions of moisture and temperature, the organism can survive for long periods of time outside the body.

Rats and mice are common carriers of *S. typhimurium* and contamination of feedstuffs by them is a common source of herd outbreaks. Salmonellae multiply rapidly in liquid or moist feeds. Milk replacer and pig feed in slurry form if mixed in batches and allowed to stand very long at room temperature will rapidly become a thriving *Salmonella spp.* culture if the organism is present. For the same reason, to prevent human infections, it's important to keep cold foods, especially those containing poultry products, refrigerated until served.

Treatment

Treatment of salmonellosis in food-producing animals sometimes presents a dilemma. The organism develops antibiotic resistance quite rapidly and a limited number of antibiotics is effective against it. Perhaps the most consistently effective is chloramphenicol, but this drug is not cleared by the Federal Drug Administration for use in food-producing animals. While this does not preclude use of the drug by a veterinarian to save the animals, it does mean that meat or milk from the animal thereafter cannot be used legally for human food because the duration of drug residue in meat or milk has not been established. Nitrofurazone is also a useful drug particularly suited for use in drinking water for mass medication but it, too, has been banned from the market entirely on the basis of suspected carcinogenicity. Ampicillin and trimethoprim are among the drugs used to treat the septicemic form of the disease. Supportive therapy such as intravenous fluids and corticosteroids to combat shock is often indicated. Treatment in view of these and other complications including the difficulty of making a positive diagnosis make this a disease best left to your veterinarian to handle.

Diagnosis Difficult

Positive diagnosis of salmonellosis in the living animal is difficult because of varying clinical signs and resemblance to many other diseases. A positive fecal culture coupled with history and clinical signs is helpful but recovery of the organism is sometimes difficult and several samples taken at different times may be necessary for a positive result. Infected but asymptomatic animals shed the organism intermittently so, by itself, a positive fecal culture may not mean much. Recovery of the organism from tissues at necropsy is more diagnostic.

Prevention of the infection also presents some problems and depends primarily on scrupulous sanitation. Commercially prepared Salmonella bacterins may help if they contain antigen for the particular species causing the trouble. Autogenous bacterins prepared from isolates from the farm would be more helpful but sanitation is still the most important component.

Salmonellosis is likely to be more of a problem in intensive rearing operations common to the veal and pork industries. For these, the "all in-all out" method allows time for adequate cleaning and disinfection of the barn before the next group of animals is brought in. Avoiding rodent contamination of feedstuffs, removing leftover feed, and thorough cleaning of feed utensils following each use are all important parts of a control program. Continuous low level feeding of antibiotics may help to keep the *Salmonella spp.* population in check but that procedure, too is not looked upon favorably by the Federal Drug Administration.

TUBERCULOSIS

At one time this was a major disease of domestic animals and man. It is caused by members of the genus *Mycobacterium* and several distinct strains, human, bovine, and avian are recognized. Of these, the human type tends to be the most host-specific, rarely being found in species other than man, although occasionally dogs contract the infection from their owners. A classic example of this occurred in New York City several years ago. A child was found to have tuberculosis but other members of the family were negative and the source of the infection was obscure. Epidemiologic investigation subsequently revealed a dog who was a neighborhood pet that customarily played with all the children living nearby. The dog was tested and found positive and its owner was found to be infected as well. The infection apparently passed from owner to dog to child.

The bovine type is least host-specific and infects not only cattle but man, swine, goats, horses, and sheep in about that order of frequency. The avian type is commonly found in older birds and readily infects swine and, to a lesser extent, cattle and sheep.

Tuberculosis is best described as a chronic wasting disease typically without overt clinical signs early in the disease. Except with the avian type in birds and swine, the initial lesions usually develop in the lung and thoracic lymph nodes. The organism slowly develops tumor-like masses called *tubercles*. These may be few or numerous and may become quite large. The center of the tubercles degenerates into a caseous or cheesy mass which may undergo calcification in long-standing cases. Although the primary lesions are usually in the chest cavity, generalized or miliary tuberculosis does occur and the organism can thrive anywhere in the body. Bovine tuberculosis in man, for example, commonly locates in the spine to cause serious spinal deformities. One of the outstanding contributions of veterinary medicine to human health has been control of tuberculosis. The precipitate decline in the disease in man during the last forty years exactly parallels the rate of eradication in cattle.

The tubercle bacilli are shed in saliva, feces, and milk from infected cows. Infection may occur by inhalation or ingestion. Because of this, the disease is more likely to occur in stabled animals than range cattle. Signs of the disease are variable depending on location. With lung involvement, a persistent cough and intermittent low-grade fever may be seen as the disease progresses. Gradual weight loss to the point of emaciation is the usual sequel, despite adequate food intake. The avian type in swine occurs primarily in the digestive tract as it does in birds and may not cause any visible signs. The principal loss in swine is through condemnation of carcasses or parts of infected carcasses at slaughter.

Diagnosis

Diagnosis of tuberculosis in animals, because of the absence of clinical signs early in the disease, is sometimes difficult. In cattle the intradermal tuberculin test is routinely used as a part of the official tuberculosis eradication program. Tuberculin is prepared from a culture of *M. bovis* and is basically a standardized culture filtrate. A small amount injected intradermally in the tail fold of a cow sensitized by exposure to the organism will cause a swelling at the injection site in forty-eight to seventy-two hours. Those with no prior exposure do not get any reaction. The test is really an allergy-type test and unfortunately exposure to other related organisms will give a similar response. The comparative cervical test, wherein both avian and mammalian tuberculin are used and the responses measured, is more sensitive. Despite this shortcoming, the tuberculin test has been a very effective tool in reducing the level of infection in cattle in this country to less than 1 percent.

Although it's frustrating to owner and veterinarian alike to see a good cow slaughtered because of a positive test and have a post-mortem report come back marked "No visible lesions," the test should not be condemned. A percentage of those may be in the early stages of infection with lesions too small to be seen. Loss of an occasional cow is a small price to pay for a healthier cattle and human population. A greater deficiency is its failure to identify cattle with advanced tuberculosis because they have lost their sensitivity.

Control

Test and slaughter is the proven effective control method for bovine tuberculosis and by the end of 1992 had reduced the number of known infected cattle herds in the U.S. to sixteen. The disease rarely occurs in sheep and goats unless they are exposed to infected cattle but the same test technique applies. In poultry the disease can be kept under control by marketing all birds at the end of their first laying period, since the disease is more of a problem in old birds. Swine can be protected by keeping poultry away from them and by keeping wild birds out of the farrowing and finishing houses.

Before leaving tuberculosis, a word of caution is in order. Non-human primates (such as monkeys and chimpanzees) are highly susceptible to and notorious carriers of tuberculosis. If you have any inclination to keep one as a pet, try to resist it because they are nothing but trouble. But if you can't resist, by all means have the animal tested for tuberculosis before you bring it home.

PARATUBERCULOSIS

This chronic disease of cattle, sheep, and goats caused by *Mycobacterium paratuberculosis* is endemic on some farms where its principal effect is unthriftiness and decreased production. The organism is related to *M. bovis* and infection with either may give a positive intradermal test reaction. The common name of the infection is "Johne's Disease" and it is seen more frequently in cattle than other species.

The incubation period is very long, with most cattle probably becoming infected as calves but not showing clinical signs until two years of age or more. Persistent diarrhea that occasionally subsides and then recurs coupled with weight loss and decreased milk production are the only clinical signs. Generally there is no fever and appetite remains normal.

Diagnosis

Diagnosis and control of paratuberculosis are difficult because not only are the clinical signs minimal but many infected animals show no clinical signs yet they shed the organism in manure and thus are a hazard to others. The **intradermal test,** an allergy test utilizing avian tuberculin or johnin, a specific diagnostic agent, is often inconclusive. It is most reliably used on animals prior to development of clinical signs but animals late in the disease may give a negative result. The **complement fixation test** utilizing blood serum is useful later in the disease. The more recently developed ELISA test has proven more sensitive and is now commercially available. Fecal culture, which may take a month or more, is good evidence of infection if culture results are positive but the organism is both slow and difficult to grow so that a single negative culture may be meaningless.

Finding typical lesions at necropsy coupled with microscopic examination of tissues from the colon and adjacent lymph nodes is the most reliable. *M. paratuberculosis* localizes in the lower digestive track, causing a thickening and corrugated appearance of the intestinal wall — particularly the lower small intestine, cecum, and colon. This thickening interferes with absorption of nutrients and especially fluids so that loose manure is common.

Control Difficult

If these tests and examinations are positive, the existence of the infection in the herd is confirmed and it can be concluded that other animals are infected that may or may not show clinical signs later on. Control of the disease is difficult at best. There is some indication that animals on a diet deficient in calcium will show clinical signs of infection more often but this remains to be proven. The organism is shed in manure and can survive under favorable temperature and moisture conditions for a year or more. It is resistant to many disinfectants but doesn't survive long in direct sunlight.

Infection occurs when the animal eats feed or drinks water contaminated with manure containing the organism. Providing feed and water free of contamination is an essential part of control. This is relatively easy, of course, by using feed bunks and water troughs, but that doesn't solve the problem of pasture contamination. Nevertheless, sanitation is important. The risk of infection from contaminated pasture can be reduced by limiting the number of animals per acre to take advantage of the dilution factor and by pasture rotation — provided the pasture at rest is clipped and manure scattered with a drag to provide maximum exposure to sunlight. But these measures, although they will reduce the rate of new infections, will not entirely prevent the disease from spreading.

Utilizing the ELISA test and fecal culture, several states offer voluntary Johne's Disease certification programs to assist farmers and ranchers who want to establish infection-free herds. Several types of vaccines have been used successfully in sheep and cattle in Europe but they are not approved for use here except in a few states by permit. Vaccination interferes with the test for tuberculosis which is considered a more important disease because of its economic and public health significance.

ACTINOMYCOSIS

This disease sporadically appears in a few cattle in the herd to cause a rarefying osteomyelitis (bone disease) especially of the facial and jaw bones. In cattle it is a disease of bone and the bony enlargement it causes gives it the common name of "lumpy jaw." Although other species are recognized, *Actinomyces bovis* appears to cause human infections. *A. bovis* has been reported to cause a serious granulomatous mastitis in sows and, with *Br. abortus,* plays a role in poll evil and fistulous withers in the horse. Generalized actinomycosis has been reported involving the lungs and abdominal organs but this form of the disease is uncommon.

Economically, the lumpy jaw syndrome is the most important form of the disease. Typically this begins as a painless lump on the jaw or cheek. It can be distinguished from abscesses or other swellings by the fact that it is hard as bone and is, in fact, a part of the bone, although there may be some soft tissue swelling around it as the disease progresses. The disease is chronic and may extend over a period of several months to a year. Infection in the bone causes erosion of bony tissue with deposition of new bone surrounding the site so that enlargement occurs. Eventually tracts develop to the outside which discharge a yellowish pus. These eventually heal, leaving an indented scar, and new tracts develop elsewhere. Abscessation and rarification of bone cause difficulty in chewing and swallowing. In advanced cases, molar teeth in the affected area may loosen and fall out. Eventually affected animals die because they can't eat.

Diagnosis

Diagnosis of lumpy jaw can generally be made on the basis of physical examination and location of the lesion. If there is doubt, the diagnosis can be confirmed by finding minute granules in the pus typical of actinomycosis. Great care should be taken in handling infective material from the lesion because it is heavily laden with the organism and it can infect man. For the same reason, animals with a discharging lesion should be segregated from all others to reduce the risk of spread.

Treatment

Treatment of lumpy jaw leaves something to be desired because the infection is in bone, where it is hard to establish therapeutic levels of drugs. In the early stages, surgical removal of the diseased area is probably the most satisfactory. Prolonged therapy with penicillin has some value. All things considered, however, except for very valuable animals the best solution is probably to remove the infected animal from the herd. This is also the most effective control method. The disease is more likely to occur when cattle are grazing coarse stubble or fed coarse forage that may cause abrasions in the mouth. It is through these that infection takes place.

ACTINOBACILLOSIS

This disease of ruminants is closely related to actinomycosis in some of the lesions it produces although in cattle it primarily affects the tongue, hence the name "wooden tongue." Onset of infection with *Actinobacillus lignieresi* is usually rather sudden with swelling particularly at the base of the tongue and of the adjacent lymph nodes. Affected cattle refuse feed, drool excessively, and make licking or chewing movements as though a foreign body were present in the mouth. The base of the tongue becomes hard and swollen and ulcers may be present on the surface. In sheep and goats the tongue is usually not affected but lesions develop in the soft tissue of the lower jaw, face, and nose. These discharge a greenish yellow pus and as the lesions progress, extensive scar tissue develops which may interfere with eating or breathing. Lymph nodes in the area commonly become enlarged.

Because it is primarily a soft tissue rather than a bone disease, actinobacillosis responds better to treatment than does lumpy jaw. Sodium iodide, penicillin, streptomycin, and the tetracyclines have all been used effectively, usually bringing relief in twenty-four to forty-eight hours.

Like actinomycosis, the infection probably occurs via abrasions in the mouth. Coarse forage likely to produce these should be removed from the diet, but prompt treatment and segregation of infected animals is essential to control spread.

LISTERIOSIS

Despite rapid progress in animal disease research in recent years, the development of some diseases remains mysterious. Listeriosis, commonly called "circling disease" and caused by *Listeria monocytogenes,* falls in that category. Although it occurs primarily in cattle, sheep, and goats, the organism has been isolated from a wide variety of domestic and wild animals, birds, fish, and man. Many normal animals carry the organism and the clinical disease occurs sporadically for reasons not well understood.

In ruminants there appears to be a causal relationship with corn silage feeding, particularly if the silage is not well preserved and has a pH above 5.5. In sheep, outbreaks commonly occur about three weeks after they are started on a full feed of silage and terminate when silage is withdrawn from the diet. It can and does

Listeriosis. Symptoms include drooping left ear, sunken eye, and tongue paralysis.

occur, however, in animals that have never been fed corn silage.

The organism is extremely hardy, surviving in manure for a year or more and readily withstanding repeated freezing and thawing. Its distribution is limited primarily to the colder climate areas and the disease is rarely seen in the South. The route by which infection occurs in nature is obscure but experimentally the disease can be reproduced by inoculating the organism in a variety of ways. Route of infection may have some bearing on the clinical signs seen.

Diagnosis

Typically, in cattle, sheep, and goats, the disease causes an encephalitis or brain inflammation. The first thing noted may be an animal standing off by itself looking rather dull and depressed. The animal may wander aimlessly and if it comes to a fence or wall, just stand there pushing against it. The animal may stand with its head and neck turned to one side — if you turn the animal's head the other way it will go back to the original position when released. A high percentage of, but not all, affected animals when they walk will move in a tight circle always in the same direction. Facial paralysis on one side with drooping of the ear, eyelid, and lip on the same side is typical of listeriosis. Commonly animals with this sign will stand with some hay or feed in the mouth, making no effort to chew or swallow. Frequently not all of these signs will be seen in the same animal especially in sheep and goats where the disease is more acute, causing death in twenty-four to forty-eight hours. Cattle tend to be more resistant and the disease may run a course of seven to ten days. Once the first case is recognized, checking temperatures of other animals in the herd may pick out those in the early stage of the disease, since fever is a consistent early finding.

Encephalitis, however, is not the only form of the disease. In monogastric animals such as the pig and occasionally in young calves, lambs and foals, the disease will become generalized, involving the liver and other viscera. Affected animals show all the signs of acute septicemia: fever, lack of appetite, increased pulse and respiration, diarrhea, and early death. It can also infect the uterus, causing abortion and retained placenta with no other clinical signs. All three forms can occur in man, although the encephalitic manifestation may be more frequent. Aborted fetuses, placenta, and vaginal discharges are highly infective and extreme caution should be taken when handling such material.

Strangely, herd outbreaks that may involve up to 10 percent of the animals usually consist of all encephalitic cases or all septicemic. Abortions may occur without any other clinical signs of disease. Except when the unilateral facial paralysis and circling are evident, diagnosis is sometimes difficult. The septicemic form looks like any other septicemia and the encephalitic form can be confused with other diseases causing brain disorders such as thromboembolic meningoencephalitis, tumors, rabies, pregnancy toxemia in sheep, and the nervous form of ketosis in cattle. Blood tests are of little value because many normal animals have a strong antibody titer against *L. monocytogenes*. Culture of the organism in the laboratory from body tissues coupled with the clinical signs is most diagnostic but special techniques may be required.

Treatment

Treatment of the septicemic form in all species and the encephalitic form in sheep and goats is worth trying but usually disappointing. By the time it is noticed, the disease is too far advanced and the sick animals die too soon. Because it runs a longer course in cattle, treatment may be more rewarding but some recovered animals may show evidence of permanent brain damage. Without treatment, mortality approaches 100 percent. In any case, prompt treatment is essential and at the first indication the disease is present, temperatures should be checked on all animals in the herd or flock. Any with above-normal temperatures should be treated immediately, using broad-spectrum antibiotics or other drugs recommended by your veterinarian. If corn silage is a part of the diet, especially for feedlot lambs, it should be removed.

Because the organism is widespread and its mode of infection is unclear, specific control measures are hard to define. Thus far, satisfactory bacterins or vaccines have not been developed. Because of the apparent circumstantial relationship, the best present recommendation, particularly for sheep and goats, is to introduce silage to the diet gradually and to avoid feeding spoiled silage entirely.

CALF DIPHTHERIA

This disease occurs sporadically on some farms in calves under six months of age although occasionally older calves may develop the disease as well. It is encountered most frequently when calves are penned together where the principal causative agent, *Fusobacterium necrophorum* is likely to be present in large numbers. This is the same organism that causes foot rot and conditions favoring development of the one disease also favor development of the other. Although *F. necrophorum* can consistently be isolated from calf diphtheria lesions, it is quite probable that other organisms play some as yet undefined role.

Types

Two types of the disease may be encountered, **necrotic stomatitis** (inflammation of the mouth) and **necrotic laryngitis** (inflammation of the larynx) but the pathogenesis is the same. Necrotic stomatitis occurs more frequently in younger calves and involves the tongue, inside of the cheeks, especially at the angle of the lips, and the soft palate. Fever and refusal to eat are the earliest signs noted followed by drooling and swelling of the tongue and cheeks. The breath has a foul odor identical to the smell of foot rot. Lesions in the mouth are readily apparent consisting of deep ulcers of the cheek and sometimes the adjacent area of the tongue which are filled with necrotic tissue debris and food particles. The lesions are painful and affected calves generally refuse feed and water of any kind.

Diagnosis

The clinical signs of necrotic laryngitis are more pronounced and severe with fever of 106°F, moist cough, labored breathing, especially on inhalation, complete lack of appetite, and painful swallowing movements. External swelling in the laryngeal area may be evident and will be painful to the touch. Nasal discharge may be present and the breath always has the typical "foot rot" odor. Necrotic laryngitis can occur as a primary disease, can occur concurrently with necrotic stomatitis, or can be secondary to it. In any case the infection may extend to the lungs, causing a severe pneumonia.

Calf diphtheria is unrelated to diphtheria in man and is not a contagious disease in the usual sense. It is primarily a wound infection, with the organism gaining entrance through mouth abrasions caused by coarse feed or erupting teeth. More than one calf in the pen may be infected, however, because infection is more likely when the environmental contamination level is high. Affected calves dehydrate rapidly because of fever and failure to drink. Without treatment the disease is usually fatal in a week or less. Fortunately, the disease responds well to treatment with several of the sulfa drugs, penicillin, and tetracycline. The sooner treatment is started the better the response will be.

A similar condition, *necrotic rhinitis* (bull-nose) is occasionally seen in young pigs. Swelling of the face, nasal discharge, sneezing, nasal hemorrhage, lack of appetite, and emaciation are typical of the disease in pigs. The infection may be severe enough to cause erosion of the nasal turbinate bones and facial distortion. Generally, only a few pigs in the herd are affected and infection is generally thought to be a sequel to clipping needle teeth too close to the gum line. The disease can be confused with atrophic rhinitis, but the latter affects more pigs, is more chronic, and causes a lateral deviation rather than a bulging distortion of the face.

The only and most effective means of preventing these diseases lies with good management and sanitation. Keeping the pens clean and dry will make their occurrence a rarity.

ATROPHIC RHINITIS

This chronic debilitating disease of swine causes considerable economic loss on some farms each year. The most obvious change when it occurs is lateral deviation or shortening of the snout due to atrophy of the nasal turbinate bones. This does not occur in all infected pigs, however, and its occurrence seems to depend upon the age at which infection occurs. The younger the pig when first infected, the more likely the characteristic "twisted" snout is to occur. Older pigs may show little, if any, change following infection.

The disease has been recognized since the early 1800s in Europe and since the early 1940s in the United States. As might be expected, over the years many agents have been suggested as the cause ranging from bacteria, viruses, and protozoa to nutritional deficiencies. The gross pathological changes in the nasal turbinates can be produced experimentally by feeding diets deficient in calcium and phosphorus, or an imbalance of the two. More recent evidence indicates that a specific organism, *Bordetella bronchiseptica*, is the primary cause. Concurrent infection with *B. bronchiseptica* and toxigenic *P. multocida* results in a more serious form of the disease. Nevertheless, elimination of *B. bronchiseptica* carriers from the herd effectively prevents occurrence of atrophic rhinitis.

Diagnosis

The earliest sign in young pigs is excessive sneezing and snuffling occasionally with discharge of mucopurulent material from the nose and eyes. In some severe cases mild to profuse nosebleed occurs. Temperatures are usually normal and the pigs continue to eat. This is not sufficient evidence on which to base a diagnosis, however; many other conditions produce similar signs. On most farms a majority of the pigs recover from these mild symptoms, although some become carriers. Especially if concurrent infection with organisms such as *P. multocida* is present, some of those infected go on to develop the turbinate atrophy and snout deviation typical of the disease. Once it occurs this deviation is irreversible and may result in reduced rate of gain and hence economic loss. The disease usually is not fatal but may be complicated by secondary pneumonia.

In the absence of obvious snout deviation, a positive clinical diagnosis cannot be made. Often, however, even though no external signs can be seen, turbinate changes can be detected when the snout is sectioned with a bandsaw at necropsy. This doesn't do much for the pig being examined but it can establish the presence of the infection in the herd. A more useful technique is laboratory culture of nasal swabs taken from representative pigs in the herd. Your veterinarian can provide this service for you to determine the presence of *B. bronchiseptica*.

Treatment

Treatment of the infection is possible on some farms using sulfamethazine in the feed or sulfathiazole in the drinking water for several weeks. It is not always successful because some strains of the organism are resistant. Treatment of the young animals is less satisfactory than treatment of older stock. Because treatment results vary, several other means have been developed to control the prevalence of atrophic rhinitis. Because spread is primarily via aerosol transmission from one generation down to the next and turbinate atrophy is more likely to occur when infection occurs early in life, a good degree of control can be obtained by removing piglets from the sow as soon as they have nursed colostrum. They are then kept separate from other mature swine and reared by hand. A modification of this is to confine the sow in such a manner that piglets are kept away from her head and have access only to her udder at feeding time. A third method is the same as that used to establish a specific pathogen-free herd. This is to take the piglets by Caesarian section or by collecting them in clean plastic bags as they are born and then rearing them in isolation from all other swine. All of these methods present obvious management problems.

Identify Carriers

The advent of a reliable, economical culture technique makes it possible to identify carrier animals so the herd can be divided into clean and infected groups. The infected group can then be treated or sold for slaughter as circumstances indicate. They must be kept separate, however, and the clean group should have two additional cultures taken to be sure that, in fact, no infected animals are in it. It should also be protected from access by dogs, cats, and rodents because these species may carry B. bronchiseptica.

All of these techniques as well as periodic herd depopulation have been successfully employed to control atrophic rhinitis. But the most promising technique may prove to be the routine use of intranasal **B. bronchiseptica** bacterin and/or P. multocida bacterin/toxoid in sows and gilts prior to farrowing.

INFECTIOUS KERATOCONJUNCTIVITIS

This disease, commonly called "pink eye," occurs frequently in young cattle and less often in sheep and goats. It is seen most often during the summer months although sporadic cases occur in the other seasons.

Clinical Signs

Onset of the disease is sudden and it spreads rapidly. The first indication of the disease is usually an excessive flow of tears and a tendency to hold the eye partially closed. Bright sunlight increases the pain of the disease and affected animals usually seek a shaded area. Within a short time an ulcer develops, almost always in the central part of the cornea. Infiltration of leucocytes (white blood cells) and swelling of the ulcerated area causes the cornea to become opaque and milky in appearance. At first this is limited to a ring around the ulcer but in twenty-four to forty-eight hours the entire cornea becomes opaque. The animal is then blind. In a majority of cases only one eye is affected but involvement of both eyes is by no means rare. The elapsed time from onset to total corneal opacity may be no more than forty-eight hours.

Without treatment the corneal ulcer may heal spontaneously but more often gets progressively worse. As the ulcer gets progressively deeper the strength of the cornea is diminished and pressure within the eye causes the front part of the eyeball to assume a conical shape. Concurrently blood vessels extend from the periphery into the cornea in an attempt to speed the healing process. In a few days the ulcer may extend completely through the cornea resulting in loss of fluid and collapse of the front chamber of the eye. Blindness is then permanent.

Adjacent structures of the eye are also involved. The blood vessels in the sclera, the white fibrous covering of the eyeball, become enlarged and there is inflammation of the lining of the lids that causes a mucopurulent discharge and conjunctivitis.

For some reason, at least in my experience, pink eye seems to be more prevalent in some years than others. This may be related to climatic conditions and fly population. I recall very vividly seeing over 200 beef calves on one farm at one time with varying stages of the disease. It was a heartbreaking sight and many of them never recovered.

The most common causative organism in cattle is *Moroxella bovis* and in all probability it is carried from one animal to the next by flies, especially face flies. Irritation by dust and tall grass increases susceptibility of the eye to infection.

Diagnosis

Diagnosis is not difficult although the condition must be distinguished from the eye lesion caused by IBR virus. Almost invariably the corneal opacity of pink eye extends from the center of the cornea outward while that of IBR extends from the periphery inward. Also, with pink eye there are usually no adverse symptoms other than the eye lesion, whereas with IBR some animals in the group will usually have fever and respiratory involvement.

The most important thing is to recognize the disease and start treatment early before too much damage is done. It responds well to antibiotic ointment instilled onto the eye or small amounts of antibiotic injected into under the conjunctiva.

Too many people turn young stock out to pasture in the spring and forget about them until fall. In the interim some may get pink eye and become blind. It pays to check them at least once a week. Incipient pink eye isn't hard to spot because there will always be evidence of tears streaming down the cheek.

Affected animals should be put in a darkened stall and treated immediately. Where this isn't feasible, as with range cattle, at least one manufacturer makes an eye patch that is fastened over the eye with adhesive after treatment with antibiotics.

As a result of considerable research, there is now a bacterin for the prevention of the disease. Vaccination, fly control, isolation of infected animals, and reduction of dusty irritating conditions insofar as possible, are the best means of prevention.

ERYSIPELAS

The organism causing this disease, *Erysipelothrix insidiosa* (rhusipathiae) is widespread in nature and persists for long periods of time in soil and water. It is resistant to freezing and drying, and can tolerate most common disinfectants. It is capable of infecting a wide variety of animal species including man, fish, and birds. It is an infectious disease in swine, turkeys, and fish, but in other species it is generally a wound infection disease.

Except for the individual turkey grower who experiences an outbreak, the disease is most significant economically in pigs. The disease may range from inapparent to acute, subacute, or chronic in pigs. The organism can readily be isolated from the tonsils of many apparently normal pigs. It is excreted in the manure, and infection in pigs occurs primarily via the oral route. Stress seems to be a factor in the development of the clinical disease and it frequently occurs following farrowing. It is usually not seen in suckling pigs under three weeks of age.

Diagnosis

Acute septicemic erysipelas produces fever ranging up to 108°F, lack of appetite, and a reluctance to move. The organism becomes generalized and among other things produces a painful arthritis. Although it doesn't always occur, the disease usually produces very characteristic skin lesions on the neck, ears, shoulders, and belly. These are raised, reddened areas that take a definite diamond or trapezoidal shape. Because of this the disease has been referred to as "diamond skin" disease. The coloration ranges from pink to an angry purple and as the disease progresses the skin lesions may coalesce to form a large discolored area. The skin lesions usually appear within twenty-four hours and are a good diagnostic sign. Death may occur two to four days later.

Mortality with the subacute form is lower and the skin lesions are the most prominent sign. Fever is not as high and although appetite may be depressed, affected pigs will usually eat. Depending on severity of the lesions, affected patches of skin may become necrotic, dry, and peel off. Occasionally the tips of the ears and tail will slough off. The underlying surface after the skin peels is raw and should be treated with antiseptics as you would treat any open wound.

The acute or subacute forms of the disease may lead to the chronic form. The chronic disease is characterized by an arthritis, especially of the hip, hock, stifle, and elbow and knee joints, which at first is hot and painful. In a few weeks the active inflammation subsides and pain is no longer a factor but the joints are stiff. A more significant lesion for the life of the pig with chronic erysipelas is vegetative endocarditis (inflammation of the heart lining) especially involving the heart valves. This is a frequent complication that may be inapparent at first but may result in sudden death due to pulmonary embolism or cardiac infarct. More extensive endocarditis causes unthriftiness and labored breathing. Affected pigs have a poor rate of gain and are unprofitable to keep.

Treatment

Erysipelas responds well to treatment with penicillin, and the earlier treatment is started the better. This disease has important implications for the productivity of the swine herd and prompt professional diagnosis based on clinical signs, necropsy, or culture of the organism from tonsils or blood is important. Annual vaccination with bacterin is reasonably but not entirely effective in preventing it.

Erysipelas also can cause problems in sheep flocks as a result of wound infection following castration or docking. Arthritis is the principal sign in lambs and the resulting production loss can be severe. Doing these operations in clean surroundings with instruments disinfected after use on each lamb will minimize the problem.

Flock outbreaks of laminitis due to *E. insidiosa* two to three weeks after dipping sheep have been reported. Infection in this case occurs via skin abrasions if the dip water is heavily contaminated with the organism. Addition of a suitable germicide to the water helps to minimize the problem.

STRANGLES

Prior to the advent of antibiotics and when horses were congregated in large numbers in stables, remount depots, etc., this disease caused by *Streptococcus equi* was rampant. Its occurrence now is limited primarily to occasions when groups of horses are assembled for summer camps, rodeos, and shows. The disease is often referred to as **distemper** or sometimes **shipping fever,** the latter because it often occurs three to four days after a group of horses are brought together. It is possible that the stress of trucking predisposes to infection if an animal in the group is carrying the infection. However, strangles bears no relationship to shipping fever in cattle and does not cause pneumonia.

Progress of the Disease
Onset of the disease is sudden, with the first signs being lack of appetite and fever as high as 106°F. These are followed by a clear nasal discharge that soon becomes purulent. A mild conjunctivitis or eye inflammation sometimes occurs concurrently. The disease causes a severe pharyngitis (inflammation of the pharynx), sufficiently painful that affected horses are reluctant to swallow and sometimes hold the neck outstretched to relieve the pain. Within a few days abscesses develop in the lymph nodes of the throat region and accumulation of pus in the guttural pouches is common. Many of these abscesses break and drain to the outside yielding a thick creamy yellow pus from which pure cultures of *Str. equi* can be obtained.

The disease affects younger animals primarily but those over five years old who have had no prior exposure to it are also susceptible. In the individual it runs a course of about two weeks but in a band of horses it may be several months from the time of the first case until the last one recovers. Mortality from strangles averages less than 2 percent but once it appears, all horses in the group generally will be affected.

Occasionally abscesses will get large enough to interfere with breathing and a tracheostomy will have to be done to save the animal's life. The possibility always exists, too, that a few organisms will be carried in the blood stream to other organs especially liver, kidney, and brain, to form abscesses in these locations as well.

Such cases usually are fatal.

Purpura hemorrhagica, an immune disease unique to the horse and thought to be due to circulating bacterial protein, is a not uncommon sequel to strangles occurring about two weeks after the initial infection. Damage to the lining of blood vessels results in swelling especially of the head and legs with varying degrees of subcutaneous hemorrhage and anemia. This is a serious complication which is fatal about 50 percent of the time.

Str. equi is a more resistant organism than the majority of streptococci and can survive, for example, in a contaminated stall for up to a month. The route of infection is primarily by inhalation or ingestion. Therefore, an infected animal should be isolated from all others and the stall where it was kept thoroughly cleaned and disinfected.

Although the disease is not as prevalent as it once was, it still exists and every precaution should be taken to avoid it. By all means, if you are taking a horse to a show, take along your own feed and water utensils. The use of community feed troughs or water buckets is an ideal way to spread the infection. Try to keep your horse isolated from others at the show as much as reasonably possible. These measures may help to prevent other infections as well.

Treatment

Treatment of strangles is quite effective if started early in the course of the disease. The organism is sensitive to penicillin, tetracycline, and the sulfonamides but relapses are common unless treatment is continued for four to five days after the initial signs disappear. Antibiotic therapy after abscesses have formed is much less valuable and some people feel it actually prolongs the course of the disease. Surgical drainage of mature abscesses may hasten recovery but if breathing becomes labored due to obstruction, tracheostomy may be required.

A *Str. equi* bacterin is available for immunization against strangles but its use is not without complications. It is given in two or three doses two weeks apart and a few horses after the second dose may develop an allergic reaction. Also, local irritation at the site of the injection is common enough to cause concern. I would recommend you follow the advice of your veterinarian on whether to vaccinate depending on local circumstances.

POLYSEROSITIS

It has been estimated that about 2 percent of the swine in the United States suffer some degree of polyserositis manifested primarily as an arthritis (inflammation of the joints). At least two distinct organisms, *Hemophilus suis* and *Mycoplasma hyorhinis*, are capable of producing the disease. Both are common inhabitants of the upper respiratory tract where they normally do little harm. But under conditions of stress, they may produce generalized infection with localization in the joints.

Polyserositis in weanling pigs due to *H. suis* tends to be more acute with fever ranging to 107°F, with a high percentage of the herd infected and death losses up to

10 percent or more. Hot, swollen, painful joints are a common part of the syndrome regardless of the cause. Infection caused by *M. hyorhinis* tends to be less acute with an incubation period of four to five days and recovery in about a month.

Mycoplasma hyosynoviae has also been shown capable of producing arthritis in older pigs. However, it is difficult, if not impossible, to determine the causative organism on the basis of clinical signs alone. Isolation of the organism from joint fluid is the only sure way.

A retrospective diagnosis can sometimes be made based on response to therapy. Infection caused by *H. suis* responds fairly well to treatment with sulfonamides and antibiotics such as tylosin and lincomycin. Infection due to *Mycoplasma spp.*, on the other hand, responds better to tylosin, lincomycin, or erythromycin.

Polyserositis is a complex disease with no specific control measures available. Older swine act as unaffected carriers and are a constant source of infection. Any degree of isolation between age groups that can be achieved will be helpful as will avoiding stress situations such as rough handling, shipping, or abrupt changes in diet. Where the problem is severe, depopulation and establishment of a specific pathogen-free herd may be the best answer. This is obviously expensive but the economic loss from reduced weight gain of infected pigs in severely infected herds is equally costly.

JOWL ABSCESS

Although they have little relevance for the life or productivity of the pig, jowl abscesses due to *Streptococci spp.* are a major cause of partial carcass condemnation at slaughter. This adds to the cost of pork, and annual losses add up to millions of dollars.

The condition is endemic on some farms with recovered animals acting as carriers to infect every new pig brought to the farm and a high percentage of those born on the premises. The organism colonizes in the tonsils and extends from there to the cervical lymph nodes where abscesses develop. These may be as large as 5–6 cm in diameter and contain a greenish-yellow pus. The majority ultimately rupture and drain on the outside. Healing takes place after several weeks but fistulous tracts often remain. Initial infection is usually accompanied by mild fever of two or three days duration but this is rarely observed.

The first indication that anything is wrong is usually swelling at the site of a developing abscess. Unfortunately, it's too late then for treatment to have much value. Streptococcal abscesses develop a thick wall or capsule with little if any blood supply to the interior. Since antibiotics are transported in the blood stream they can't get to the site of infection.

Prevention is by far the best course to take. Your veterinarian can help you to design a control program which may include vaccination and/or incorporation of low levels of antibiotics in the feed. While reasonably effective, legal constraints on the type and level of antibiotics used make the latter procedure less effective than it could be.

VIBRIOSIS (CAMPYLOBACTERIOSIS)

Bovine genital campylobacteriosis is a true venereal disease of cattle being spread at the time of coitus or by breeding cows artificially with untreated semen from infected bulls. Generally, the only evidence of infection is infertility and irregular heat period intervals. Early embryonic death is an important feature of the disease but passage of the embryo in cervical and vaginal mucus is rarely observed. Abortions later in gestation due to *Campylobacter (Vibrio) fetus* var. *venerealis* occasionally occur.

When the disease first appears in the herd there is usually a history of recent additions to the herd, a new source of untreated bull semen or a new bull bought or borrowed. The disease is particularly troublesome in range cattle, where natural service is commonly practiced. Since there are no clinical signs, several months may go by before it becomes apparent that cows are not conceiving. The resulting delay in the calf crop can be disastrous. The prudent manager will not only do everything possible to prevent the disease but will have the cows examined for pregnancy sixty days after the bulls are put with them to be sure that conception rates are satisfactory.

Bovine vibriosis is self-limiting in the cow if the source of infection is removed, with the infection in a majority of cows clearing up in two or three months. Most cows develop sufficient immunity to conceive in about four to six months but a few carry the infection through a normal pregnancy and remain carriers and a source of new infections. A mild endometritis (inflammation of the uterus) may result from the infection, which responds reasonably well to infusion of the uterus with streptomycin. Young bulls tend to be resistant to infection but, nevertheless, mechanically carry the organism from an infected cow to others in the herd. Bulls upwards of five years of age are more likely to become infected and to remain carriers for life. Treatment of these bulls is not consistently satisfactory and following a course of treatment they should always be test-mated to a couple of virgin heifers and the heifers then examined by the mucus agglutination test.

Diagnosis

Diagnosis of vibriosis in the herd presents a challenge to the veterinarian and cattle owner. The history when infection is first introduced is one of greatly reduced conception rates and prolonged calving interval without other clinical signs and with occasional abortions. This history tends to set the disease apart from others affecting reproduction, assuming the bull is fertile or the semen of good quality. Diagnosis is more difficult in subsequent years when most of the herd has become resistant and the problem is limited to susceptible older cows and those added to the herd. The disease must be distinguished from others causing infertility or abortion such as trichomoniasis, IBR, BVD, and leptospirosis.

Several diagnostic tests have been developed, all of which require the services of a veterinarian and a good diagnostic laboratory. Among these are the mucus agglutination test, culture of cervical mucus, preputial washings, or an aborted fetus, fluorescent antibody test, and test-mating of bulls to virgin heifers. Where the history indicates vibriosis as a possibility, a single negative test may be misleading and in these cases the testing should be repeated. The laboratory must be careful to distinguish between *C. fetus* var. *venerealis* and *C. fetus* var. *intestinalis.* The latter is a common fecal contaminant that rarely produces abortion in cattle. A laboratory report, therefore of *"C. fetus positive"* is not sufficiently specific for diagnostic purposes.

Control
Vibriosis will not appear in a herd where all breeding is done artificially with properly antibiotic treated semen, and artificial insemination is a strongly recommended control procedure. An alternative with slightly more risk is to use only virgin bulls on the herd but this may limit herd improvement since the genetic potential of virgin bulls is not proven. A vaccine is available that, when given annually, produces a reasonably good immunity. Its use is more practical in the beef herd where artificial insemination is not feasible. Annual booster vaccination about a month prior to the breeding season is recommended. Vaccination and treatment with dihydrostreptomycin are useful to treat infected bulls.

Sheep and Goats
While *C. fetus* var. *intestinalis* is insignificant for the cow, it is a cause of abortion in sheep and goats but unlike vibriosis in cattle, transmission is by ingestion. Abortion late in pregnancy or birth of weak lambs is the principal sign. There are usually no other clinical signs and no warning an abortion is about to occur. Lesions are confined to the fetus and consist of edema and necrotic areas in the liver. Other diseases can produce similar lesions, however, so the most definitive diagnosis is by culture of the organism from the fetus.

Because the infection spreads orally, it is important to isolate all aborting animals and promptly dispose of any aborted fetuses. Infection produces immunity lasting several years following the initial abortion. Administration of penicillin and streptomycin, incorporating tetracycline in the feed and repeated vaccination with bacterin have all been used with some success to control outbreaks.

SWINE DYSENTERY

There are many causes of diarrhea in pigs, including salmonellosis and colibacillosis to name a couple. But the term **swine dysentery** is reserved for a specific severe mucohemorrhagic diarrhea complex due primarily to *Treponema hyodysenteriae.* It is often referred to as **vibrionic dysentery** although the role *Campylobacter coli* plays in causing it is unclear. Other names are "black scours" and "bloody scours."

The disease is most prevalent in young growing pigs, although it can affect piglets and adult hogs as well. Up to 90 percent of the weanling pigs on a farm may be affected at one time and reports of 30 percent mortality are not unusual. The disease is spread by ingestion of feces from sick pigs or from recovered or unaffected carriers. Initial outbreaks are most common in late summer or fall and can usually be correlated with addition of new pigs to the herd. Once it appears, recurrences tend to be cyclical with new cases occurring every month or so. Many, but not all, recovered pigs become resistant to further infection. Severity of the disease is related to the size of the infecting dose, stress, and the age of the pig. Swine are the only known reservoir of *T. hyodysenteriae* and carrier swine are the source of infection. Once infection appears in a herd, recurrences can be expected.

Symptoms

Diminished appetite and soft mucoid feces are the first signs of infection. Body temperature may rise slightly in the early stages but more often is normal. The diarrhea rapidly becomes worse and frequently bloody. Dehydration and weight loss accompany the severe diarrhea. Mucus and bits of intestinal lining tissue often appear in the feces as the disease progresses. The course is variable, ranging from two days to a month. In some cases it looks like the animals are recovering, but in a few days or weeks they are as bad as ever. Recovered pigs are frequently stunted and unthrifty, making this one of the economically most important diseases of swine.

Control Difficult

Control of the infection is difficult because carrier swine cannot readily be identified with currently available methods. Certainly additions to the breeding herd of pigs of unknown origin or pigs from herds where the health status is unknown should not be made. This admonition is not so easy to follow for the feedlots, where feeder pigs commonly come from random sources. Hygiene, sanitation, and isolation are all important to reduce fecal contamination and spread of disease. The disease can be transported from one pen to another or one farm to another on dirty boots and feeding utensils. The risk of spreading this and other diseases is the reason most swine growers prefer not to receive visitors in the barns.

Where the infection is present on the farm, a degree of control can be achieved by adding medication to the feed or drinking water. A variety of antibiotics, sodium arsanilate, and carbadox have been used with success. However, *T. hyodysenteriae* develops antibiotic resistance quite rapidly and therefore medication must be changed frequently. The same drugs can be used for treatment but must be given individually where possible or in drinking water because sick pigs won't eat.

Control through medication alone is not only a continuing expense but is rarely successful. It must be coupled with sound hygienic husbandry practices. Thus far, a vaccine for control of this disease has not been developed.

WINTER DYSENTERY

This baffling disease occurs primarily in stabled dairy cattle during the winter months and is more prevalent in the Northeast than elsewhere. Although beef cattle can be affected, it is seen mostly in the dairy breeds and rarely in young stock. It appears suddenly, rapidly affects the majority of the herd, and disappears as quickly as it came. Older texts state unequivocally that it is caused by *Campylo-*

bacter (Vibrio) jejuni, but attempts to reproduce the disease with the organism have been unsuccessful and its rapid spread indicates that other agents must be involved. Recovery seems to confer some immunity because once it appears in a herd a recurrence is not likely the following year. Where the infectious agent stays between outbreaks is unclear, nor are the precipitating factors well understood. *Campylobacter jejuni* is known to be a cause of severe diarrhea in man and it is not unusual for an episode of diarrhea to appear in the household concurrent with that in the barn.

Symptoms

Abdominal discomfort, uneasiness, and slightly depressed appetite are the earliest clinical signs. These are followed in a few hours by a profuse watery explosive diarrhea having a fetid odor. The diarrhea is so profuse and forceful that it behooves one to be very alert when walking behind cows with the disease. An effective range of ten feet is not unusual! Temperatures are usually in the normal range and in some cases the diarrhea becomes quite bloody. Dehydration caused by the fluid loss may be severe and a milk production decline of 50 percent is not unusual. Mortality is low if there are no complications. In a very few cases, intestinal hemorrhage accompanying the diarrhea may necessitate blood transfusion and where the disease is unduly prolonged, acidosis may contribute to death.

Treatment

A great variety of intestinal astringents and protectives have been used to treat the disease but their value is difficult to assess. It has been said that the uncomplicated case of winter dysentery recovers in seventy-two hours with treatment; otherwise it takes three days. There is little doubt that oral medication with any of the currently available drugs recommended coupled with electrolytes given orally and intravenously will help to minimize the effect of the disease, particularly on milk production. But with half or more of the herd to be treated at one time the labor requirement to do so may not be justified. This does not apply, of course, to the few individuals whose symptoms are so severe that vigorous treatment is necessary to save their lives. The normal course of the disease in the individual is about three days and on a herd basis the whole unpleasant episode usually passes in two or three weeks. For the dairyman and his cows, however, those weeks are messy, unpleasant, and costly in terms of milk production.

Prevention

Because the causative agent and mode of transmission are not well defined, specific preventive measures are elusive. Circumstantially it appears that the agent can be carried on boots, clothing, and vehicles from farm to farm. Many instances have been observed where the disease appeared in herds successively down the road about two days after a visit by an inseminator, drug and feed sales representative, cattle dealer — or veterinarian. Although there is no scientific basis for it, many veterinarians report that a degree of immunity can be achieved by vaccinating the herd with mixed bacterin at sixty-day intervals beginning in October and extending through March. Purchase of replacement animals during the season when winter dysentery is likely to occur is an obvious risk. Thus, at present, the best recommendation that can be made is to avoid overcrowding, keep the barn well ventilated, keep the barn as clean as possible, and, perhaps most important, keep new animals and new people out.

PYELONEPHRITIS

This is a serious but fortunately sporadic infection of the urinary tract most commonly encountered in mature cattle and more often in cows than bulls. The causative organism, *Corynebacterium renale,* can also infect horses and sheep but such infections are rare.

Pyelonephritis is generally referred to as an ascending urinary tract infection — that is, infection enters the tract via the urethra and proceeds upward to the bladder then via the ureters to the kidneys. The probable sources of infection are vulvar contact with contaminated bedding or tail switching, and spreading contaminated urine droplets from one cow to another. The use of unsterilized urinary catheters is an excellent way to spread the infection. The disease is seen more often in cows during advanced pregnancy or under the stress of inclement weather.

The organism thrives in urine and causes inflammation of the walls of the urethra, bladder, and ureter. In the kidney it causes destruction of functional tissue and small abscesses, eventually destroying so much kidney tissue that the animal dies from uremia. This occurs over a period of weeks or months.

Symptoms

The typical history is a gradual loss of appetite and weight with no fever. The animal may have intermittent periods of colicky abdominal pain due to restricted urine flow evidenced by kicking at the belly, frequent urination, and straining. The urine usually has flakes of pus and clots of blood in it, which makes the diagnosis at that point relatively easy. The entire urinary tract and kidneys will be greatly enlarged and detection of this enlargement by rectal palpation helps to confirm the diagnosis. The organism is quite easy to culture from urine samples.

Other than good sanitary practices and isolating infected cows, there are no specific preventive measures to be taken.

Treatment

If the damage already done is not too great, the infection responds well to treatment with penicillin. However, relapses following apparent recovery are common, so that overall the prognosis is guarded. It's well known that once infection appears in a herd, occasional additional cases are likely to occur. For that reason it seems prudent to remove the first case from the herd as soon as possible in hopes of preventing further cases from occurring.

Disease in Pigs

A closely related organism, *C. suis,* causes pyelonephritis in sows. The disease in pigs is a bit different in that clinical signs are not so pronounced. Apparent sudden death may be the only clinical sign — if that can be called a sign. Necropsy of infected sows will show an enlarged thickened bladder and ureter containing pus and blood. There is another difference in the swine disease, too. It occurs most commonly three to four weeks after breeding, leading to the possibility that it is a venereally transmitted disease in pigs.

Because there is a strong possibility of venereal transmission, boars that have been used on sows that developed pyelonephritis should not be used again until cultures of preputial swabs and semen are negative for *C. suis.* Fortunately, the disease is not common in pigs or cattle and is of relatively little economic significance except in the few herds where it is endemic.

CASEOUS LYMPHADENITIS

This disease, most important in sheep and goats, is caused by another member of the *Corynebacterium* genus, *C. pseudotuberculosis.* In these species it is characterized by chronic abscesses of the superficial lymph nodes. It rarely infects cattle, but in the horse may cause an ulcerative lymphangitis (disease of the lymph glands) with enlargement and nodule formation in the subcutaneous (under the skin) lymphatics of the lower leg. In the horse it's important that the disease be distinguished from a much more significant equine disease, glanders. The latter has been eradicated from the United States but could reappear.

Caseous lymphadenitis in sheep and goats is a wound infection. The organism gains entrance through an abrasion, especially following shearing, and is carried to the lymph nodes, where it colonizes to develop abscesses that may not be apparent until several months after the actual infection occurred. Although the disease causes pain and fever in the horse it is relatively innocuous for sheep and goats except in the rare instance where abscesses develop in vital organs such as the liver or kidneys.

The disease is important economically in sheep, however, because affected carcasses or parts thereof are condemned at slaughter. In goats the disease is unsightly and particularly troublesome to exhibitors of purebred animals. While wool hides the lymph node enlargement in sheep, the enlarged nodes are readily apparent in goats, particularly where they rupture to drain a caseous (cheesy) greenish pus and then heal, leaving an unsightly scar.

Prevention

Once it appears in a herd or flock, prevention of further cases is difficult. Vaccines have not been effective and none is commercially available. Draining abscesses discharge the organism onto the ground, thereby contaminating the premises and increasing the possibility of further infections. An important control procedure for the goat herd is to isolate any animals with draining abscesses, preferably in an area with an impervious floor that can be readily disinfected. The same advice is valid but usually impractical for the sheep flock, since detection of infected sheep is so difficult. Serologic testing for the disease has no value. The best procedure for the sheep flock is to use the shears carefully and disinfect them frequently. Shorn sheep should not be held in a corral, where the concentration of the organism is likely to be high, but should be turned out to pasture immediately to take advantage of the natural dilution factor.

If detected early before abscesses form, the infection responds well to penicillin. The drug, however, will not reach bacteria inside an abscess. In goats the ripe abscesses should be surgically drained and medicated as an open wound to promote healing with minimal scarring.

PERIODIC OPHTHALMIA

This eye disease of horses and mules was much more prevalent at one time than it is now. The common name is "moon blindness," given to it many years ago because of its characteristic of recurrent acute attacks which some people felt coincided with the phases of the moon. Periodic recurrences are typical, each causing additional damage eventually resulting in total blindness, but the moon has nothing to do with it.

Symptoms

Onset of the disease is sudden with profuse lacrimation (flowing of tears) and the eyelids held closed to protect the eyes from light. Slight swelling of the orbital area due to conjunctivitis is common. Usually only one eye is affected at a time but both can be involved. Some degree of corneal opacity may be present and contraction of the pupil is a rather consistent finding. Toward the end of an acute attack a yellowish exudate can often be seen at the bottom of the anterior chamber. The acute attack generally subsides in a few days, only to recur at intervals ranging from a few weeks to a year. Tags of fibrin and exudate tend to remain in the aqueous and vitreous humor of the eyeball that can be detected between acute attacks with the aid of an ophthalmoscope. Examination for soundness of a horse should always include a careful ophthalmoscopic examination.

Prevention

The cause of periodic ophthalmia is still debatable. It has been produced experimentally by infecting horses with *Leptospira pomona* and vaccination with *L. pomona* bacterin is a helpful preventative. But the disease is encountered more frequently in horses where the diet is marginal and the standard of husbandry poor. Supplementing the diet with riboflavin also gives a good degree of protection. Last, some researchers feel the disease is not a specific infection at all, but a localized allergic reaction to some other infection or toxemia.

Regardless of the cause, the disease is serious for the future eyesight of the horse and requires prompt veterinary attention. Antibiotics and corticosteroids relieve the acute signs minimizing damage to the eye at the time of that attack. Your veterinarian can suggest ways to reduce the possibility of future attacks.

THROMBOEMBOLIC MENINGOENCEPHALITIS (TEM)

This disease, commonly called TEM for convenience, is an acute infectious, highly fatal disease limited almost entirely to feedlot cattle. It occurs rarely in cattle at pasture or in dairy cattle. Generally fewer than 10 percent of the cattle in the group are affected but mortality of 95 percent is common.

Onset is sudden with high fever, stiffness, and reluctance to move. This is followed rapidly by normal or subnormal temperature, staggering, prostration, coma, and death. Death usually occurs anywhere from one to forty-eight hours after clinical signs are first observed. The disease seems to be occurring with increased frequency in recent years.

The organism thought to be responsible is *Hemophilus somnus* but little is known about its mode of transmission. The primary lesions produced are in the brain but it produces extensive damage to blood vessels and causes thrombi in other organs as well.

Prevention

Because the mode of transmission is unclear, it is difficult to make definitive recommendations for prevention. Vaccinating with *H. somnus* bacterin, decreasing concentrate intake and increasing roughage may help. The disease affects cattle near the end of the finishing period in the 800–1000 pound range, raising the possibility of minimizing losses by marketing cattle early when an outbreak occurs. Early treatment with antibiotics is effective, but the emphasis must be placed on *early*. Just a few hours can make the difference between survival and death. In the event of an outbreak, addition of tetracycline or chlortetracycline to the feed or water may reduce the number of new cases.

EXUDATIVE DERMATITIS

The most obvious effect of this disease affecting pigs up to a month of age is the appearance of moist, crusty, weeping skin lesions that sometimes combine so that the entire body is covered. The appearance of the skin gives the disease its common name: "greasy pig disease." Although sporadic occurrence is more common possibly because of colostral immunity, up to 90 percent of a litter may become infected and mortality ranges from 5–90 percent. Very young pigs are more severely affected and are less responsive to treatment than those in the older age range. At first glance the condition closely resembles parakeratosis due to zinc deficiency, but the latter disease is rarely, if ever, seen in pigs as young as a month old.

Symptoms

The first indication of imminent greasy pig disease is listlessness, and dullness of the skin and haircoat. Depression and complete lack of appetite follow but fever is not common. Concurrently, the skin thickens and reddish spots appear on the ears, back, and belly. Serum exudes from these, providing a medium for secondary infection, which contributes to the obnoxious odor characteristic of piglets with

"Greasy" pig disease.

this disease. Conjunctivitis (inflammation of the inner surface of the eyelid and adjacent tissue) is common, as is a purulent inflammation of the external ear. Frequently, blister-like lesions develop on the snout and heels. These rupture and the resulting infection leads to erosions and occasionally sloughing (shedding off) of the hoof. This type of vesicular lesion is characteristic of some viruses, leading to the belief that greasy pig disease may not be solely a staphylococcal infection but may be triggered by an as-yet-unidentified virus.

Treatment

The disease is contagious and infected piglets and litters should be immediately segregated from others in the farrowing house. However, it is basically a wound infection disease with the organism gaining entrance through skin abrasions. Occasionally the urinary tract as well as the skin is involved, and such cases terminate fatally.

Given early, antibiotics are helpful in relieving the clinical signs, but as a group the staphylococci develop antibiotic resistance quite readily, so several different antibiotics may have to be tried. Severely affected piglets can be bathed in warm soapy water to remove the crusts and debris and then antibiotic ointment can be applied to the skin. These measures will help to save many piglets that would otherwise die.

Prevention

Skin abrasions are the primary route of infection. Scraped knees from rough concrete floors and bites and scratches incurred in the daily struggle for a place at the dairy bar are the common source of wounds that subsequently become infected. Reducing the level of environmental contamination through good sanitation will help to prevent infection. Abrasions from rough floors can be prevented by covering the floor of the pen with rubber mats or even indoor-outdoor carpet. Very smooth concrete floors, although good from the standpoint of reducing knee abrasions, are undesirable because they are slippery and contribute to the functional problem known as "spraddle-leg." On farms where greasy pig disease is a major problem, extreme sanitary precautions must be taken. When outbreaks appear, giving antibiotics to all pigs in the litter even before they show signs may be helpful.

PYODERMA

This is a non-specific and non-contagious disease occasionally seen in all species but most commonly in the horse as a sequel to saddle sores. By definition the name means "pus in the skin," and it is usually due to one or more species of staphylococci. The infection starts initially in the hair follicles to cause swelling and extreme sensitivity. It may remain superficial or go into the deeper layers of skin to cause abscessation and fistulous tracts. Involvement to this degree may cause fever and other signs such as lack of appetite, depression, and enlargement of regional lymph nodes.

Treatment

The superficial infection responds well to local treatment with antiseptics. Scabs and crusts should first be softened with wet packs or ointments and gently removed before applying the antiseptic. Deeper infection with fistulous tracts underlying the skin is much more difficult to treat and surgical drainage may be required in addition to local and systemic treatment.

Cleanliness and frequent careful grooming will do much to prevent this condition from occurring.

NAVEL ILL

The common name given to this septicemic infection of the newborn of all species implies that the route of infection is always via the navel. This is not necessarily so. Infection can also occur by ingestion of bacteria with subsequent invasion through the digestive tract. The navel is frequently the site of infection and invasion by a variety of bacteria which produces a septicemia (bacteria and their products in the blood) that is especially serious and common in animals that have not received colostrum.

Symptoms

Depending on the organism and the animal species involved, a variety of symptoms can result but the disease is perhaps most dramatic in the foal. Lethargy and diminished strength are frequent symptoms. If the organism invades the central nervous system, convulsions may be seen and death may occur in as few as twelve hours. In animals that live longer, arthritis, pneumonia, peritonitis, and diarrhea may be seen. A specific bacterium encountered in navel ill of foals, *Shigella equirulis,* is responsible for the condition known as "sleepy foal disease." It com-

Suppurative arthritis secondary to navel infection.

monly causes kidney disease and uremia.

Arthritis is a common sequel to navel infection in calves, pigs, lambs, and kids, but other clinical signs vary according to the organs affected by the particular invading organism. Umbilical abscess is a frequent complication in calves. Since umbilical hernia is common in this species also, don't undertake to open an umbilical abscess yourself unless you are certain of your diagnosis.

I had a client one time who did just that and found himself with a handful of intestines. The variety of possible symptoms makes the diagnosis, especially of the causative organism, difficult at times. Where the disease is occurring as a herd problem, isolation of the organism from infected tissues and an antibiotic sensitivity test is very helpful as a guide for treatment of future cases.

Treatment

A variety of antibiotics has been used successfully to treat early cases of navel ill. Treatment of long-standing cases is much less rewarding. Choice of antibiotic depends on the organism involved, but large doses of streptomycin and penicillin are a good starting point. Other symptomatic treatment is helpful. For example, if diarrhea is present electrolytes intravenously and orally are indicated. Where the value of the animal warrants, blood transfusion is very effective.

Prevention

Since navel ill is both common and serious, measures to prevent it are most important. First, be sure that the area where the animal is to be born is clean and as sanitary as possible. Then dip the navel in tincture of iodine as soon as the umbilical cord separates. **Simply swabbing iodine on the navel is not sufficient.** The best way is to fill a wide-mouth jar half full, hold it firmly against the body wall with the stump of the navel in it and slosh it around. This method insures adequate penetration of the iodine solution, which kills all bacteria present. The alcohol in the tincture of iodine also has an astringent effect that helps to seal the umbilical blood vessels. Next, be sure the animal gets a meal of colostrum within the first hour after birth. If it won't or can't nurse, bottle feed it. Strict adherence to these suggestions will make navel ill a rare occurrence.

LYME DISEASE

This disease, named for the locality where it was first diagnosed is caused by a spirochete, *Borrelia burgdorferi*. It is transmitted by ticks and principally affects humans and dogs, but has been occasionally reported in horses and cattle. The principal host for the immature tick larvae is the white-footed mouse and for adults, the white tailed deer. The disease has been reported in most of the continental U.S. and infections occur most frequently in summer and early fall when tick activity is at its peak.

Symptoms

In horses and cattle the primary signs are fever and lameness caused by arthritis particularly involving the joints of the foreleg. The affected joints feel hot, swollen, and are painful. The arthritis may be transitory or it may become chronic. The clinical signs are not sufficiently definitive to provide a positive diagnosis. A tentative diagnosis can be confirmed by an ELISA test of blood serum.

Prevention

As with all disease, prevention is preferable to treatment; however, the disease does respond to early treatment with antibiotics such as ampicillin, penicillin, and tetracycline. Prevention consists of those measures which keep animals and ticks separated. Fence off brush areas or cut the brush where ticks reside and keep pastures clipped. During the high-risk season examine animals daily and remove any ticks found. Frequent use of acaricidal dips or tick repellents is helpful.

POTOMAC FEVER

More properly called equine ehrlichial colitis, this disease causes an acute diarrhea in horses. The causative organism, *Ehrlichia risticii*, is a member of the rickettsiae group most of which are transmitted by insects. Occurrence sporadically and primarily in summer and early fall indicates that this disease is carried the same way, although a specific vector has not been identified.

Symptoms

Lack of appetite, depression, fever, and increased intestinal motility are followed in 24 to 48 hours by profuse watery diarrhea. The disease closely resembles acute salmonellosis. It may be complicated by colic and laminitis. Severity varies and only one or two horses in a herd may be affected but mortality may reach 30 percent. The symptoms coupled with a positive ELISA or FA test generally provide a positive diagnosis.

Prevention

Other than protecting horses from biting insects little can be done to prevent Potomac fever. Fortunately only a few will be affected at a time and it doesn't seem to spread from horse to horse. But it is a serious disease requiring prompt therapy with antibiotics such as oxytetracycline and IV fluid.

Diseases Caused by Viruses

VIRUSES, AS PATHOGENS, differ in many respects from bacteria. Physically, virus particles are very much smaller than bacteria and cannot be seen with the ordinary optical microscope. With the magnification afforded by the electron microscope, virus particles can be seen as symmetrical geometric shapes without a nucleus or cell wall. The lack of a cell wall assumes importance in their response to antibiotics because many antibiotics exert their effect by disrupting the integrity of the bacterial cell wall. Consequently, these drugs have no effect whatsoever on viruses and at the present time we have very few drugs available that will substantially influence the course of a viral infection. Treatment of viral diseases, therefore, depends on symptomatic therapy, prevention of secondary bacterial infection, and immunologic techniques such as administration of antiserum or gamma globulin from previously immunized animals.

Although most viral infections follow a recognizable pattern of symptoms, confirmation of the diagnosis by culture of the pathogen is not as easy or reliable as it is with bacterial infection. In general, viruses will not survive long outside the animal except under special conditions such as freezing, and attempts to isolate viruses from sick or dead animals frequently fail. Laboratory diagnosis of viral infections, therefore, depends heavily on serologic technique such as a rise in serum antibody titer concurrent with clinical signs or specialized tests such as fluorescent antibody (FA) or agar gel immunodiffusion (AGID). Because of the special techniques required, some of which are quite time-consuming, laboratory diagnosis of viral diseases tends to be more expensive than other diagnostic testing procedures.

Although there are exceptions which will be pointed out, most viral diseases tend to spread with great rapidity through the herd with all susceptible animals becoming infected in a short time. With some viral diseases the carrier state is quite common. As a general rule of thumb, viral infections are characterized by sudden onset, fever, depressed white blood cell county (leucopenia), absence of pus formation, and lack of specific response to drug therapy. For these and other reasons, some viral infections assume great importance in animal and human medicine.

RABIES

In terms of death losses, animal or human, this disease in the United States is almost inconsequential at present. Because of the anxiety and worry it causes and the actual discomfort thousands of people undergo each year from antirabies therapy, however, it must be considered an important disease.

The rabies virus is capable of infecting all mammals and the virus is transmitted in saliva via bite wounds. At one time this was thought to be the only route of infection. However, there is good evidence now of transmission in bat colonies via aerosol dispersion, through the air. This probably has significance, however, only for bats and for spelunkers who explore caves where bats reside. Rabies is a reportable disease that is almost invariably fatal, and all of the state health departments and the federal government maintain records of prevalence of the disease. Skunks, foxes, raccoons, and bats are statistically the most important wildlife reservoirs of the virus but the infected dog or cat, because of its close association, is the greatest threat to humans.

Progress of the Disease

Rabies is a neurotropic virus that follows the nerves from the point of virus inoculation (bite wound) to the brain. The incubation period of the disease is usually less than ten days, with the interval between infection and onset of clinical signs being determined in part by the proximity of the bite wound to the brain and the species of animal under consideration.

Skunks and bats can remain asymptomatic carriers for many months, unlike other species where the disease is consistently fatal. Incubation periods up to six months have been reported in man but this is exceptional. Immune status of the individual, the size and location of the infective dose, and individual resistance also play a role in determining the length of the incubation period. Although the disease is invariably fatal for domestic animals and must generally be considered so for man, there is a record of a human case in which the individual survived. The odds against survival are so great, however, that rabies must be considered a public health hazard with serious potential.

Rabies in livestock occurs in the United States as a result of a bite by an infected animal — usually a dog, fox, coyote, raccoon, or skunk. In Central America, vampire bats are important vectors of the disease. Furthermore, its occurrence is generally limited to those areas where the disease is known to be endemic in wildlife. Thus, geographic distribution is a help in separating rabies from other neurological disorders. However, when the clinical signs indicate, rabies should always be considered.

Symptoms

The earliest sign of rabies common to all species is a change in normal behavior. Usually there is loss of appetite and a pattern of obscure clinical signs easily confused with such things as indigestion, inability to swallow, foreign objects in the mouth, and so on. Early in the disease normally sociable animals may seek solitude and wander off by themselves, whereas others, normally shy, will become unduly friendly. Reports of rabid foxes, raccoons, and skunks walking into the barn or even the house are not unusual.

Within about forty-eight hours either an **excitatory** or a **paralytic stage** begins to develop. The mention of rabies usually conjures up in most people's minds the image of a dog frothing at the mouth running down the street biting anything that moves. This does occur and in livestock species as well. Cattle with the excitatory stage of rabies will urinate frequently, strain, and run aimlessly in the pasture, bellowing as they go, with their tails in the air. While the ruminants, cattle, sheep, and goats are less prone to bite, rabid horses and pigs will, and one should exercise great caution in their presence.

The **paralytic** form of the disease follows the premonitory directly in some individuals, while in others the excitatory stage may precede it by a few hours to a day or two. The earliest indication of the paralytic stage is inability to swallow. The drooling that results gives rise to the expression, "frothing at the mouth." This pharyngeal paralysis is easily confused with the signs produced by a foreign object caught in the mouth or throat. The first inclination is to open the animal's mouth and reach in to see if anything is there. Where the possibility of rabies exists, don't do it! The promising career of a good friend and colleague came to an early end some years ago indirectly as a result of failure to heed this admonition. The paralytic stage proceeds rapidly to total collapse, coma, and death.

Treatment

There is no economically feasible or effective treatment for rabies in livestock, and because of frequency of failures the temptation to try post-exposure immunization should be avoided. Animals bitten by a known rabid animal should be destroyed immediately. In case of bites by an animal not known to be rabid, the bitten animal should be confined and carefully observed for a minimum of fourteen days.

In case of an animal showing signs of rabies, call your veterinarian immediately. He will advise you what to do and will notify the appropriate health authorities. Generally, infected animals should be allowed to die or be humanely destroyed **without damaging the brain.** Brain tissue is necessary for laboratory diagnosis to confirm the disease.

Prevention

Rabies is best prevented by area control procedures, including mass immunization of dogs and control of susceptible wildlife populations, especially foxes. With few exceptions immunization of livestock is usually not necessary.

An exception would be when the prevalence of rabies in an area is high, with proportionate risk of infection.

Vaccines

Several types of vaccines are available for immunization against rabies that are reasonably safe and effective when properly used. However, their use should not be taken lightly. A modified live virus vaccine used on the wrong species of animal occasionally will induce clinical signs of rabies. Because of the seriousness of the disease, anything to do with rabies — diagnosis or immunization — should be left to your veterinarian.

BOVINE VIRUS DIARRHEA (BVD, MUCOSAL DISEASE)

Based upon serologic testing surveys, this may well be the most prevalent viral infection of cattle. Positive antibody titers indicate that upwards of 75 percent of our adult cattle have encountered the virus and become immune. Fortunately, only a small percentage of these ever show clinical signs of the disease.

Two distinct forms of the disease are recognized, which at one time led to the belief that BVD and mucosal disease were separate entities. The term "mucosal disease" was given to a disease that affected many cattle but with low mortality. It occurs primarily in feedlot cattle. The other form sporadically affects few cattle, primarily yearlings, but with high mortality and is seen more often in dairy cattle. Further research has established that the two diseases are caused by the same virus. The difference in clinical signs may be a reflection of stress at the time of infection, immune status of the animal, or viral mutation.

Virus Easily Spread

Widespread distribution of the virus makes it apparent that it can be carried from farm to farm by many routes, probably including carrier animals, contaminated clothing and vehicles, as well as by other animals and perhaps birds. Experimentally, infection can be produced by administering virus orally, intranasally, or by injection. Most naturally occurring cases probably result from ingestion of virus.

Symptoms

The earliest clinical sign is high fever and loss of appetite occurring four to seven days following infection. The virus has an affinity for epithelial and lymphoid tissue, and typical lesions are small erosions on the lips, dental pad, tongue, and palate. At necropsy the same lesions may be seen throughout the digestive tract. The erosions may coalesce to form a larger lesion in some areas but they tend to heal quickly. When present, they help greatly to confirm the diagnosis, but, unfortunately or fortunately, depending on one's point of view, they do not occur in all cases. Concurrent with onset of fever, a profuse watery

Bovine virus diarrhea.

diarrhea develops, sometimes accompanied by violent straining. Extreme dehydration and rapid weight loss accompany the diarrhea. In cases of a few days' duration, the diarrhea subsides to be followed by periodic expulsion of small amounts of black tarry stool. Lacrimation (shedding of tears) and an ocular discharge sometimes occur and the muzzle is frequently crusty, with the nostrils partially plugged with sticky mucus. Lameness due to laminitis (inflammation of the tissue inside the wall of the hoof) is not uncommon, and on some animals the skin in the neck region will get scruffy and wrinkled.

Those that recover generally show improvement in four or five days but apparent recovery followed by periodic bouts of diarrhea and unthriftiness lasting a period of several months is not unusual. Mortality, however, is high and death may occur anywhere from three days to a month or more after the onset of clinical signs. In recent years the disease has been seen more frequently in yearling cattle and is generally limited to those in the group that are unthrifty for unrelated reasons. Although the preceding description may seem perfectly straightforward the actuality is somewhat different. These symptoms will usually be seen in different animals in the herd but usually not all in the same animal. The clinical signs observed in infected animals range from none to death depending on the pathogenicity of the particular virus, age of the animals, stage of pregnancy, and immune status.

Causes Abortion

While the clinical signs of the disease occur infrequently, they may only be the tip of the iceberg as far as the economic importance of BVD is concerned. The virus can cause abortion at any stage of gestation and when the fetus becomes infected during the first three to six weeks of gestation, cerebellar (part of the brain) development is arrested. Many of the calves that survive to term are born with physical incoordination due to cerebellar hypoplasia. If they can stand at all, they move with a peculiar jerking gait and stand with legs outspread to keep from falling. Cataracts of one or both eyes often accompany this condition. It's entirely possible that many of the unexplained early embryonic deaths and abortions that occur in cattle each year are the result of inapparent BVD virus infection.

Diagnosis

Better diagnostic tools would help to resolve this question. Clinical signs and lesions at necropsy usually define the cause of death without difficulty. It is not so easy in those with minimal lesions that survive. In these cases, diagnosis must be based on a rise in antibody titer that occurs between the time of initial infection and three weeks later. This diagnosis requires two separate blood samples and is retrospective — by the time a laboratory report is received, the animal is either dead or better. Its chief value is to establish the presence of the virus in the herd. This can serve as a guide for future vaccination programs.

Vaccine

An effective modified live virus vaccine is available singly or in combination with IBR for the prevention of BVD. When given to animals six months of

Tongue erosions. Bovine virus diarrhea.

age or older, it provides immunity of long duration. It can be given earlier but if so should be repeated later because of possible interference from maternal antibody. The vaccine does have drawbacks, however. If given during pregnancy, some cows may abort. Also, it is a live virus and there is an element of risk in using it on animals that are under stress because a few may develop serious illness.

This presents a difficult choice for the feedlot operator. At the time they enter the feedlot, cattle are under the stress of shipment, change in diet, and new surroundings. These factors combine to make them good candidates for a variety of infections and poor candidates for vaccination at that time. In consultation with their veterinarians, many operators will weigh the odds and accept a few vaccine-induced illnesses in preference to the possibility of a larger number of natural infections. A killed virus vaccine is available for BVD which produces adequate immunity with less risk.

INFECTIOUS BOVINE RHINOTRACHEITIS (IBR, REDNOSE)

IBR is a common upper respiratory infection of cattle that is more prevalent during the fall and winter than during other times of the year. Symptomatically, the typical case is not unlike a severe head cold in man — with fever, coughing, eye and nasal discharge, and depressed appetite.

The first indication of the disease is usually a dry, hacking cough involving just a few animals. This cough is accompanied by fever, lack of appetite, and a clear nasal discharge, which later in the disease becomes mucopurulent. The disease affects cattle of all ages and is occasionally fatal for young calves. Unless complicated by secondary pneumonia, IBR is rarely fatal for adult cattle, and its principal economic effect is lost production during the acute attack. However, like BVD virus, it will cause abortions, usually beginning about three weeks after the episode passes. In the individual animal, recovery takes place in about four to seven days. However, the virus spreads rapidly through the herd by aerosol dispersion and it may be two months before all signs of the disease disappear from the herd.

Eyes Involved

While the foregoing symptoms may be considered a description of typical IBR, the effect of the virus can be quite variable. Concurrent with an acute attack, a few individuals may develop a corneal opacity easily confused with pink eye. With pink eye, the opacity spreads *outward* from a central ulcer of the cornea, while with IBR in most cases the opacity spreads *inward* from the periphery and there is no ulceration. With eye involvement the sclera or white part of the eye becomes reddened. The term "red nose" developed from the appearance of the white nose of Hereford cattle in the feedlots. Just as we get a reddened sore nose when we have a bad head cold, so do cattle, and this is most striking in cattle with a white muzzle. In a herd outbreak, a few animals may develop raised, whitish plaques on the lining of the vagina and nostrils.

These lesions, if present, are good evidence that IBR is the problem.

Occasionally a more severe genital infection called infectious pustular vulvovaginitis occurs in cattle. It is caused by the same IBR virus and is spread primarily during breeding. Whether the virus affects the respiratory system or the genitalia seems to be determined by the route of infection.

IBR virus can be very insidious. It may pass through a herd without any observable clinical signs, but a month or two later a rash of unexplained abortions may occur. Careful necropsy of an aborted fetus may reveal lesions suggestive of IBR. If the tissue is fresh, the fluorescent antibody test can be used to confirm the diagnosis. Testing the dam's blood serum for antibody has limited value. If it is negative, then the abortion was probably not due to IBR. If the sample is positive, it means only that sometime in the past the cow was exposed to IBR. That exposure may be entirely unrelated to the abortion.

Transmission

Once infected with this member of the herpes virus group, some cattle will harbor the virus for indefinite periods and shed virus particles intermittently, particularly during periods of stress. This shedding serves as a source of infection for new animals added to the herd and for contact animals at fairs and shows. It is also a concern of bull stud managers because it has been shown that the virus can be transmitted in semen, although such transmission is uncommon. Nevertheless, bulls in the reputable studs are routinely tested for IBR and many stud managers will not buy bulls that have been IBR vaccinated because the vaccine virus antibody titer confuses test results.

Treatment

Like all virus diseases, there is no effective treatment for IBR. Antibiotics are routinely used, however, to prevent secondary infection. The best way to handle the disease is by protection through vaccination. Both killed and modified live virus vaccines are available and provide good immunity when properly used. The killed vaccine must be used annually, while the MLV will provide much longer immunity. Because of the risk of vaccine virus-induced abortion, the latter should not be used on pregnant cows. It is available singly or in combination with BVD vaccine. If given to all calves at six to eight months of age, an immune herd can be maintained.

IBR is the first cattle disease for which a vaccine has been developed that is administered by intranasal instillation (spraying into the nostrils). It must be repeated annually but has the advantage of producing rapid local immunity in the respiratory tract with little, if any, adverse side effect. The variety of vaccines available makes the choice difficult for an individual without the training and experience to make an intelligent decision. For that reason, an immunization program worked out with the advice of your veterinarian and designed for your herd circumstances is more likely to be successful. By all means, don't do as I have seen many farmers do — wait until a few cows start coughing before deciding to vaccinate. Vaccination when the infection is already present has little if any value and may actually make a bad situation worse. The time to vaccinate is before the need arises while the cattle are still healthy.

EQUINE INFECTIOUS ANEMIA (EIA, SWAMP FEVER)

In terms of the number of animals affected, EIA is not the most important viral disease of horses and other members of the horse family, although the consequences for the infected individual are generally serious. It is a disease marked by confusion and misunderstanding on the part of some horse owners and occasionally by heated emotion when state regulatory programs enter in.

Spread

EIA is spread from one horse to another by transfer of a droplet of blood from an infected horse to one that is susceptible. For all practical purposes, this is the only means of spread, although intrauterine infection of foals from infected dams has been reported and the possibility does exist of virus transfer during copulation if there is any bleeding. In nature the virus is transferred from one horse to another by biting insects, especially the horse fly. Transfer of infection depends on the level of virus in the blood and the volume of blood transferred. Since volume is a factor the biting flies are of more concern than mosquitoes. Because horse flies are the principal natural vector and they rarely range more than a few hundred yards, spread of the disease is slow. It has been recognized for over a hundred years, yet just a small percentage of the horse population is infected.

Spread of the disease is more rapid and dramatic in stables where contaminated hypodermic needles or surgical instruments, even dental floats, have been used successively without sterilization between horses.

Symptoms

Symptomatically three forms of the infection are recognized: inapparent, acute, and chronic. EIA virus attacks red blood cells and the acutely affected horse will have a fever, marked anemia, signs of jaundice, and occasionally edema or swelling of the lower part of the abdomen and the legs. The pulse rate and the respiratory rate will be high due to the reduced oxygen-carrying capacity of the blood. The acutely affected horse will be weak, depressed, and may die in a day or two or may apparently recover.

Those that recover from the initial attack remain infected for life and usually suffer periodic recurrences during the stress of heavy work or other illness. The majority of horses chronically infected with EIA virus lack the stamina for racing or other competition events. Sooner or later (which may be years) most of them die from the effects of the disease. A few horses become infected and never show any clinical signs of the disease. Nevertheless, they do harbor the virus and can serve as a source of infection for others. All evidence to date indicates that every infected horse carries the infection for life although the level of viremia varies from time to time, being highest at the time of the acute attack.

Periodically, EIA has had devastating effects where large numbers of horses were congregated, such as at racetracks, with disastrous economic effects. Recognizing this, the Standardbred industry and the State of New York supported research at Cornell University that led to the adaptation of the agar gel immunodiffusion test (AGID) by Dr. Leroy Coggins for the diagnosis of EIA. This was a major breakthrough in control of the disease, and after several years of extensive testing the AGID or Coggins test was adopted by the state governments and the U.S. Department of Agriculture as the official test for EIA. In capable hands this has proven to be the most accurate serologic test ever devised for any disease. Prior to the AGID test the only reliable diagnostic tool for EIA was inoculation of test ponies or horses with suspect blood, a very time-consuming and expensive procedure.

Control Possible

The advent of a reliable diagnostic test has made control of the disease a practical possibility and many states now have official regulatory programs in effect. In general, these programs provide for a test when the animal is moved off the home premises. If the initial test is positive, it is confirmed by a second test. If both are positive, the animal is identified by a permanent freeze brand and quarantined to the farm.

These programs have aroused strong emotions in some people, which is not hard to understand. Horses are livestock, but for many people they are pets as well and part of the family. How do you explain to the tearful girl that although her horse appears normal it carries EIA virus, is a danger to other horses, and therefore must be quarantined to the farm or destroyed? It isn't easy. Yet EIA is a disease that could be totally eradicated in a relatively short time if the decision were made to devote the resources to the effort. Only a small portion, probably not over 2 percent of the total population is infected; the disease spreads very slowly; and a good economical diagnostic test is available. In New York State, for example, where 50,000 to 60,000 horses were tested annually between 1973 and 1978, the rate of positives dropped from over 3 percent to 0.6 percent.

No Treatment

There is no specific treatment for EIA and there is no vaccine available despite intensive research. It behooves the prudent horse owner to do everything possible to prevent infection. Those with a single horse that never gets near other horses have little to worry about. The greatest risk is in commercial stables, at racetracks, and at shows where there is considerable traffic in horses. Requiring that every horse brought in have evidence of a negative Coggins test will go a long way to protect the others. Beyond that, a good fly control program, and careful cleaning and scrubbing of curry combs, brushes, and other paraphernalia between successive uses will help. Perhaps most important is sterilization of hypodermic needles and surgical instruments, including dental floats and hoof knives.

PARAINFLUENZA

The significance of this disease of cattle due to a myxovirus, *parainfluenza-3* (PI$_3$), is not clearly understood. The virus is widely distributed in the cattle population where by itself it causes little if any clinical disease. However, in conjunction with *Pasteurella multocida* under conditions of stress it is a factor leading to the contagious pneumonia called shipping fever.

Shipping fever is a major disease and in an effort to provide the best vaccines possible to control it, several vaccine manufacturers now market vaccine containing killed or attenuated PI$_3$ virus. There is mixed opinion among virologists on how effective the PI$_3$ component is, but it apparently does no harm and anything that may help to prevent shipping fever is all to the good.

BOVINE RESPIRATORY SYNCYTIAL VIRUS

Like PI$_3$ virus, the significance of this virus as a component of the respiratory disease complex in cattle is uncertain. Serologic testing indicates that a high percentage of the cattle population has been exposed to it. It can produce mild or acute respiratory disease but present indications are that stress factors coupled with secondary bacterial infection are necessary for acute disease to result.

Pulmonary edema is a complicating factor in respiratory disease where this virus has been incriminated. BRSV antigen is included in some vaccines for prevention of respiratory disease in cattle.

BLUETONGUE

This is an important disease of sheep, cattle, and goats that, thus far, is limited primarily to the western states. The disease is seasonal in occurrence, a reflection of the fact that it is spread by biting insects, especially midges, and is seen concurrent with peak populations of these insects. Many different serologic types have been identified worldwide and six types have been found in the United States. Each is antigenically distinct and vaccination against one type will not protect against the others.

Symptoms

Of all ruminant species, sheep appear to be the most susceptible. After an incubation period of about a week they develop fever, labored breathing, loss of appetite, and depression. Ulcers and erosions of the lips, tongue, and dental pad are commonly seen and in advanced cases the tongue becomes swollen and cyanotic (bluish) hence the name "bluetongue." The saliva may be blood-tinged and frothy due to the mouth lesions. A secondary pneumonia is not uncommon and mortality may range up to 30 percent of a flock. Swelling and cracks at the coronary band, in the interdigital space and at the bulb of the heel causing severe lameness is not unusual. The principal effect of bluetongue virus is exerted on capillaries resulting in loss of blood supply to the area served by the affected blood vessel. The result is tissue necrosis in that area. This is most dramatic in cattle, where patches of skin may die and slough. The same thing may happen to one or more digits on the feet with the horny part actually sloughing off. Animals thus affected lose weight rapidly because the pain of moving about to graze is more than they can stand.

Sloughing digits. This can be caused by ergot poisoning, and bluetongue, among other things.

Abortion is a common sequel to bluetongue infection and this coupled with severe weight loss, damage to the fleece, and death loss make bluetongue a serious economic matter when many animals in the flock are affected. Because of its economic importance, countries that do not now have the disease, such as Australia, prohibit importation of sheep from countries where the disease is present. Canada has imposed a negative bluetongue test requirement on cattle from the United States prior to importation.

Treatment

Treatment of the disease other than good nursing care is of little value. Affected animals should be housed and fed good quality hay if they will eat. Isolation of infected animals is of little or no value, since the disease is not directly transmissible. Recovery confers a solid immunity and lambs born of immune ewes will have a passive immunity lasting about six months.

Insect control will help reduce the spread of bluetongue but vaccination is the most satisfactory control procedure. Annual vaccination of sheep in the age range of six months to three years is commonly practiced in the endemic areas. Older sheep are generally immune. The vaccine should be used cautiously in pregnant ewes during the first six weeks of gestation since abortions and deformed lambs have been reported following vaccination. Unfortunately, the vaccine currently available is not wholly effective since it protects against only one serotype of virus and it is not approved for use in cattle or goats. A polyvalent vaccine has been reported highly successful in South Africa but a similar vaccine has not yet been licensed in this country.

Bluetongue is a serious disease. If you have reason to suspect it in your flock or herd, call your veterinarian immediately.

Equine Viral Arteritis

This specific viral disease of horses can be readily confused with influenza and equine viral rhinopneumonitis (EVR). It is caused by a herpes virus and produces an illness characterized by rapid onset, acute upper respiratory distress, and abortion in pregnant mares. Unlike EVR, however, abortions occur concurrent with clinical signs whereas with EVR, the abortions occur several weeks or months after infection takes place. The disease tends to be more severe than either influenza or EVR and laboratory confirmation is generally required to make a definitive diagnosis.

The incubation period ranges from one to six days and, although the clinical signs of the disease may be quite severe, recovery usually begins in about a week. Fever is the first sign, followed rather quickly by a clear nasal discharge which may become purulent. Conjunctivitis (inflammation of the inner eyelid) and congestion of the nasal mucous membranes are common. Coughing and labored breathing due to pulmonary edema may occur. A few individuals may develop a severe diarrhea.

One of the lesions that distinguishes this from other equine viral infections is damage to the lining of the smaller arteries and arterioles. The resulting interference with blood circulation in some cases causes edema or swelling of the legs especially in horses that are stabled. Edema of the prepuce and sheath of stallions and geldings is common.

Despite the vascular damage that can occur, mortality from this disease is not high provided the sick horse is given complete rest and good nursing care. No specific treatment is indicated but antibiotics are usually given as a precautionary measure to prevent secondary infection. Spread of the disease is generally thought to be via direct contact so it's important that sick horses be completely isolated from all others, especially during the acute phase of the disease. A modified live virus vaccine is available but because of the hazard of reversion to virulence, its use is carefully regulated.

Equine Encephalomyelitis (Sleeping Sickness)

Several viruses are capable of causing encephalitis in horses. These are classified as **arboviruses** because the virus is transmitted by arthropod insects such as mosquitoes, which are the principal vectors or carriers of equine encephalomyelitis. Although the clinical signs produced by the several viruses are similar, the viruses are antigenically slightly different. Also, their distribution with some exceptions is generally limited to specific geographic areas and from this they are variously designated as Eastern, Western, St. Louis, California, and Venezuelan encephalitis virus. At the present time, only Eastern and Western are of major significance in the United States.

Diagnosis

Occurrence of the disease is sporadic and seasonal. In areas where the disease is endemic, outbreaks can be anticipated a week or two following the peak mosquito population. In the northern areas this is generally late August and September. The seasonality of the disease is an aid to diagnosis, although occasional cases may occur earlier or later. In the horse the disease is characterized by fever, lack of appetite, drowsiness, partial or complete blindness, aimless, wandering, incoordination, staggering, paralysis, and death. With Eastern encephalitis, mortality ranges up to 90 percent but is somewhat less with the Western type.

There is no specific treatment for viral encephalitis but supportive therapy and good nursing care help to reduce mortality. Serologic testing has limited value in diagnosis because many horses die before antibody develops. Isolation of virus from brain tissue confirms the presumptive diagnosis and provides a logical basis for vaccinating other horses in the area and all horses in subsequent years. A vaccine incorporating antigen for both Eastern and Western types is available. This is given in two doses initially, with an annual booster in the spring every year thereafter. The vaccine is relatively safe and gives a good immunity. Anyone who cares about his horses should have them immunized.

From a professional standpoint, Eastern equine encephalomyelitis is a very interesting disease. Birds are the principal reservoir of the virus but are rarely affected themselves. Eastern encephalitis has, however, caused serious losses in flocks of pheasants raised in captivity. Mosquitoes are the vector by which the virus is transmitted from birds to horses — and to man. Horses are actually a dead-end host for the virus since most of them die and the virus dies with them. In that sense, the term "equine" encephalomyelitis is really a misnomer. It is really a disease of birds causing inapparent infection that accidentally gets transmitted to horses by mosquitoes. Whether horses get the disease or not is a matter of chance. First, there must be birds in the area carrying the virus. Second, there must be mosquitoes available to bite the bird. Then sufficient time must elapse for the virus to replicate in the mosquito salivary gland to reach an infective dose level and then the mosquito must bite a susceptible horse. When all these factors come together in the right sequence, the disease appears. Remove any one of them and disease will not occur. Mosquito population control and vaccination of horses therefore are valuable tools in preventing this disease.

Venezuelan Encephalitis

Although symptomatically, Venezuelan encephalitis is similar to Eastern and Western, it differs in two important respects. Mammals other than birds can be unaffected carriers and there is evidence the virus can be transmitted by aerosol transmission between horses in addition to transfer by mosquitoes. This disease has appeared sporadically for years in the northwestern countries of South America but during 1969 and 1970 it progressed northward through

Central America and across Mexico and was reported in the United States in June of 1971 in Texas. An intensive and expensive control program kept it confined to that state but several thousand horses died from it. No new cases have been reported in this country since December of that year and the virus has apparently disappeared from this country.

All three types of equine encephalitis virus are capable of infecting humans and the disease must be considered a public health hazard. During the Texas outbreak a number of human cases developed and the symptoms were reported to be similar to influenza. The Eastern and Western types, however, cause an encephalitis in humans similar to that produced in horses — with equally serious implications. In humans, as in horses, mosquitoes are the vector.

Control

Because of its fatal potential for horses and people, every effort should be made to control equine encephalomyelitis. The most logical approach is through vaccination of members of the horse family about a month before the mosquito season starts and again four months later. Where mosquitos are active all year round, annual vaccination is indicated.

PAPILLOMATOSIS

This impressive-sounding name is the medical term for the common skin condition seen in most species called **warts.** The most dramatic of these are the large cauliflower-like lesions seen most frequently on the skin of the head and neck of cattle. These may occur singly and reach the size of a softball or they may be smaller and quite numerous. Warts of this type, although they are unsightly, do not seriously impair the health of the animal. They do bleed easily and profusely if torn at the base and do provide a good site for screwworm infestation in areas where the screwworm is endemic.

Smaller warts occur on the teats of cattle and often interfere with milking. These may be broad-based or rather long and pedunculated. Warts are rare in sheep but do occur in goats and particularly around the muzzle of young horses. A particular type of wart, fibropapilloma, occurs occasionally on the penis of young bulls and in the vagina of heifers. These are particularly troublesome because they often bleed during coitus and even a small amount of blood is lethal to sperm cells.

Wart tissue is an overgrowth of epithelial basal cells that enlarges and erupts through the epidermis. This overgrowth is stimulated by papillomatosis virus and virus is present in wart tissue. Fibropapillomas occasionally occur in the mouth, pharynx, and even the esophagus of cattle. Warts in the esophagus, although rarely reported, may interfere with swallowing. There is some indication these may be due to papular stomatitis rather than wart virus.

Wart virus is quite hardy and readily spread by hypodermic needles, tattoo instruments, and tagging pliers. In nature, spread is probably via direct contact or indirectly by rubbing against a post or wall where infected cattle have recently rubbed themselves.

Warts are most common in young animals and may disappear spontaneously as they get older. This is especially true of the large proliferative type seen on the skin. It's a common observation, too, that surgical removal of one or two hastens disappearance of the others. Commercially available wart vaccine given in repeated doses at monthly intervals is an aid to removal of warts in cattle. Wart virus, however, is host-specific and the cattle vaccine has little if any value when used on other species. When warts are a herd problem, an autogenous vaccine prepared from wart tissue taken from an animal in the herd may be more effective than commercial vaccines. Your veterinarian can arrange to have an autogenous vaccine made for you.

The small "seed warts" commonly found on the teats are less responsive to vaccine. If the base is broad, surgical removal is probably the best bet. Those with a narrow stalk or pedicle can frequently be twisted off or snipped off with sharp scissors.

Since antiquity, a variety of concoctions for topical application have been recommended for removal of warts. With the possible exceptions of silver nitrate or caustic potash carefully applied to small warts, these have little value. Vaccine or surgery is the best approach.

While prevention of warts through vaccination is possible, it is usually not feasible because of the need for repeated doses, short duration of immunity and cost as well as the minimal effect of warts on animal health.

EQUINE RHINOPNEUMONITIS (EQUINE VIRUS ABORTION)

This is a common upper respiratory infection of young horses caused by a virus belonging to the herpes group. It is a major problem where large numbers of horses are brought together. Although the upper respiratory infection is bad enough, its major economic significance is that it causes abortion in mares pregnant in late gestation, usually without producing any signs of illness in the mare.

The upper respiratory infection in young horses is characterized by fever, clear discharge from the eyes and nose, coughing, pharyngitis, and lack of appetite. Secondary bacterial infection is common and may cause the nasal discharge to become mucopurulent. The clinical disease runs a course of about ten days, although the cough may persist longer. Mortality is low but infection of yearlings generally disrupts training schedules. On breeding farms or at training stables the entire episode may span several months from the time of the first case to the complete recovery of the last. Treatment will not alter the course of the viral disease, but it may help prevent secondary complications.

Equine herpes virus I (EHV-1) is but one of several that contribute to what is often referred to as the equine respiratory disease complex. Influenza, parainfluenza, and occasionally arteritis, may all produce similar respiratory signs. Several other viruses are known to produce respiratory disease in horses but the extent to which they are a factor is unknown at present. In each case the primary mode of transmission is probably by aerosol dispersion.

Where the upper respiratory tract involvement is the only sign noted, a definitive diagnosis must be based upon serological tests. However, if abortions in otherwise normal mares follow an episode of respiratory infection in young horses on the same premises by anywhere from one to four months, you can be reasonably sure you are dealing with EHV-1. Characteristic lesions, especially in the liver of the aborted fetus, help to confirm the diagnosis. A variety of laboratory tests can make it unequivocal. In some outbreaks a few horses may develop neurological signs ranging from mild incoordination to paralysis.

Vaccination

The disease can be prevented or its effects at least minimized by vaccination. The necessity for vaccination depends somewhat on circumstances. On one hand, the pet horse kept in the backyard and rarely in contact with other horses will probably never encounter the virus and vaccination would be needless expense. On the other hand, horses on the show circuit or at the racetracks will almost certainly be exposed. Those under three years old should routinely be immunized with modified live virus vaccine. Those in the older age brackets tend to be resistant through prior exposure and are less likely to show clinical signs. The resistance of the pregnant mare, however, may not be sufficient to protect her foal; mares, depending on exposure risk, should be vaccinated using inactivated vaccine. On breeding farms, particularly when outside mares are brought in for service, all horses on the premises should be vaccinated annually.

Occasional adverse reactions to the vaccine have been reported but these have not been sufficiently frequent or severe to preclude its use when necessary. Vaccination coupled with good isolation and quarantine procedures for new arrivals are the best available means for controlling the disease at present. It should be emphasized that efforts to control this disease by vaccination alone will be disappointing. A vaccination program must be accompanied by sound management practices.

INFLUENZA

This is among the most interesting of viral diseases for the number of species it affects, including man, and for the variability and adaptability of the viruses that cause it.

Equine Influenza

Among livestock, equine influenza is the most economically significant. Two myxoviruses, designated A-equi-1 and A-equi-2, are responsible for most cases in horses in the United States. Symptomatically in the horse the disease closely resembles human influenza. The incubation period is short, usually one to three days, and the onset is sudden with high fever, coughing, weakness, and lack of appetite. Duration of the acute signs is generally only several days but the cough and weakness, aggravated by exercise, may last much longer. The disease spreads rapidly through the herd, and rapid spread is one of the characteristics that helps distinguish influenza from other equine respiratory ailments. Severity of the clinical signs is influenced by degree of immunity, age, debility, and stress.

Spread of the disease is by aerosol dispersion or by contact with horses in the early stages of the disease. Therefore, as with rhinopneumonitis, the risk of infection is greatest in situations where large numbers of unrelated horses are brought together. Influenza in the horse is a serious disease readily complicated by secondary bacterial infection. Absolute rest, good ventilation in the stable, and a nourishing diet help to speed recovery. Antibiotics, although routinely used to prevent secondary infection such as strangles, have no effect on the influenza virus. It is sometimes necessary to control persistent high fever with aspirin or other antipyretics. This, coupled with rest and good nursing care, is usually all that can be done or is necessary once the disease occurs.

A vaccine is available for prevention of influenza in horses which should be used routinely to immunize horses at risk.

Swine Influenza

While the myxovirus causing equine influenza is host-specific, the cause in swine influenza is not. In fact, there is evidence to indicate that the swine influenza virus, belonging to influenza virus Type A, originated with man during the great influenza pandemic of 1918–1919. While this particular strain of virus has since disappeared from the human population, it has stayed with the pigs. An exception was a few cases of influenza at Fort Dix in New Jersey identified as swine Type A virus during early 1976. This aroused some medical and great political concern that a repeat of the 1918 epidemic was in the making for 1976–77. This concern culminated in a federally financed mass-immunization campaign that proved to be a fiasco. It did serve at least two purposes, however. It alerted millions of people to the interrelationship between animal and human disease and it helped demonstrate once again that medicine and politics don't mix!

Swine influenza is most prevalent in the Midwest, where swine are concentrated. It is a disease that occurs primarily during the inclement weather of fall and winter, indicating that stress is a factor in the appearance of the clinical signs of fever, lack of appetite, coughing, muscular weakness, depression, and death of 1–2 percent of affected pigs. The disease spreads rapidly through a herd with sudden onset involving most of the herd and disappearance of the more conspicuous signs in three or four days. The principal loss is economic through stunting and reduced weight gain.

The mystery in swine influenza is where the virus survives between outbreaks. Since these occur primarily in fall and winter and the life of a pig from birth to slaughter is only about six months, the usual concept that a virus particle requires living cells to survive wouldn't hold true. Of course, there is no problem with that theory where breeding stock are kept over from one year to the next. The problem arises on farms where swine influenza is endemic but only feeder pigs are kept.

Part of the answer lies in intermediate hosts. At the time of acute attacks, the virus infects the swine lungworm. Eggs of the lungworm containing virus are passed out in pig feces and in turn are ingested by earthworms. The earthworm population thus becomes infected and months later when new pigs out on pasture eat infected earthworms they also get a dose of virus. The virus in the pig then remains more or less dormant until the pig's resistance is lowered by the stress of chilling and especially by concurrent infection with *Hemophilus suis.* This accounts for the characteristic rapid spread of the disease in the herd. It is as much simultaneous activation of latent infection as it is spread from one pig to the next.

Fortunately, swine influenza is not a major problem in pigs because prevention is difficult due to the mode of transmission. Buying only SPF breeding stock or feeder pigs and keeping them in paved feedlots would help, but it is not practical in all situations. Antibiotics in feed or drinking water and reduction of stress to minimize weight loss during an outbreak are usually the best bet.

MALIGNANT CATARRHAL FEVER (MCF, MALIGNANT HEAD CATARRH)

This is an infectious, sporadically occurring disease of cattle that is usually fatal. Generally only a small percentage of cows in the herd is affected but in some herds the disease may persist to cause significant losses over a period of time. Sheep are apparently unaffected carriers of the virus and the majority of cases occur in herds where the cattle are kept in close proximity to sheep.

Symptoms

The signs of MCF are variable but typically onset is accompanied by high fever, lack of appetite, and a clear discharge from the eyes and nose. The nasal discharge soon becomes mucopurulent and dark with encrustation of the nostrils. Conjunctivitis, inflammation of the eyelid, is commonly seen and breathing may become labored. Dehydration is a consistent complication contributing to the high (90 percent) mortality. Encephalitis (inflammation of the brain) and blindness may occur. On the basis of clinical signs alone in the individual cow MCF can easily be confused with bovine virus diarrhea, acute shipping fever, or a foreign animal disease, rinderpest.

A few cases develop a profuse diarrhea with severe straining which, when accompanied by signs of encephalitis, may be suggestive of rabies. The incubation period may range from several days to several months, and in its most acute form the disease is usually fatal in ten days or less. Occasionally affected cows live longer but recovery, if it occurs at all, is a slow process.

Malignant catarrhal fever. Note drooling, crusty muzzle and facial dermatitis.

No Vaccine

No vaccine is available to prevent the disease and, considering the relative infrequency of its occurrence, it's doubtful that the potential market would justify the cost of vaccine development and licensing. Similarly, presently available drugs do little to influence the course of the disease and past experience indicates destroying the animal may be the most humane course to take except in the case of valuable purebred animals, where the cost of vigorous therapy including intravenous fluids, blood transfusion, and antibiotics can be justified.

Keeping sheep and cattle completely separated is the best method of preventing the disease and, of course, isolating any infected cattle from the herd.

"Foothill" Abortion (Epizootic Bovine Abortion)

This abortion disease of cattle confined thus far to the western states, especially California, Oregon, and Nevada, is caused by one of several viral pathogens carried by an insect vector, the soft-shelled tick. *Chlamydia spp.* is the most likely cause, although there is still some question about this. Abortion is the only clinical sign, and the disease gets its name from the frequency of occurrence in cattle pastured in the foothills. The mode of transmission is not known but its restriction to a particular terrain and isolation of the organism from ticks and rodents suggests that it is a vector-borne disease. Also, that abortion typically occurs only during the first pregnancy or in cattle newly introduced to the area indicates that infection confers some degree of immunity. Abortion rates as high as 75 percent in susceptible cattle have been reported. Abortion usually occurs about the middle of gestation and retention of the placenta is a common sequel.

The disease produces characteristic lesions in the fetus that are useful in making a diagnosis. Isolation of the organism from fresh fetal tissue is far more reliable to confirm the diagnosis than serological testing at present.

Enzootic Abortion of Ewes

A similar, if not identical, disease called for want of a better name, enzootic abortion of ewes (EAE), occurs in sheep. In sheep, it is believed, infection occurs at lambing time through ingestion of the organism present in aborted fetal membranes or contaminated forage and remains latent until conception occurs. Isolation of aborting ewes and proper disposal of aborted fetuses therefore is an important control procedure. Interestingly enough, it's not unusual for only one lamb of a set of twins to be affected. In some case the lambs are not aborted and become mummified. Ewes carrying mummy lambs from whatever cause often show signs of systemic illness such as rapid weight loss. As in cows, however, abortion is generally the only clinical sign. The disease has not been reported to be a problem in goats. However, that it occurs in both cattle and sheep leads one to believe that it could occur in goats as well, and it should be considered as a possible cause of unexplained abortion in goats in the endemic areas.

At the moment, isolation of aborting animals until all vaginal discharge ceases and disposal of aborted fetuses by deep burying or burning is probably the most practical control. Broad spectrum antibiotics such as tetracycline in rather high doses will control the disease but administration under range conditions is difficult. Inactivated vaccine given prior to breeding is helpful in controlling this disease in sheep but does not provide absolute protection.

HOG CHOLERA

At one time this was by any measure the most costly disease of swine in this country, with annual losses running into millions of dollars. In addition to the direct losses, many foreign countries, free of the disease, refused to import United States pork products because of the risk of introducing infection. The hog cholera virus can survive several months in pickled pork and for years in frozen pork. Thanks to an intensive state-federal eradication campaign and the cooperation of swine producers, the disease appears to have been eradicated. No cases have been reported in the United States since the summer of 1976. This should not be cause for complacency, however, because prior to that episode, the disease had not been seen for almost two years.

Symptoms

Hog cholera is an acute highly contagious disease of swine causing high fever, lack of appetite, constipation followed by diarrhea, incoordination especially in the young, prostration, coma, and death in a high percentage of cases. With an incubation period sometimes as short as two days and very rapid spread, it was not uncommon to hear of a producer being literally wiped out

Typical scene when hog cholera was rampant.

overnight. Mature swine tend to be more resistant, with an incubation period sometimes as long as thirty days and recovery more common. Even then the economic loss through reduced rate of gain and abortion was highly significant.

Vaccination

With such an important disease it's not surprising that vaccination played an important role in its control. The earliest attempt, which was used at great cost for many years, was the simultaneous administration of live virus and antiserum at two different sites. The theory, which worked most of the time, was that the live virus would stimulate immunity but the antiserum would control its replication so disease would not result. Breaks were not unusual, however, due to improper administration or antiserum of inadequate potency. **Use of live virus in any immunization program guarantees perpetuation of the disease.**

The next development, never totally satisfactory, was the use of live virus inactivated with crystal violet. Unfortunately the inactivation was occasionally incomplete and vaccine breaks occurred. With improved knowledge of virology techniques, attenuated or modified live virus vaccine became available and was widely used until the early 1970s. Despite occasional vaccine breaks, it helped to reduce the prevalence of hog cholera to a manageable level. When it became feasible to eradicate the disease all vaccination was stopped by law because at that time most of the cholera being seen was due to vaccine failures and, in fact, the last outbreak in New England was traced to illegal use of vaccine. A stockpile of vaccine is maintained under federal control in case of emergency.

It's interesting that the hog cholera virus and the virus causing BVD in cattle are antigenically related. In the laboratory, pigs vaccinated with BVD vaccine withstood challenge by hog cholera virus. However, as a control procedure, use of BVD vaccine never found much favor.

Caution

Hog cholera can be diagnosed on the basis of clinical signs, fluorescent antibody test, and virus isolation. The disease is so important, although it appears to be eradicated, that anyone with a pig having a fever as part of the clinical picture should isolate the pig and call a veterinarian immediately. Although the majority of veterinarians today have never seen a case of cholera, they do know the clinical signs and have access to epidemiologists and laboratories to aid in the diagnosis. There is always the possibility that, if not hog cholera, the disease could be African swine fever, an equally devastating foreign animal disease that resembles cholera.

BOVINE MAMMILLITIS

Fortunately this disease is rare in the United States because it can cause considerable grief for the dairy cow and the person who has to milk her. As an illustration of the importance of analyzing statistics, one could legitimately say there has been a threefold increase in the prevalence of the disease in recent years. To the best of my knowledge that is true, but represents only three herd outbreaks, one in Minnesota and two in New York.

Lesions of herpes mammillitis.

In the New York herds, lesions were confined to the teats and udder, starting as reddened, thickened areas which soon developed into vesicles or blisters. These slough, leaving denuded areas ranging in size from a dime to larger sections involving the whole side of the teat or the teat end. These heal rapidly in the dry cow, but in the lactating cow healing is delayed due to the constant irritation of milking. The raw areas left after the skin sloughs are painful and the response of affected cows when milking is attempted is, as one might expect, a swift kick.

The virus causing mammillitis is a member of the herpes group and in other countries causes thickened lumps on the skin of the neck and back as well as the lesions described on the teats and udder. It could easily be confused with lumpy skin disease, a serious cattle disease we don't have, or, when the lesions are confined to the teats and udder, it resembles a severe case of pseudocowpox.

The source of the virus in the few domestic outbreaks is unknown as is the mode of transmission. There may be a mild febrile reaction early in the disease but generally the skin lesions are the only clinical sign noted. The skin lesion coupled with a rising serum neutralization antibody titer are diagnostic.

Management of the disease is largely symptomatic. Affected cows should be isolated from the rest of the herd or at least milked last. Antibiotic ointment applied to the teats help to reduce secondary infection and to keep the scabs soft. Where the teat end is involved, infusion of antibiotics into the quarter will help prevent mastitis as a secondary complication.

PSEUDORABIES

Swine are the natural host of this viral disease that is endemic in the major swine-producing states. Adult swine may be unaffected carriers and clinical signs are generally limited to suckling pigs. Since 1976 the disease has been reported much more frequently in the upper Midwest.

The disease spreads via contact with nasal and oral secretion from carrier animals and the clinical picture in piglets is one of fever, paralysis, coma, and death in as little as twenty-four hours. The virus is a member of the herpes group and, typical of this group, latent infection may be activated in adults to cause abortions or stillborn pigs.

Most other animal species are susceptible and in these the symptoms are much more dramatic and consistently fatal. While encephalitis occasionally occurs in pigs, it is common in species such as cattle, sheep, goats, and dogs. The clinical picture in these is primarily intense itching, so much so that infected animals literally rub or lick themselves raw prior to death. This behavior gives the disease its common name, "mad itch."

At necropsy typical lesions can be seen microscopically. Diagnosis can further be confirmed by virus isolation and serologic testing. Serologic tests can be used to identify carrier swine and many states now require a negative test as a prerequisite to importation.

Outbreaks in species other than swine can be prevented by keeping them away from swine. In the swine herd itself serologic testing and removal of reactors from the herd may be necessary. Herd replacements should be from herds known to be free of the disease or should be negative to serologic test. A vaccine is now available for use in states where the disease is endemic. Vaccination with either attenuated or inactivated vaccine will prevent clinical signs of the disease but will not prevent infection, and infected vaccinates may intermittently shed the virus to infect others. Vaccination may confuse the issue when serologic testing is done as part of an attempt to build a negative herd or to meet shipping requirements.

SCRAPIE

Although uncommon in the United States, this disease of sheep and goats is an enigma in many respects. The causative agent is believed to be a virus, although virus has not been isolated from affected sheep. Nevertheless, the disease has been reproduced in test animals by inoculation of brain suspension from those showing clinical signs, indicating that it is a transmissible disease. Second, it appears in certain bloodlines of sheep more than others, especially in the Suffolk breed. Third, it doesn't appear until sheep are two years old or more and it is more likely to occur in the progeny of those who later develop the disease. The mode of transmission in nature is unknown and onset is slow and insidious.

The earliest sign may be excitability with almost imperceptible tremor of the head and neck. As the disease progresses, there may be a peculiar high-stepping gait or even convulsions in response to external stimuli. One of the more obvious clinical signs, reminiscent of pseudorabies, is intense itching sufficient to interfere with eating or sleeping. The wool may come out in patches where the animals rub themselves. The clinical signs intensify over weeks or months, eventually terminating in death.

Similar disease has been reported in mink, mule deer, elk, and cattle but in most cases the disease has occurred only when these species were in close contact with sheep. A worrisome exception occurred in England in 1991–92 where a major outbreak in cattle is thought to have resulted from feeding processed animal protein to dairy cattle. In cattle the disease is called bovine spongiform encephalopathy.

At the moment, the disease is not prevalent enough to cause concern but the sheep grower should be aware of its existence and know the clinical signs. Scrapie is a legally reportable disease and the established control program, once a diagnosis is made, is quarantine and slaughter of all affected and exposed animals. While this may seem radical, with a disease such as this with low prevalence, unknown epidemiology, and fatal consequences, it is the most logical approach.

CONTAGIOUS ECYTHEMA (SORE MOUTH)

The virus causing this disease has an affinity for the lips of lambs and kids. Mature animals rarely show lesions with the exception of ewes nursing infected lambs, which, unless solidly immune, may develop lesions on the teats and udder. The disease occurs worldwide and most outbreaks in the northern hemisphere occur in late summer, fall, and early winter.

The infection spreads primarily through contact with the lesions. However, the virus is highly resistant to drying and other influences. Dried scabs falling to the ground may remain infective for years so that once the disease appears on a premise, additional cases may be expected in subsequent years.

Contagious ecythema lesion on the udder of a ewe.

Symptoms

Small reddened papules (pimples) on the lips are the first clinical sign. These soon become vesicles (blisters) which rupture, becoming pustular prior to scab formation. Adjacent vesicles may coalesce to become rather extensive lesions involving the entire lip. Occasionally similar lesions occur inside the mouth. With extensive involvement, the lips and mouth become quite sore. Some affected lambs are reluctant to nurse and as a consequence lose weight and become weak. A few may actually die from starvation. The problem is compounded if the disease is transmitted to the ewe when the affected lamb tries to nurse. The lesions on her teats may be so sore that she won't allow the lamb to nurse. Occasionally lesions develop on the feet, causing lameness.

Contagious ecthyma can readily be confused with a much less common viral disease of sheep called *ulcerative dermatosis*. The latter, however, causes actual ulcers on the lip, muzzle, feet and, unlike sore mouth, also on the prepuce and occasionally the penis of rams. Both diseases can be complicated by secondary bacterial infection and screwworm infestation.

Vaccine

Contagious ecthyma is preventable by vaccination; however, vaccination against this disease is actually planned infection using a suspension of live virus. Therefore the vaccine should not be used on farms where the disease has not appeared before. The usual procedure is to apply virus suspension to a lightly scarified area on the inside of the thighs of lambs when they are about a month old. Repeating the procedure several months later provides a more solid immunity. Recovered animals are solidly immune.

Treatment of the disease is of questionable value. Antibiotic ointments or antiseptic solutions may prevent secondary infection and promote earlier healing but the labor requirement in a commercial flock may be more than the effort is worth. In the majority of cases the lesions are completely healed in a month or less.

Caution

A word of caution is in order when handling infected animals or vaccine. The disease is transmissible to humans, causing lesions on the hand and face not unlike those in sheep. In humans the disease is referred to as "orf." Because contact is the mode of transmission to man as well as animals, it's prudent to wear rubber gloves when handling lesions or vaccine and to scrub thoroughly with soap and water when through.

VESICULAR STOMATITIS

Cattle, horses, and swine as well as a number of wild animals are susceptible to this vesicular disease and human cases have occasionally been reported. This is one of a group of viral diseases referred to as "vesicular" diseases because of the blister-like vesicles which the virus produces. Several serious foreign animal diseases, foot and mouth, swine vesicular disease, and vesicular exanthema produce identical lesions, so prompt accurate diagnosis is important.

Symptoms

Vesicular stomatitis occurs sporadically in all parts of the United States, usually during the warmer months and is recognizable by fever and development of vesicles on the lips, tongue, on the nostrils and muzzle of cattle, and frequently in the interdigital space and on the bulb of the heel in cattle and swine. In fact, lameness may be the first sign noted in swine. Excess salivation and drooling usually are a sequel to the mouth lesions. The incubation period is up to five days and the disease may spread rapidly through the herd by direct contact, since the vesicular fluid is teeming with virus, and probably also via insect vectors. Appetite is depressed due to soreness when mouth lesions are present. The disease is self-limiting, usually with complete recovery in about two weeks. Recovered animals are immune to further infection for about a year. Dairy cows may develop vesicles on the teats and udder and when the teat end is involved, secondary mastitis may occur.

The disease occurs sporadically with several years elapsing between outbreaks in a given area and the natural reservoir of the virus is unknown. Because of the commonly long interval between outbreaks, the use of vaccine is indicated primarily to protect animals at risk when an outbreak occurs.

Treatment

No specific treatment is available although topical application of antibiotic ointments may reduce the complication of secondary infection. The disease is generally not of sufficient importance or sufficiently common to warrant special precautions to prevent introduction to the herd other than the usual caveat, "Raise all your own replacements."

The chief importance of vesicular stomatitis is its similarity to the much more serious foreign vesicular diseases. Diagnosis can be confirmed by serologic test or virus isolation but animal susceptibility is the classic and perhaps most certain way of distinguishing between them. Table 8-1 shows the varying susceptibility of different animals to each disease.

TABLE 8-1

Disease Susceptibility

	Horse	Cow	Pig
Vesicular stomatitis	+	+	+
Foot and mouth	–	+	+
Vesicular exanthema	–	–	+
Swine vesicular disease	–	–	+

BOVINE LYMPHOSARCOMA
(BOVINE LEUKEMIA, BOVINE LEUKOSIS)

This disease is undergoing intensive study as a model for further understanding of the pathogenesis of leukemia in humans. Bovine lymphosarcoma is a viral-induced neoplastic disease of cattle that in adults is slow in onset and eventually fatal. There is evidence to indicate infection occurs *in utero* or via colostrum and becomes manifest months or years later. Also, familiar predisposition is a factor. The disease is more prevalent in dairy cattle than in beef cattle.

Diagnosis

A consistent finding of elevated white blood cell count, principally lymphocytes with many immature forms, is typical of the disease. This leucocytosis may precede clinical signs by months or years. The most readily recognized clinical sign in adult cattle is enlargement of the superficial lymph nodes. Enlargement of the thoracic or abdominal lymph nodes may cause clinical signs which mimic other diseases such as respiratory distress or digestive dysfunction. Diagnosis in these cases is usually an accidental finding during rectal palpation or exploratory surgery.

Although the primary lymphosarcoma is to be found in lymph nodes, metastatic tumors may develop in a variety of locations including liver, kidney, spinal cord, and brain in which case clinical signs are those to be expected due

Lymphosarcoma. Posterior paralysis the result of a tumor compressing the spinal cord.

to pathological change in the organ involved. Otherwise, unexplained decline in milk production and weight loss are reason to suspect lymphomatosis. Occasionally lymph nodes back of the eyeball will enlarge, forcing the eye outward to give the cow a pop-eyed appearance. Once tumors appear, the condition of the animal deteriorates over a span of weeks or occasionally months with fatal termination. The disease occurs occasionally in young calves causing generalized lymph node enlargement, lymphocytic infiltration of bone marrow, and anemia prior to death.

Better understanding of the disease, including its viral etiology, has led to development of a specific serological test. Interpretation of test results requires some discretion, however. A positive test indicates only that the animal has encountered the virus at some time and has circulating antibody, not that it has lymphosarcoma. Several surveys based on serologic testing indicate that 20 percent or more of our dairy cattle have been exposed but prevalence of the clinical disease is probably less than 1 percent. There is no present evidence of any relationship between enzootic bovine leukosis and leukemia in humans.

Prevention

Several northern European countries have initiated test and slaughter programs based on high leucocyte counts in an attempt to eradicate the disease, with moderate success. For the individual dairy farmer, prevention is difficult at best. Certainly any clinically affected animals should be removed immediately from the herd. Where the disease is a herd problem it is possible that a combination of a positive blood test and a high leucocyte count could be used to identify incipient disease and provide a logical basis for removing these animals from the herd. The same criteria could be applied to prospective herd replacements to keep the disease out of the herd.

TRANSMISSIBLE GASTROENTERITIS (TGE)

This is a major disease of swine, most prevalent in the swine-producing areas of the Midwest during winter and early spring. Although swine of all ages can be affected, its effect on piglets under two weeks of age can be devastating.

Profuse, watery diarrhea preceded sometimes by vomiting and very rapid dehydration are the principal signs in very young pigs. The incubation period may be only a matter of hours in some outbreaks and very rapid spread through adjacent litters in the farrowing house is a common characteristic. Mortality in young pigs can range up to 100 percent after an illness of one to five days. Less severe diarrhea without the early vomiting characterizes the disease in older swine. After several days' illness, older swine generally recover but they may continue to shed virus in the feces for a couple of months after all clinical signs have disappeared. These virus shedders are a source of infection for susceptible new pigs added to the herd and, if sold into other herds, carry the virus with them.

TGE should be suspected whenever a rapidly spreading diarrhea affecting all ages but fatal only to the very young occurs. The virus causes a physical change in the intestinal lining that results in rapid fluid loss. This in turn produces an extreme dehydration that even very young pigs try to counteract by drinking copious amounts of water. The diagnosis can be confirmed in the laboratory by fluorescent antibody techniques or by virus isolation.

Treatment and Prevention

Treatment is of very limited value because of the peracute nature of the disease. Antibiotics generally don't have much effect on the outcome. Antidiarrheal drugs such as carbadox and oral electrolytes by drench or added to the drinking water may save a few pigs that would otherwise succumb.

Prevention is generally more rewarding than treatment. A number of techniques have proven helpful. Avoiding introduction of the virus to a clean herd is highly desirable. The feces of infected pigs are highly contaminated with virus and the virus can be mechanically carried from one farm to another on equipment, dirty footwear, and by dogs, rodents, and wild birds. The first step then is to keep all unnecessary traffic — human, avian, animal, and vehicular — away from the pigs and particularly away from the farrowing house. To isolate the most susceptible population further, separate cleaning and feeding equipment, boots, and coveralls should be kept and used only in the farrowing house. And, of course, new breeding stock should be kept isolated from the remainder of the herd until danger of disease transmission has passed. These measures will help to prevent other contagious diseases as well.

While these measures are ideal, under some husbandry conditions they may not be practical, and other measures must be taken to cope with TGE. When the disease has occurred on the farm or the risk of infection is high, immunization can be useful. Immunization through planned infection was used prior to the advent of a vaccine and is still widely practiced. Deliberately exposing sows to virus in dead pigs during early pregnancy will stimulate antibody transferable in milk to piglets when they are born. This will protect many but small losses may still occur. Vaccination of sows increases antibody in colostrum to protect newborn pigs.

VIRAL DIARRHEA OF CALVES

Viruses belonging to the two groups, rotavirus and coronavirus, have been identified as the cause of a contagious diarrhea seen in some herds. The original virus isolations were from herds in Nebraska.

Rotavirus infection affects calves primarily in the one- to three-day age bracket, while coronavirus is more common in those a few days older. Much is yet to be learned about the significance of these viruses as they relate to the calf diarrhea complex. Both are apparently capable of causing pathological changes in the intestinal epithelium that result in rapid fluid loss, dehydration, and death of some calves with or without concurrent bacterial infection. It's possible, however, that the most severely affected calves are those with concurrent infection due to other pathogens such as *E. coli*.

A third virus group, parvovirus, must be added to the list of viruses capable of inducing diarrheal disease. First identified as a cause of severe frequently fatal diarrhea in dogs, it is possible that members of this virus group may also play a role in diarrhea of neonatal livestock, particularly swine.

Transmission as far as is known is by direct contact and the calf hutch or elevated tie stall system of housing helps control spread of disease.

Vaccine

A vaccine for the calf rotavirus and corona virus is commercially available but mixed reports follow its use. To be effective at all it must be given immediately after birth. When used this way, some herd owners report a marked decline in calf diarrhea problems; others report no detectable difference. From this it must be concluded that the vaccine may be useful in those herds where calf diarrhea due to rotavirus is endemic, but the vaccine is not the answer to the entire calf scours complex. Since the specific etiologic agent is rarely identified early in outbreaks of calf diarrhea, ensuring that the calf gets colostrum right after birth is still the most effective recommendation to be made.

CHLAMYDIAL POLYARTHRITIS (SEROSITIS)

Distribution of this disease, caused by a large-particle-size virus of the genus designated *Chlamydia,* thus far seems limited to the upper Midwest and West. The disease occurring in lambs, calves, and swine causes primarily an arthritis (inflammation of the joints). The organism, in addition to joint fluid, can be found in urine, feces, and eye discharges as well. The disease does not occur commonly, but herd or flock outbreaks can involve half or more of the young animals.

Lambs show varying degrees of lameness and, if checked, some of them will have a moderate fever. This helps to distinguish the disease from other conditions causing stiffness or lameness such as white muscle disease.

Calves, in addition to fever and lameness, frequently develop diarrhea as well. Swelling of the joints is usually more noticeable in calves than in lambs and is quite noticeable in pigs. The disease in pigs is often complicated by nasal congestion, sneezing, labored breathing, and conjunctivitis.

History, clinical signs, and joint lesions seen at necropsy all must be considered in arriving at a diagnosis but laboratory confirmation may be required. The principal effect of the disease is economic, through reduced rate of gain or outright starvation, when lame animals are so reluctant to move because of pain that they won't nurse.

Although little work has been reported on the pathogenesis of the disease, it's reasonable to assume that carrier animals perpetuate the infection from one season to the next and introduce it to new herds. Broad-spectrum antibiotics are useful in treating it and daily low level antibiotic feeding in the feedlots helps to control it. This practice, however, is under scrutiny by the Federal Drug Administration and may be banned.

POX DISEASES

Almost every species from human being to mouse is subject to infection by pox viruses. The viruses tend to be host-specific, with some exceptions, although, except for sheep and goat pox, they are clearly related. Sheep pox causes a very severe, frequently fatal disease, transmissible by inhalation — much like smallpox in humans. Fortunately, sheep and goat pox do not exist in this country. Horse pox, although it may exist, is rare. Pox infections of cattle and swine are those most commonly encountered.

Symptoms

In cattle and swine the disease is spread by contact appearing first as a small raised red area on the teats and udder of cattle and the belly of swine. These are variable in size and soon develop into vesicles that rupture, leaving a crater-like lesion which generally scabs over and heals uneventfully. The disease tends to be localized with no general effects. However, secondary bacterial infection may occur which delays healing. Lesions on the teats and udder, of course, interfere with milking of dairy cows.

Cowpox

Although swine have a specific pox virus of their own they are susceptible to cowpox as well. Animals that recover are immune to further infection. Immunologically there is an interesting historical note to cowpox. It is transmissible to humans, causing a disease referred to as "milker's nodule." Many years ago when smallpox was ravaging Europe, it was noted that those who had had cowpox or milkers nodule were immune to smallpox. This became the basis for the smallpox immunization still in use today. People are infected with cowpox (vaccinia) by placing a suspension of virus on a lightly scarified area. This immunizes them against smallpox (variola) and cowpox. Because of the presence of live vaccinia virus, people recently vaccinated against smallpox should not go near cows until the vaccination site is healed because they could infect cows. With the eradication of smallpox from the United States and most parts of the world, routine vaccination during childhood is no longer done.

True cowpox does not occur anymore in this country. However, a disease very similar in appearance called **pseudocowpox** is a common occurrence in dairy cattle. It is less severe than cowpox and there is some indication it may be a manifestation of papular stomatitis. It is transmissible to humans, as is cowpox. However, people vaccinated against smallpox are immune to cowpox.

Control

Control efforts for both diseases in cattle are aimed at reducing further spread by segregating infected cows and milking them last. The virus is readily transmitted on milking equipment and the milker's hands. Treatment is generally not necessary, although antiseptics applied to the lesions may hasten healing. Ointments applied after each milking help to soften the larger scabs, making the milking process less traumatic for the cow. Topical application of an antiviral drug such as acyclovir may hasten healing in those cases where the cost of the drug can be justified.

PORCINE PARVOVIRUS

There is a growing body of evidence that this virus is widespread in the swine population. It is a very small and resistant virus that tolerates wide ranges of pH and temperature. Although it is capable of infecting any body cell it exhibits a preference for embryonal and fetal tissue.

Serological studies indicate that up to 80 percent of sows have antibody to the virus indicating prior infection but the percentage of exposed gilts is not as high. The virus has been isolated from boar semen. Considering its adaptability to a variety of tissues and its wide distribution in the swine population, it is probable that the route of infection is oral or nasal and perhaps venereal.

The only outward sign of parvovirus infection in swine is reproductive failure. Infected animals appear to be healthy. The significance of the infection is its effect on the embryo or fetus and the resulting infertility it produces.

Infection of the embryos at about 12–20 days after conception results in embryonal death and a delayed return to heat. Infection at 21–35 days when the fetus is larger results in fetal resorption and pseudopregnancy. Typically, a sow may be diagnosed as pregnant but fail to farrow. Later infection, 35–55 days, produces a high percentage of mummified fetuses. If the entire litter is infected, abortion may occur. Infection occurring at 55–80 days may produce mummies and stillborn pigs although a few in the litter may survive. Infection after the 80th day of gestation does not seem to be as much of a problem.

The economic implications of parvovirus infection, which is a part of the SMEDI complex, are obvious. Reproductive failure can be a disaster for the swine producer.

Although vaccination of gilts is recommended, management for prevention is of paramount importance. Maintaining a closed herd is most desirable. The alternative is planned infection at a time when litters will not be affected. This means exposing new boars and gilts to older sows which may be carriers at least two weeks prior to breeding. This allows time for them to develop antibodies and become immune without endangering subsequent litters.

There is no treatment for parvovirus infection. It should be considered whenever reproductive failure occurs in a swine herd. Diagnosis can be confirmed by laboratory examination of fresh mummified fetuses or placenta. A positive antibody titer in blood samples from sows in the herd will confirm presence of the virus but will not establish parvovirus as the cause of the problem.

Diseases Caused by Yeasts, Molds, and Fungi

WITH A FEW EXCEPTIONS the majority of organisms in this category are not pathogenic and cause disease only rarely as secondary invaders. The exceptions, however, deserve some discussion.

RINGWORM

In terms of frequency of occurrence this is by all odds the most important fungal infection of livestock. Several species of the genus *Trichophyton* are responsible for most cases and the disease is seen most frequently in cattle, horses, swine, goats, and sheep — in that order.

If you have studied biology you may recall that fungi grow with many branching hyphae and reproduce by sporulation. Infection occurs within the surface layer of the skin and hyphae extend down into the hair follicles and sometimes into the hairs causing the hair to break off or fall out.

Symptoms

Ringworm in cattle is more common in calves and yearlings than in adults and is more prevalent during the winter months although it can occur throughout the year. The face and neck are the most frequent sites of infection in cattle and the early lesions appear as small slightly raised areas with the hair roughened rather than smooth. This hair falls out, leaving grayish circumscribed areas varying in size from almost imperceptible to large patches three or more inches in diameter. It is not unusual to see a gray ring completely around the eyes of cattle.

Ringworm in pig (left) and calf (above).

The lesions in the horse are somewhat similar but are more inclined to be moist and weeping and located where parts of the harness rub. In swine the lesions appear more like ringworm in humans, starting as a reddened area that gradually enlarges with the center healing as the disease progresses outward. This leads to lesions that appear as circles, which gave rise to the superstition years ago that the infection was caused by a "ringworm." Although the name has stuck, we now know it is not caused by a worm at all but by a fungus. Although it causes itching and discomfort, ringworm is not a serious disease and tends to be self-limiting, although it may persist for months. Nevertheless, it is unsightly and, most important, is contagious to man. Effort should be made therefore to control and treat it.

Prevention

Prevention of ringworm through the usual isolation and quarantine procedures applied to infectious diseases is not very effective. Spores of *Trichophyton spp.* are ubiquitous and the majority of animals carry some spores on the skin all the time with no evidence of infection. The disease is more likely to occur in the presence of filth, when nutrition is marginal, and when sunlight is lacking. Calves kept in dark, damp, filthy pens on a marginal diet almost invariably develop ringworm. Ultraviolet rays from the sun help to reduce development of ringworm spores and particular attention should be paid to vitamin A content of the diet to be sure it's adequate because this vitamin plays an important role in maintaining resistance of epithelium. Frequent grooming is helpful especially for horses, using clean brushes and curry combs. These should be cleaned and disinfected after each use to help prevent spread of infection.

Diagnosis of ringworm is generally not difficult because of the characteristic nature of the lesions. However, if there is any question, microscopic examination of deep skin scrapings in the laboratory will generally reveal the typical hyphae of the organism. It can also be cultured on selective media but this takes considerably longer.

Treatment

Treatment is not as easy as the diagnosis. The organism is susceptible to a variety of drugs if the drugs reach it. The single most important thing in treatment is to remove the scabs with soap, water, and a stiff brush because the organism is in the skin. Simply painting the lesions with iodine or similar solution without this important first step usually gives disappointing results. Many different drugs are effective, including copper napthenate, tincture of iodine, and even ordinary household bleach such as Clorox. When the lesions are extensive, these simple remedies may not be practical. In these cases, high pressure sprays using fungicides such as lime sulfur or Captan may be required. The latter is not cleared by the FDA for use on food-producing animals, however. Before embarking on a heroic treatment plan such as spraying or dipping, the advice of your veterinarian would be a good investment.

MYCOTIC ABORTION

Abortions due to mold infection of the fetus and placenta occur sporadically in all species but perhaps most commonly in the cow. Mold species such as *Aspergillus spp.* or *Mucor spp.* are generally responsible. In most cases the mold spores are probably introduced at the time of breeding although some researchers believe occasional infections occur when spores are conveyed via the circulatory system to the placenta. Frequently, aborted fetuses will have skin lesions that look like ringworm and the placenta is always greatly thickened, with evidence of necrosis, especially in the cotyledons.

Although mold infections are a very minor cause of abortion, they contribute to the overall problems of reproduction, and effort to prevent them will help to improve breeding efficiency. For this and other reasons, moldy feed should be avoided insofar as possible. The cleanest technique possible should be used when breeding either by artificial insemination or natural service. Scrub the vulva and surrounding area thoroughly with soap and water and wipe it dry prior to inserting the insemination pipette. This helps reduce risk of introducing other miscellaneous infections as well. The same procedure applied to the prepuce and sheath of the bull will help improve conception rates by natural service. Equine stud managers have learned by experience that cleanliness at breeding time is essential and the same applies to other animal species.

Sporotrichosis

This skin disease, caused by a fungus, is seen primarily in horses. The condition takes the form of multiple small painless nodules on the skin that discharge small amounts of pus. Initial infection probably occurs via wound contamination. The disease does not spread rapidly and the lesions usually heal in three to four weeks. Outbreaks are more likely to occur when horses are stabled due to a higher concentration of mold spores in the environment.

The disease responds well to treatment and most cases can be prevented by careful disinfection of cuts and abrasions.

Mycotoxicoses

This name is given to a group of disease conditions caused not directly by molds themselves but by poisons called **mycotoxins** they produce.

A mycotoxin is a fungal metabolite that exerts a deleterious effect on a biological system. For example, most of the antibiotics are mycotoxins, which, as therapeutic levels, are more toxic for bacteria than for animals. Historically, ergot was the first known mycotoxin. Epidemics of dry gangrene and nervous derangement in humans, undoubtedly due to ergot, were recorded as early as the eleventh century. The source was contaminated rye used in bread. Interest in mycotoxins has paralleled the interest in antibiotics and accelerated since 1940.

Over 100 molds are known to produce toxic metabolites under certain conditions of temperature, moisture, oxygen tension, pH, and type of substrate. Of these, 25 to 30 have been associated with animal disease. They produce a wide variety of effects, some clinically dramatic and others clinically unrecognizable. Toxins may be produced by molds on the standing crop or in stored feeds. Mycotoxin, when present, may be in the mold itself or diffused into the substrate. It is visually unidentifiable.

There is considerable species variation in susceptibility to mycotoxins. Swine and poultry are quite susceptible, followed by horses, cattle, and sheep. Humans and fish are near the top of the list. Similarly, some feedstuffs favor the growth of toxigenic fungi more than others. Aflatoxin, for example, is commonly found in peanuts, cottonseed, copra, corn, grain sorghum, barley, and apple juice. Many mycotoxins are heat-stable and survive canning, pelleting, and other such processes.

Detection of mycotoxins in feeds is difficult. It is possible to have grossly moldy feed without any mycotoxin present. Conversely, feeds without obvious mold may contain mycotoxins. Distribution of mycotoxin in stored feeds is rarely uniform and detection presents a problem. Black light screening for mold fluorescence is a moderately good rough method but it is most effective only when the mold is living and does not indicate the presence of mycotoxin. Chemical analysis is the most satisfactory detection method. Unfortunately, few laboratories are equipped to do it and those that will accept samples for analysis are generally set up to test for only a few of the known mycotoxins.

With a few exceptions the clinical signs of mycotoxicoses in animals have not been well defined. Much of the available data are from experimental work with laboratory animals that has been extrapolated to livestock. Therefore, it is difficult to say with certainty that a particular syndrome is attributable to a specific mycotoxin.

AFLATOXIN

The best known of the mycotoxins in stored grain is aflatoxin from *A. flavus* and *A. parasiticus*. The aflatoxins are a group of toxic metabolites that vary in their toxic and carcinogenic potential. The susceptibility of different animal species to aflatoxins also appears to be variable. Acute aflatoxicosis causes hepatitis, hepatic cell necrosis, and prolonged clotting time. Affected animals often die with severe hemorrhages and feeds containing as little as 1 p.p.m. can cause acute poisoning in some animals. In subacute poisoning the changes in the liver are those of cell destruction, regeneration, and repair with areas of scar tissue formation and bile duct proliferation. Growth rate and protein formation are depressed but the animal may or may not die. Chronic poisoning in addition to retarding rate of growth lowers resistance to disease and, in turkey poults has been shown to impair the immune response to vaccination. Chronic poisoning results in icterus and liver cirrhosis. Prolonged consumption of as little as 0.5 p.p.b. is carcinogenic in some animals.

RUBRATOXIN

Rubratoxins are potent hepatotoxic, hemorrhage-inducing metabolites of *P. rubrum* and *P. purpufogenum*, common soil fungi that frequently contaminate animal feeds. The role of these substances in naturally occurring disease is suspected but has not been demonstrated definitively.

OCHRATOXIN

Ochratoxin A from *Aspergillus ochraceous* causes hepatic and renal damage in rats. It also causes fetal resorption and abortion in pregnant rats. Similar signs have been seen in livestock fed moldy feeds, although in these cases ochratoxicosis has been diagnosed retrospectively.

ZEARALENONE

The effect of F2 or zearalenone from *F. roseum* and related species on swine is well known. It is a potent estrogenic substance producing characteristic sexual changes such as swelling of the vulva, enlargement of the mammary glands and uterine hyperplasia. Stunting of male and female swine has also been observed following consumption of *F. roseum* contaminated corn. Evidence exists that the fungus produces several interrelated substances that may affect animals synergistically, inasmuch as contaminated corn has a much greater effect on pigs than does an equivalent amount of purified F2 toxin. Other fungal metabolites associated with vomiting and feed refusal have been found in *F. roseum* contaminated corn that cause significant economic effects.

T-2 TOXIN

F. tricinctum is consistently the most toxigenic fungus isolated from moldy corn. Its principal effect is that of necrosis of the skin, oral mucus membrane, intestine, and liver. Fatal doses can be absorbed through the skin with large necrotic areas developing at the point of absorption. Sublethal doses produce a hemorrhagic syndrome similar to that of other mycotoxicoses. The death of seven out of thirty-five cows in a Wisconsin herd was attributed to T-2 toxin in 1971.

Fescue foot, a progressive lameness of cattle with heat, swelling, pain, and later, gangrene has long been recognized as a hazard of grazing on pastures containing tall fescue. More recent evidence indicates that the condition is not due to the fescue itself but to a mycotoxin form mold growing on the fescue. The clinical signs strongly resemble those produced by *F. tricinctum* toxin.

ERGOT

Ergot poisoning is due to the alkaloids produced by the fungus *Claviceps purpurea*. There are two forms of ergotism commonly observed in domestic animals: a convulsive form and a gangrenous form. The convulsive form is characterized by vertigo and muscle spasms of the hindlimbs, followed by temporary paralysis. The gangrenous form is characterized by lameness, which can be followed by loss of the limbs, tail and ears. In cattle and sheep, in addition to lameness, the animals commonly have decreased rate of gain and increased body temperature and respiratory rate. In swine, although there are reports of decreased rates of gain and feed efficiency, the most common sign is agalactia (lack of milk) and dead pigs at birth. There is some evidence that ergot interferes with reproduction.

TREMORTINA

This toxin from several species of *Penicillium* induces tremor, ataxia, and tonic, clonic convulsions when administered to animals. In experimental work 2.5 mb/kg was sufficient to cause clinical signs. The first sign of toxicity in calves was a fine tremor that increased in severity with forced movement or excitement. With continued consumption the tremors became more severe; the calves stood with legs stiff and spread apart and swayed rhythmically. When forced to move, their gait was stilted and they were ataxic (dizzy). In the most severely affected, there was lateral recumbency with paddling, intermittent extensor rigidity, opisthotonos, (head and neck arched back), and severe tremors.

SLAFRAMINE

This mycotoxin from *Rhizoctonia leguminacola* found in red clover has been identified as the cause of excessive salivation and reduced milk production and body weight in dairy cattle. Salivation is the most consistent sign, followed by lacrimation, diarrhea, frequent urination, and anorexia.

It is probable that some unexplained disease syndromes in livestock may be in fact due to a mycotoxicosis; however, we should avoid the temptation to attribute every obscure syndrome to mycotoxins. Fortunately, except for fatalities, the effects of most of the mycotoxicoses are reversible once the toxin is removed. The prudent course is to avoid the use of moldy feeds, but if moldy feeds must be used, they should be fed cautiously to a few animals to observe the effects rather than fed to the entire herd at the outset. Since the effect of mycotoxins is dose related it may occasionally be possible to salvage moldy feed by diluting it with feed which is not.

YEAST INFECTIONS

Infections with organisms of this group, especially *Candida spp.*, often follow prolonged indiscriminate antibiotic therapy. Yeast mastitis in cattle and goats causes an acute inflammation with fever, swelling of the udder, change in milk consistency to almost a creamy pus, and virtually total cessation of milk flow. Treatment other than symptomatic is of little avail. In most cases recovery occurs in about two weeks but some cows never return to full production.

Almost invariably the infection is introduced during faulty udder infusion technique or via contaminated medication. Serious herd outbreaks have occurred when mastitic cows were treated with "homemade" antibiotic mixtures that became contaminated. Penicillin actually favors the growth of *Candida spp.* and contamination of multiple dose vials can readily occur. Always disinfect the top of the vial with alcohol prior to use and sterilize syringes after each use. Failure to do so may cause trouble with yeast infection. It is not unusual where herd yeast infections are a problem to recover pure cultures from the syringe used to treat the cows for mastitis.

Prolonged use of oral antibiotics can also promote overgrowth of yeast in the intestinal tract causing chronic enteritis in young animals. Yeasts are essential microflora in the gut which can become pathogenic when people unwisely interferes.

Diseases Caused by Protozoa

ALTHOUGH, AS A GENERAL RULE, protozoan diseases are more of a problem in the tropics, several species of pathogenic protozoa are economically significant in the United States. Protozoa are single-cell organisms, much larger than bacteria, that are widely distributed in nature. Those that are pathogenic tend to be host-specific (survive in only one animal species) and about half of them require the assistance of a vector to spread from one animal to the next.

COCCIDIOSIS

This is the most common protozoan disease in the United States affecting virtually all species of animals. Its effects are serious in cattle, sheep, and goats, occasionally in swine and much less commonly in horses.

Symptoms

Coccidia have an interesting life cycle that has bearing on the characteristics of the disease they produce. The principal clinical sign in all species is profuse, often bloody, diarrhea. Clinical signs follow ingestion of infective oocysts that have been passed out in the feces of other animals that may or may not have been clinically ill themselves. Infective oocysts contain sporozoites that escape from the oocyst and invade intestinal cells, where they develop into schizonts. These divide asexually into merozoites, which invade additional cells to cause extensive intestinal inflammation. After several of these asexual cycles a sexual generation occurs with development of micro- and macrogametocytes, ultimately forming a zygote that becomes encapsulated as an oocyst and is passed out in the feces. At this point, the oocyst is not infective and must undergo further development outside the body. Under favorable moisture and temperature conditions, sporazoites form in the oocyst in about a week and they are then infective. Typically an initial acute attack of coccidiosis will subside only to recur in one or two weeks. The apparent recovery occurs when the oocysts are forming and before reinfection with the sporulated oocysts occurs.

Eimeria and *Isospora* are the two most common pathogenic genera of coccidia and there are many species within each genus. The species tend to be quite host-specific. *E. zurnii*, a common bovine coccidium, rarely infects other animals. While infection of aberrant species may occur, it is usually transitory and inconsequential.

Coccidiosis is a disease primarily of young animals. Mature animals, although commonly infected, usually have developed sufficient immunity so that clinical signs do not develop. They periodically shed oocysts however and are probably the source of infection for younger generations on the farm.

The effect of acute coccidiosis can be quite devastating, with diarrhea, rapid dehydration, and sufficient blood loss to require blood transfusion to save the animal's life. The history, clinical signs, and microscopic identification of the organism in the feces are sufficient to confirm the diagnosis. A single negative microscopic finding may be misleading since in the early stages oocysts may be present in the feces only in very small numbers. This goes back to the life cycle explained above and a couple days later overwhelming numbers of oocysts may be seen in a fecal sample.

Treatment

Left untreated, mortality of calves, lambs and goats may range up to 10 percent or more and those that recover from the acute attacks undergo a long recuperative period that reduces weight gain and growth rate. Furthermore the debility caused by the disease often leads to further complications such as pneumonia. Therefore treatment early in the disease is important. Blood transfusion when indicated and sulfonamides orally or intravenously are the usual effective treatments. Individual treatment is most desirable but in a flock or herd outbreak the labor requirement may make this impossible. In such cases medicated feed or drinking water may be the only feasible route. Lasalocid, one of a new group of drugs called ionophores, has recently been approved as a feed additive for prevention of coccidiosis in lambs. It also has the advantage of improving feed conversion efficiency in beef cattle as well as in lambs.

Prevention

As with every other disease, prevention is far more rewarding than treatment. Since infection occurs by ingestion of oocysts and these originate in manure of infected animals it follows that overcrowding of animals in a given area will increase the concentration of oocysts on the ground. This is the reason coccidiosis is more of a problem in beef and lamb feedlots. The problem is obviously greater when animals are fed on the ground where feed rapidly becomes contaminated. The same thing happens when the only source of drinking water is pools or streams. To reduce the risk of infection by coccidia and other internal parasites, don't overcrowd pastures, rotate pastures frequently and, in confinement such as feedlots, put feed in bunks or troughs protected from fecal contamination. In feedlots where coccidiosis has been a problem, some operators have found it advantageous to begin medication of animals when they arrive as a prophylactic measure during the stress period until they become adapted to the new surroundings and diet. On the dairy farm rearing calves in individual hutches described earlier will almost completely eliminate the problem.

ANAPLASMOSIS

There is disagreement among taxonomists whether the organism responsible for this disease, *Anaplasma marginale,* is a protozoan or whether it more properly should be classed with the rickettsia. For our purpose it makes little difference. Suffice to say that it is a blood-borne parasite causing anemia in cattle, sheep, and goats that is a major problem especially in the Gulf and Pacific Coast states. Isolated cases have been identified in the north central and northeastern states but the disease is not endemic in those areas.

The effect of anaplasmosis on the animal is variable depending on age, resistance, and possibly, the size of the infecting dose. Unlike most diseases, young animals are more resistant to anaplasmosis than adults. With most infectious diseases it is usually the other way around, with adults having sufficient immunity through prior exposure to be resistant.

Symptoms
The incubation period may be as long as three weeks and onset of clinical signs is marked by persistent high fever, lack of appetite, and depression. The organism attacks red blood cells causing anemia which in turn results in rapid pulse and respiration, pale mucus membranes, dehydration, and weight loss. Exertion may result in collapse of the animal due to hypoxia. The disease may be peracute, with death in one or two days, acute lasting ten days to two weeks, or chronic. A few animals never recover completely and remain thin and unthrifty. In adult cattle, especially range cattle where the disease may not be recognized and treated early, mortality up to 50 percent may occur.

In nature the organism, *A. marginale,* is spread from infected to susceptible cattle by biting insects, particularly ticks and biting flies. Of these ticks are the more important vector and the organism may survive in the tick for several months. In the United States prevalence of the disease tends to parallel the natural distribution of the several ticks serving as vectors. Anaplasmosis is not transferable through direct contact but requires mechanical transfer of a droplet of infected blood. On occasion man has done this more effectively than insects. Serious herd outbreaks have occurred when animals were vaccinated with the same contaminated needle. In endemic areas it's important to sterilize surgical instruments, hypodermic needles, tattoo instruments, tagging pliers, and other implements after each use. Recovered animals commonly remain carriers for life.

Treatment
When the disease is detected early, infected animals respond fairly well to treatment with broad spectrum antibiotics such as chlortetracycline and oxytetracycline. Elimination of the carrier state requires therapy with these drugs for thirty to sixty days. Several different serologic tests are available to confirm the diagnosis but during the acute illness microscopic examination of a stained blood smear usually reveals the organism at the margin of red blood cells.

Prevention
Prevention of the disease depends on vector control through spraying or dipping with insecticides, careful disinfection of surgical instruments, and vaccination. A killed vaccine is available that does a reasonably good job in preventing new infections.

BABESIASIS

Several species of *Babesia* infect horses, cattle, sheep and swine in various parts of the world, but in the United States at the present time only *B. caballi* causing infection in horses is of importance and, thus far, only in Florida. This was not always the case and cattle babesiosis, also called **Texas fever** or **cattle tick fever,** at one time was a serious threat to the beef industry in the Southwest. Babesiosis is spread by ticks and eradication of the specific tick responsible for Texas fever from the United States through quarantine and cattle dipping programs early in the century was a major milestone in the history of veterinary medicine.

Symptoms
Like anaplasmosis, *Babesia spp.* invade red blood cells causing anemia and sometimes jaundice. They also cause red cells to swell with a resulting sludging of cells in the capillaries. When this is severe enough circulatory impairment occurs and symptoms associated with organ dysfunction, such as hepatitis and nephritis, result. Severity of signs is a function of the size of the infecting dose and resistance of the animal. In horses the disease is called piroplasmosis and clinical signs include high fever, jaundice, anemia, subcutaneous edema, rapid pulse, and general weakness. Many infected horses develop petechial (pinpoint size) hemorrhages in the conjunctiva and some show signs of colic. The disease may be acute, with death occurring in less than forty-eight hours; subacute, with apparent recovery in about two weeks; or chronic, in which case the animal fails to gain weight and lacks the stamina for hard work.

Prevention

At the moment, prevention is basically a matter of keeping infected ticks and susceptible horses apart by daily grooming and application of insecticides to the horse or, if prevalence warrants, area spraying. The latter is not widely used due to adverse effect of insecticides on other insects. Similarly some of the most effective insecticides cannot be used legally on animals because of their environmental persistence. Although it would be possible technically to eradicate this disease in Florida through vector eradication as was done with Texas fever, it is highly unlikely that such a program will be undertaken because of possible adverse effects on other insects and wildlife. It should be remembered that like anaplasmosis and other blood-borne diseases, equine piroplasmosis can be spread by contaminated surgical instruments.

EPERYTHROZOONOSIS

The significance of this disease of swine is not clearly understood. It is capable of causing fever, weakness, lack of appetite, anemia, and all the usual signs associated therewith. However, the infection is usually mild and recovery is the rule. The organism, *E. suis*, invades red blood cells and appearance of the disease primarily in the summer suggests biting insect transfer but this has not been proven. The clinical signs coupled with microscopic examination of a stained blood smear generally confirm the diagnosis.

Treatment with broad spectrum antibiotics is helpful. The mode of transmission is unclear but based on what is known, control of the biting fly population using residual sprays on the premises, screening the farrowing and finishing houses and sterilization of surgical instruments between each use are the best means of control.

TOXOPLASMOSIS

The protozoan *Toxoplasma gondii* is capable of infecting all mammalian species, although among livestock it is most significant in swine and sheep. Sows may be infected without showing any signs of illness and may transmit the organism to their piglets in the uterus or via milk. Clinically affected piglets may show evidence of pneumonia, enteritis, hepatitis, and nephritis. The clinical infection is not common but occasional serious outbreaks have been reported. Some individuals involved in an outbreak may show signs of encephalitis.

Toxoplasmosis is an important cause of abortion in sheep in some parts of the world. Ewes themselves rarely show signs of illness but fetal tissues and the placenta are apparently quite susceptible. Although not a significant problem in the United States, that *T. gondii* is widely prevalent makes the infection a possibility in otherwise unexplained flock abortion problems. Correlation of characteristic microscopic lesions in the fetus with positive serologic tests on the ewe would confirm the diagnosis.

The mechanism by which toxoplasmosis spreads is not clearly defined. *In utero* transfer, ingestion of contaminated meat and milk, and inhalation of infective droplets are all possible routes. With so many routes of infection and others probably unknown, control recommendations other than the usual recommendation for good sanitation are difficult to make. The fact that the organism is widespread and the clinical disease uncommon leads one to believe that specific control procedures are probably unnecessary. A word of caution is in order, however. Toxoplasmosis also infects humans and is particularly hazardous for the unborn infant. Although the family cat has been implicated in human infections far more often than livestock, persons handling known infected animals should be cautious and, at the very least, scrub thoroughly with soap and water when through.

TRICHOMONIASIS

Trichomonas fetus causes a true venereal disease in cattle resulting in early embryonic death or abortion and pyometra (pus in the uterus). Irregular heat periods at long intervals are characteristic of the disease. Infection of the bull is inapparent and persists for the life of the animal. The disease is spread to the cow at the time of coitus and if the cow is given complete sexual rest, the disease will generally disappear after several months. The principal effect is economic loss through delayed breeding. Occasionally there will be some discharge of pus from the vagina but other clinical signs of illness are rarely noted.

Trichomoniasis is a problem only in herds where natural service is used. Artificial insemination presents infection because dilution of semen and in most cases, freezing, reduces the number of trichomonads to a very low or nonexistent level. Artificial insemination is the single most important means of preventing the disease.

Diagnosis

Trichomoniasis is an insidious disease and the entire herd may be infected before its presence is realized. Diagnosis is based on history and identification of the organism either by direct microscopic examination of vaginal mucus or preputial washings or by fluorescent antibody test using the same fluids. The organism may also be found in fluids from the placenta and stomach fluid of an aborted fetus. It is not easy to find, however, and a single negative sample can be misleading. Fluids from a number of cows in the herd should be checked and where the history is compatible, finding a single trichomonad confirms the diagnosis.

Once the diagnosis is made, steps can be taken to eliminate the infection from the herd. It may take a year or more to accomplish. The first essential step is to stop all natural breeding and use artificial insemination exclusively. The disease is self-limiting in the cow, provided the source of infection — the bull — is removed. A few cows develop sufficient resistance to carry a calf to term despite infection, which only confuses the history and diagnosis. Infected bulls remain that way and the best place for them is the slaughterhouse. Although infected bulls can be treated, treatment is laborious. It must be repeated several times, and samples must be checked over a period of several months to determine effectiveness of treatment. Even then, there is a chance that the last organism may not be killed and the infection will recur once the treatment and surveillance procedures are stopped. Nationwide, prevalence of the disease is low and it isn't worth the risk of perpetuating it by trying to salvage infected bulls.

Prevention

Prevention of trichomoniasis is easily accomplished by using artificial insemination exclusively. If a bull must be used, select as herd sires young virgin bulls that have never bred cattle before. And for added insurance, mate them with a couple of virgin heifers first before putting the bull with the herd. If the heifers become pregnant, confirmed by rectal examination, you can be reasonably sure the bull is not carrying trichomoniasis. You will also have the added assurance that the bull is fertile.

Parasitism

TECHNICALLY SPEAKING, any organism that lives at the expense of its host is a parasite. Under this definition, pathogenic bacteria, viruses, yeasts, molds, fungi, and protozoa are parasites. In common usage, however, when we speak of parasites in animals we are referring to several types of worms (internal parasites) and insects (external parasites). There is also a third category, wherein the larval stage of an insect becomes an internal parasite. A good example of the latter is the stomach bot of the horse.

Internal Parasitism

All species of animals including humans are susceptible to a variety of internal parasites. Among livestock, sheep, horses, goats, and cattle are most susceptible to parasitism. Although there are exceptions, some general statements can be made about internal parasitism that will be helpful in designing a parasite control program suitable for your circumstances.

First, most internal parasites are host-specific and those that thrive in one species — the swine ascarid, for example — will not infect other animal species except perhaps for brief periods. Second, most internal parasites have direct life cycles — that is, they develop to maturity in the intestinal tract, lay eggs that are passed out in manure, contaminating pastures and drinking water, and infect other animals when they consume the contaminated feed or water. Last, it is virtually impossible under farm or range conditions to raise parasite-free animals. Generally, the best that can be hoped for is to keep parasitism at a low enough level so that the effect on the animal is minimal.

There is a school of thought among many competent parasitologists that a low level of infection may actually be desirable because it stimulates some immunity (premunition), thereby protecting the animal from overwhelming exposure. This has been demonstrated with haemonchosis in sheep. The premunition concept is being actively pursued and in the not too distant future we may see vaccines cleared for use in this country which will prevent major worm infestations. Such products are in limited use in Europe now.

Control

Given the generalities above, it is possible to devise programs that will keep parasitism to a minimum. The one favored by the drug companies is frequent therapeutic use of anthelmintics or continuous low-level feeding of anthelmintics (worm medicine). Most of the newer anthelmintics work by destroying the adult worms or rendering them sterile so that fertile eggs are not passed out in the manure. If other control measures are not adopted concurrently, this method has two obvious disadvantages. It is a continuing expense for medication and some species of worms become tolerant to the anthelmintic after prolonged exposure. Also, in food-producing animals, the range of drugs that can be used legally is limited.

Where the need for control of intestinal worms is not acute, management methods will in most cases prove more productive and economical. Remember that eggs are passed out in the manure and that reinfection is by ingestion. Anything that reduces the concentration of eggs will reduce the level of reinfection. The corollary to this is that high concentrations of infected animals will cause greater ground contamination and higher infection rates. Conversely, contamination can be reduced by weekly pasture rotation, periodic plowing and reseeding of pastures, paving holding areas and cleaning them daily, and protecting feed bunks and water supplies from fecal contamination. Pulling a drag over the pasture at weekly intervals helps distribute manure piles, thereby exposing worm eggs to the destructive effects of sunlight. Some species of intestinal worms go through a period of embryonation in the egg stage lasting several days before they become infective. This process is facilitated by conditions of warmth and moisture. It is helpful, therefore, to keep pastures mowed short so tall grass doesn't trap moisture, favoring egg development.

All of the foregoing are really methods of sanitation, which is the key to control of most internal parasites. Sanitation is especially important in controlling the swine roundworm, a major destructive parasite of baby pigs. A proven effective method is to worm the sow prior to farrowing, keeping her in a paved yard or pen that can be hosed down periodically for the next few days. Then scrub her thoroughly with soap and water to remove all traces of dirt and manure before putting her in the farrowing crate or pen. If the piglets are destined for pasture at weaning, trucking them to a clean pasture rather than having them walk over contaminated ground helps to ensure that roundworms will not be a problem. This procedure, known as the McLean County system, was effective long before the advent and popularity of anthelmintics.

Physical Condition

Another important generality that can be applied particularly to the stomach and intestinal worms is that they are most prevalent in and detrimental to the animal that is in poor physical condition for some other reason, the major one being malnutrition. The biological interrelationship of living things, whether it be mutualistic, commensalistic, or parasitic, is complex, interesting, and sometimes even logical. In the case of parasitism, a delicate balance is maintained in nature between the welfare of the parasite and its host. All other things being equal, the parasite will persist in numbers sufficient to maintain its race but not in numbers lethal to the host. Since the parasite must have a host to survive, destruction of the host would be self-defeating. Among wild animals, internal parasitism is universal and rarely fatal. Among domestic animals parasitism is also universal but is frequently fatal because people, either through lack of knowledge or lack of caring, upset the delicate host/parasite relationship. A well-nourished animal not under stress can withstand a parasite burden far in excess of what would kill one that is half-starved.

Sheep Most Susceptible

Of all livestock species, sheep are the most susceptible to infection with gastrointestinal worms and the principal genera affecting sheep, goats and cattle are *Haemonchus, Ostertagia, Trichostrongylus, Oesophagostomum, Bunostomum,* and *Cooperia.* Of these, *Haemonchus* is perhaps the most pathogenic for sheep. It and *Bunostomum* are blood-sucking worms and the

"Bottle jaw" from parasitic anemia. Note edema under the jaw.

major sign of serious infection is anemia and edema particularly of the submandibular region, giving rise to the term "bottle jaw." Under certain conditions, haemonchosis in sheep can give the impression of a peracute infectious fatal disease. Sheep grazing a heavily contaminated pasture a few days after a warm rainfall can undergo massive infection, resulting in rapid death with no other clinical signs noted. The warm rain favors egg maturation so that large numbers of worm larvae are infective all at the same time.

General Symptoms

Watery diarrhea, rough hair coat, and general unthriftiness are typical signs of infestation with the other gastrointestinal parasites. If the worm burden is moderate and nutrition is adequate, external evidence of parasitism will usually be lacking. Diagnosis is generally confirmed by identification of worm eggs in manure samples using concentration techniques and the microscope. A tablespoonful of fresh manure is an adequate sample and egg concentration is usually expressed in terms of eggs per gram. The technique is simple and inexpensive. Your veterinarian can readily check samples for you and a routine check of samples from several animals in the herd at least twice a year is a good precaution. If the count trend is upward it indicates a break in control procedures somewhere that must be corrected to prevent trouble. Some people have the false impression that if they don't see worms in the manure it's because the animal doesn't have worms. Similarly, if they don't see worms after giving the animal an anthelmintic, they think the drug didn't work. Both assumptions are false because the worms we have named thus far are extremely small and rarely can be seen without a magnifying glass. Ascarids common to swine and foals are an exception. These are large worms approaching the diameter of a pencil and occasionally an adult worm will be passed in the manure. If you see one you can be sure there are many more.

Control

Control of these common gastrointestinal worms depends on sanitation, management, and judicious, timely use of proper anthelmintics. A number of good medications for use orally, topically, or by injection are available but these alone will not do an adequate job. Accurate diagnosis is important because worm life cycles and season of the year influence the effectiveness of the anthelmintic. Your veterinarian can help you devise a control program compatible with your circumstances that will reduce the detrimental effect of these parasites to a minimum.

Thus far we have been talking primarily about the gastrointestinal worms that affect sheep, goats, and cattle. It's convenient to lump them together because their life cycles are similar and their response to anthelmintics is similar. There are, however, other internal parasites, equally or more important, that differ substantially and deserve special mention.

Ascarids (Roundworms)

The swine roundworms, *Ascaris suum,* and the horse ascarid, *Paracaris equorum,* are the most important species affecting livestock. The adult worms are large and easily recognized. Except where they are sufficiently numerous to mechanically block the intestine or bile duct, however, they do little harm to the animal. It's the migrating ascarid larvae that do the most damage. Adult female ascarids lay up to a quarter million eggs a day. These are passed out onto the ground in the manure where they readily withstand freezing, drying, and chemicals so that ground contamination reaches high levels rapidly and persists. The eggs become infective in two to three weeks and when ingested, the larvae emerge in the intestine. These penetrate the intestinal wall and are carried in the blood stream eventually to the liver where they migrate around and develop further. As development progresses they are carried in the blood to the lungs where they emerge into the alveolar spaces, eventually getting to the bronchi. From there they are coughed up and swallowed, ending up in the small intestine to become adults.

Symptoms

With this pattern of larval migration it's not surprising that the symptoms of ascarid infection may bear little relationship to those we generally associate with worms. The migration to the liver may take a circuitous route, and larvae migrating in the sow or mare can cross the placenta and infect foals or piglets prior to birth. That's why it's important that pregnant animals be as free of ascarids as possible and be confined to areas that are relatively uncontaminated. Visceral larva migrans is a serious disease of children caused by migrating canine ascarids. It can cause blindness and brain lesions. In foals and piglets larval migration causes damage to the liver, leaving lifetime scars. In pigs the white spots and streaks in the liver resulting from larval migration are cause for liver condemnation. Extensive infestation may cause enough liver inflammation to result in jaundice. Blockage of the bile duct by adults has the same outward effect. Verminous pneumonia is not unusual in heavily parasitized swine causing labored breathing and all the other signs associated with pneumonia.

In foals and young pigs a "pot" belly, rough hair coat, unthriftiness, failure to gain weight, and frequent coughing should lead one to suspect roundworms as the cause. Roundworms respond well to administration of anthelmintics such as piperazine but the life cycle illustrates why a single oral dose of the drug has no lasting value. It may kill all the adults but many larvae will be inaccessible to the drug and will soon come back to the intestine to become adults. Many other drugs, diclorvos, levamisole, and pyrantel to name a few, are effective against ascarids. A new drug, ivermectin, given subcutaneously shows great promise in eliminating migrating larvae. Treatment with oral anthelmintics must be continuous or repeated frequently and reinfection must be prevented using the principles of the McLean County system outlined earlier.

STRONGYLES (BLOODWORMS)

The large strongyles, *Strongylus vulgaris, S. edentatus,* and *S. Equinus* are perhaps the most important equine internal parasites and of these, *S. vulgaris* heads the list.

Development

Adult strongyles inhabit the large intestine, where they lay eggs that are passed out in the manure. The eggs undergo several development stages in manure or soil until they become infective third-stage larvae, which migrate upward in water films on grass, stable walls, and so on. When ingested, these larvae pass through the stomach to the large intestine. There they penetrate the intestinal wall, become a fourth-stage larvae in about a week, and enter the walls of nearby small arterioles. Their migration continues in the walls of progressively larger blood vessels until the majority end up in the wall of the anterior mesenteric artery, the principal artery supplying blood to the intestines. A few go beyond to the aorta. This migratory period lasting a couple months results in arterial inflammation, thrombosis, and embolism.

Eventually the larvae are carried in the arterial supply back to the small arterioles in the intestinal wall from which they emerge and undergo final development in nodules about the size of a pea. When sexually mature the adults leave these nodules to enter the large intestine, lay eggs, and repeat the cycle. The complete cycle requires six months or more.

Considerable physical damage is done to the arterial vessels through which the larvae migrate. Thrombi in the smaller vessels decrease blood supply to the intestine until collateral circulation can develop. Recurrent colic is a clinical sign associated with strongylosis. A more serious complication occurs when an aneurysm (ballooning of the arterial wall) develops ahead of an anterior mesenteric thrombus. As the aneurysm increases in size its wall gets thinner until it eventually bursts and the horse dies rapidly from internal hemorrhage.

Control

Unfortunately, during the most damaging phase of their life, strongyles are beyond the reach of common oral anthelmintics. It is necessary therefore to adopt control programs coupling prevention of reinfection with regular routine anthelmintic treatment. Worming all horses on the premises regularly every six to eight weeks will help to keep the strongyle population down, but it will not eradicate it. A number of good drugs are available, among them piperazine, phenothiazine, thiabendazole, mebendazole, coumaphos, and ivermectin. To prevent worm resistance from developing, drugs should be alternated. Strongyle control is an essential component of an equine health program.

PINWORMS (OXYURIS EQUI)

These are a plague shared by humans and horses. They have little significance as far as the health of the animal is concerned but are an annoyance.
Adult female pinworms lay their eggs in masses at the anus and their activity
causes an intense itching. Affected horses switch their tails and rub their back-
sides against anything handy, fence posts, walls or anything else that offers
relief. In so doing they may rub their tail head raw.

Anthelmintic treatment is not generally necessary, but the problem can be
solved by washing the anal area with warm soapy water as part of the daily
grooming procedure.

LIVER FLUKES
(FASCIOLA HEPATICA, DICROCELIUM DENDRITICUM)

Flukes are unique parasites in that part of their life cycles must be spent in
snails. *F. hepatica* undergoes several developmental stages in an aquatic environment and in the snail, without which it cannot become infective. Ruminants, especially sheep, are their chief victims but fortunately they are not a
problem in most herds or flocks because control is difficult at best.

Life Cycle

Eggs of the common fluke *F. hepatica* after about a week in water hatch
into free-swimming miracidia, enter snails where they encyst in the tissue, and
undergo further development during the next few weeks. Eventually they
emerge as cercariae and later become affixed to grass as encysted metacer-
cariae, which are then eaten by sheep along with the blade of grass. In the
intestine they emerge from the cyst, penetrate the gut wall, and wander
through the peritoneal cavity until they find the liver. They penetrate the liver
and migrate in it until they find the bile ducts, where they develop to adults.
The duration of the life cycle is shorter in hot weather, longer in cold weather,
and ceases in freezing weather. Most infections occur during the summer
months. *D. dendriticum* is slightly different, in that it utilizes a terrestrial
rather than an aquatic snail. Cercariae are in slime balls produced by the snail.
Ants eat the slime balls and sheep in turn eat the ants along with grass and
become infected.

Effects

The effects of liver flukes on sheep and cattle may be acute or chronic. The
acute disease occurs when there is massive invasion of the liver by the developing flukes. Symptoms include abdominal pain, lack of appetite, reluctance
to move, and death. Chronic fluke disease is characterized by gradual weight
loss, anemia, weakness, and edema. Liver damage caused by flukes predisposes to the rapidly fatal "black disease" caused by *Cl. novyi*.

Control

Control of flukes is difficult. Reduction of the snail population through use of molluscicides such as copper sulfate is helpful but usually runs afoul of environmental protection laws. Fencing sheep out of wet areas or draining the areas is helpful where practical. None of these methods is practical in areas where pastures must be irrigated.

Several drugs, such as albendazole and clorsulon, are available for removal of adult and immature flukes in sheep, but proper precautions must be observed in their use. With the limited control procedures available, it's not surprising that in some areas where the fluke population is high it is simply not profitable to grow sheep.

LUNGWORMS

Dictyocaulus viviparous in cattle and *D. filariae* in sheep and goats develop to maturity in the lungs. Other parasite larvae such as *Ascaris suum* may invade the lung and reside there temporarily. *Metastrongylus spp.* infect swine and play a role in the transmission of swine influenza.

Adult lungworms lay eggs in the lung which are coughed up and swallowed with mucus. The embryonated eggs pass out in the manure and hatch in two to three days and are then ingested by animals. The earthworm is an intermediate host for *Metastrongylus* and pigs get infected when they eat earthworms. The larvae thrive in moisture and warmth. Although most infections occur during the pasture season, serious outbreaks have occurred in winter when stabled calves lick walls wet with condensation where infective larvae congregate. Ingested larvae penetrate the intestinal wall and are carried via the lymphatics to the lung where they mature.

Except under unusual circumstances, lungworm infections do not reach serious proportions and may even be self-limiting. Young animals are more susceptible than old. Clinical signs when they occur include chronic cough, unthriftiness, and abnormal lung sounds. Secondary bacterial pneumonia is not unusual.

Control by vaccination of young animals is widely practiced in Europe but as yet a vaccine has not been licensed here. Several drugs are available for treatment when necessary, but because diagnosis is not easy, it would pay to consult your veterinarian. Infestation in pigs can be minimized by keeping them in paved feedlots where they won't contact earthworms.

TAPEWORMS

Tapeworms in livestock are in most cases relatively innocuous as far as the animal is concerned and clinical disease due to tapeworm is rare in this country.

The "beef tapeworm" and the "pork tapeworm" are really human tapeworms that spend their larval stages in cattle and hogs. Animals get these worms when they ingest feed or water contaminated by human feces. Prevention therefore is dependent on improved sanitary habits by humans. In societies where people are less fastidious and live close to their animals so that human and animal fecal contamination occurs readily, these parasites cause significant health problems.

KIDNEY WORM (STEPHANURUS DENTATUS)

This unique worm of swine occasionally causes problems in some herds. The larvae when ingested migrate for several months, particularly in the liver, and eventually terminate their wanderings in cysts in the kidneys, ureters, and surrounding tissue. Eggs are passed out in the urine. Migrating larvae can infect piglets in the uterus.

The entire life cycle takes upwards of a year and a half, which lends itself to a control procedure by management alone. Since the life cycle is so long, slaughtered hogs go to the market before any eggs are laid. If breeding is confined to gilts using young boars and they are slaughtered when the litter is weaned, there is no opportunity for the kidney worm life cycle to be completed. Following this procedure for several years should render the premises free of kidney worm provided no swine over two years of age are retained. Drugs are not effective in controlling this disease.

HABRONEMIASIS (SUMMER SORES)

Habronema spp. and *Draschia spp.* are relatively innocuous stomach worms of the horse. However, when their larvae are transferred by flies from manure to moist or abraded skin they invade the skin to cause a chronic red, weeping sore that becomes thickened and bleeds easily. The lesions itch and the horse keeps them raw from rubbing. Treatment with the usual antiseptics alone usually fails. Larvae carried by flies to the eye may migrate in the lacrimal discharge to the conjunctiva and establish a chronic infection there.

Fly control and protection of wounds with fly repellents help to prevent habronemiasis. When infection occurs, local treatment with antiseptics coupled with systemic insecticides such as ronnel, thiabendazole, or ivermectin is helpful.

HORSE BOTS

These are not worms such as we have been discussing but are the larval stage of one of several species of flies belonging to the genus *Gasterophilus*. They are included here because the larvae are parasitic.

Life Cycle
The adult *G. intestinalis* lays its eggs on the hair particularly of the lower foreleg. These are cream-colored, slightly smaller than a pin-head and cemented on so tightly that it is impossible to brush them off. They remain there

until, under the stimulation of warmth and moisture from the animals licking, they hatch. The larvae then ride on the tongue to the mouth where they embed themselves in the mucosal surface of the gums, cheeks, and tongue. *G. haemorrhoidalis* deposits its eggs on the hairs around the mouth and they hatch without stimulation. *G. nasalis* deposits its eggs in the throat region.

After a month or so in the mouth, the larvae travel to the stomach where they attach themselves to the stomach wall and slowly enlarge over the next eight to nine months. When the larva is ready, it releases its hold on the stomach wall, passes out in manure, pupates and finally emerges as a fly. The whole cycle takes about a year — yet the fly lives only about two weeks.

The adult flies are annoying to horses, causing them to run or seek shelter in the brush or shade. But the most damaging aspect is when the bots are in the stomach. Digestive disturbances and colic are not infrequent with heavy infestations, although a few bots in a well-nourished horse usually do not cause any difficulty at all. Rarely mature bot larvae in the pyloric end of the stomach may be sufficiently numerous to cause physical obstruction, leading to recurrent bouts of acute indigestion.

Control

Control of bots on an individual owner basis is very difficult. The flies travel considerable distances and unless practiced by every horse owner in the area, bot fly control is of little value. The assumption, usually correct, is that all horses have bots and treatment of bots is routine in all well-managed stables. The best time to treat for bots is late in the fall when, in most of the United States, frost has killed all the flies and the larvae have completed their migration to the stomach. A number of drugs is available but the favorite of many veterinarians and horse owners is still carbon disulfide given via stomach tube. It's an old remedy and dangerous if misused, but it works well. It is gradually being superseded by products such as dichlorvos, trichlorfon, and ivermectin.

External Parasites

LICE

Of all the external parasites of animals, lice are perhaps the most adaptable in terms of survival and are ubiquitous. They can afflict all livestock species and human beings anywhere in the world. They have been known for centuries as a pest of man and beast.

Lice are divided into two broad classes, those that suck and those that bite. The sucking lice actually suck blood from the host while the biting lice feed on cellular debris and exudate on the skin. Many different louse species exist but fortunately those that thrive on one species of animal generally will not colonize on another. If they did, most livestock owners would themselves have lice! Host specificity is helpful when considering control procedures.

Effects

As far as the effect on the animal is concerned, the one thing all lice, biting or sucking, have in common is that they make the animal itch. The itching is so intense at times that animals rub themselves raw. Sucking lice are occasionally sufficiently numerous on an animal to cause anemia and, in extreme cases, death.

Diagnosis

Diagnosis of pediculosis is not difficult and a presumptive diagnosis can often be made from some distance away. For example, if you see bits of hair or wool stuck on posts, rails, wire, or trees in the barnyard, you can be sure the animals have lice or mange and the odds favor lice. If on the animals themselves you see patches of hair pulled out or areas where the hair is broken off from rubbing, you are probably dealing with lice. If you part the hair at the periphery of these patches and look closely in good light you will probably see lice on the skin or their eggs, called nits, stuck on the hairs. A magnifying glass makes observation easier and more certain. In cattle, horses, and goats, lice are more likely to be found along the topline from the tail head to the withers. The head and feet are frequent sites of infestation in sheep. Nits, smaller than a pinhead and grayish white in color, will be found in great numbers attached to the hair near the skin. Finding these, even without seeing any adult lice, is adequate justification for a control program. Problems with lice are more likely to be encountered in winter than summer and when animals are kept in close confinement.

Control

For the owner of an individual horse or two, lice are not likely to be a problem if the animals are groomed daily, and brushes are used on your animals only. The herd or flock problem is a different situation requiring mass treatment methods such as spraying or dipping. Dustbags and backrubbers laced with insecticide and placed where cattle have to use them are helpful.

Insecticide powders dusted on the top line of stabled cattle help to keep the louse population under control and systemic insecticides help control sucking lice. Except on lactating cattle or goats, ivermectin has proven to be a useful injectable drug for treatment of pediculosis. But when many animals are showing clinical signs of pediculosis, dipping or high pressure spraying are the only answers. There are many good insecticides on the market that will kill lice. Very few of these may legally be used on dairy cattle and dairy goats. In fact, the legal restrictions on the use of insecticides are so voluminous that they will not be listed here. The regulations would probably be changed again by the time this manuscript is converted to print, anyhow.

Suffice to say the livestock owner should follow the label warning on whatever insecticide he ultimately uses. Failure to do so could result in milk or tissue residues, which, if detected, could result in condemnation of the product and legal proceedings against the producer.

Last, whatever product is used as a spray or dip should be repeated in about two weeks to allow time for the eggs to hatch. Insecticides do not affect the nits but a second treatment will get those recently hatched. And, since lice commonly spend time off the host, it's important to spray the stable area as well.

MANGE

All classes of livestock are susceptible to mange, which is a dermatitis caused by one of the several species of microscopic mites. *Sarcoptes* is the mite found often affecting horses and swine. Intense itching, especially around the head and neck, papule and vesicle formation, acute dermatitis, and wrinkling of the skin characterize this form of mange. It spreads rapidly on the animal and to other animals. Left untreated, the disease can be sufficiently debilitating to be fatal.

Chorioptic mange is the type usually encountered in cattle. Like sarcoptic it causes intense itching but starts most commonly around the tail head, escutcheon and down the inside of the hind legs. Cattle mange is often called "barn itch."

Psoroptes is the other major genus of mange mite generally associated with sheep. However, any of the three, *Sarcoptes, Chorioptes* and *Psoroptes,* can infect any animal species. Distinction can be made between them on the basis of clinical signs and morphologic characteristics when examined under the microscope. Psoroptic mange is particularly serious in sheep because it causes the wool to fall out in ragged patches ruining the fleece and causing

Sheep scabies.

great economic loss. Because of its seriousness, psoroptic mange is a legally reportable disease.

A fourth type of mange, *demodectic,* is of minor importance in livestock. The organism does not spread rapidly and colonizes in the hair follicles. It may occasionally cause small papules or nodules filled with cheesy material. Demodectic mange is frequently self-limiting and treatment is of little avail.

Treatment

Treatment of the other three types of mange is essential for the comfort and productivity of the animal. Dipping or high-pressure sprays are the preferred application methods but here again, choice of insecticides is severely restricted by law. Nothing is superior to lindane for mange mites, or lice for that matter, but it cannot be used except in special circumstances by permission of livestock officials. Where permitted, thiabendazole given orally effectively controls demodectic mange. Ivermectin injectable is also effective but may not be used on lactating dairy cattle. For food-producing animals, the USDA recommends dipping in 1 percent warm lime sulfur solution. This must be repeated several times at weekly intervals. If you have reason to suspect mange in your herd or flock, I'd strongly recommend that you have your veterinarian help you work out a treatment procedure that is practical.

SHEEP KEDS

The ked, *Melophagus ovinus,* is an important blood-sucking parasite of sheep. It spends its entire life cycle on the sheep, and the female, rather than laying eggs, gives birth to a larva which attaches to the wool and pupates. The life cycle spans a period of about four months.

Keds become quite numerous in winter and early spring and the irritation of their feeding causes sheep to rub and bite, particularly around the shoulder, flanks, and rump.

Dipping is the most effective way to treat sheep and the best time is immediately after shearing. Unless a residual insecticide can be used, dipping will have to be repeated to get the keds which haven't yet emerged from the pupal case.

TICKS

Although ticks themselves are parasites depending on a blood meal for their survival, their primary importance may be as vectors of diseases such as tularemia, Rocky Mountain Spotted Fever, Q fever, and babesiasis.

Life Cycle

The typical tick life cycle involves mating on the host, and engorgement of the female with blood. At that time she drops to the ground and begins laying eggs which hatch in about two weeks into larvae or "seed ticks." These crawl up on vegetation and brush and remain there as long as eight months waiting for an animal to come by. When the animal brushes up against the plant, the larvae hop on for a ride and a blood meal. These then drop to the ground to become nymphs and the process is repeated. Ultimately the nymphs develop into adults, which also wait in the vegetation for a blood meal to walk by. The animals attacked by larvae, nymph, and adult may be all the same species or different and man may be one of them. A few ticks spend their life cycles on a single host. Adult ticks are most likely to be seen on animals in late summer and early fall.

A few ticks, although they suck blood, are usually tolerated by the animal. However, heavy infestations cause severe irritation and anemia, with affected animals being very uncomfortable as well as lethargic and unthrifty. The spinose ear tick prevalent in the Southwest crawls into the ear canal to cause pain and irritation.

Treatment

A few ticks on an animal can be removed manually, taking care not to break off the mouth parts by which the tick is attached. Gentle traction is generally all that is required but an old trick may accelerate the process. Light a match, blow it out, and apply the hot head to the body of the tick. This usually encourages it to let go in a hurry. This method is obviously impractical if many ticks are present, in which case dipping or spraying is the only resort. The same problems and precautions apply to use of insecticides for ticks as apply for lice and mange.

FLIES

Several different flies are important to livestock for the annoyance they cause, because they are vectors of other diseases, or because they are parasitic. Since the attack of a fly is quick and transitory, control is generally based upon repellents incorporating insecticides rather than upon insecticides alone.

Horse flies, deer flies, stable flies, and **horn flies** are all blood-sucking flies that cause great annoyance to livestock and consequently reduce productivity. The bite of the first three is painful, and when these pests are about, animals will run trying to get away from them. Horse flies are important vectors of equine infectious anemia and any of the biting flies can transmit anaplasmosis. Efforts to control these pests are time well spent but not always very successful. The tabanids — horse flies and deer flies — are particularly hard to control. Their feeding habit is to swoop in, get a quick suck of blood and take off again, leaving little time for exposure to insecticides. Where it can be done practically, the best way to protect livestock from these pests may be to allow them to run inside out of the sun. The tabanids don't care much for shade and they usually stay outside when animals come in.

Control

Stable flies (and houseflies) breed in manure and decaying vegetable matter. An essential part of their control is good housekeeping, keeping manure from accumulating around the barn. Residual sprays inside and outside the barn are also helpful. What may become the most important manner of control is feeding insecticides to the animal that are carried through in the manure so that the manure is toxic to fly maggots. Horse flies, since they stay on the animal, are more susceptible to locally applied insecticides. Both back rubbers and dustbags give good control. These can be supplemented with insecticide impregnated plastic ear tags or similar devices attached to the halter on horses.

Myiasis is the term given to invasion of animal tissues by fly larvae, and there are several flies capable of doing this. History records the practice at one time of deliberately placing fly maggots in wounds to clean up the cellular debris. The most dramatic myiasis is that caused by the *screwworm* in the Southwest. Adult screwworms deposit their eggs in open wounds — or anywhere there is a drop of fresh blood. These hatch and the larvae burrow into living tissue, feeding as they go. Left untreated, a colony of screwworm larvae can literally eat an animal alive.

For years, prevention of wound infestation with repellents or bandages and frequent inspection and treatment of animals when necessary was all that could be done to prevent losses. A quirk in the screwworm fly's breeding habits has made it possible to almost eradicate this pest. The female mates only once and the males can easily be sterilized by irradiation. USDA is raising flies by the millions, sterilizing and releasing them in the endemic area. When the female mates with a sterile male, no viable eggs are produced. This program has been spectacularly successful and is being extended to northern Mexico to create a buffer zone where no screwworms are present.

While the screwworm is the only fly maggot that regularly eats living flesh, the **wool maggot** occasionally gets that voracious. These are blow fly larvae which hatch from eggs deposited in the wool next to the skin, particularly under the tail and between the hindlegs where the wool is most likely to be soiled and damp. The maggots start out feeding on the wool but as they progress toward the head they begin to develop an appetite for skin and subcutaneous tissue. Such activity can be rapidly fatal to a sheep. "Tagging," shearing, dipping, spraying and use of repellents on wounds have all been used to prevent "fly strike."

Cattle grub

Several flies spend part of their life cycle as parasites of animals. Of these the most dramatic is the cattle grub, *Hypoderma spp.* Two species, *H. bovis* and *H. lineatum,* are recognized. The adult flies, which resemble small bumblebees, only live about a week during which they lay eggs on the hair of the lower legs of cattle. These hatch and the larvae penetrate the skin and begin a migration that takes almost a year. Larvae have been found in connective tissue

Ox warbles.

throughout the body but particularly around the esophagus and spinal cord. After six months or more of apparently aimless migration, the larvae localize in the subcutaneous tissue along the topline. Then they encyst and bore a hole through the skin for a breathing pore. They gradually enlarge as spring wears on and by May and June in the northern states have reached the size of about half an inch in diameter and an inch long. At this time they emerge, fall to the ground, pupate, and become flies.

In yearlings there may be 100 or more of these large lumps on the back each containing a heel fly larva but the numbers decrease in subsequent years as cattle get older. The principal economic effect of these grubs is through damage to the hide. The breathing pores leave scars, making that section of hide useless for fine leather.

Several systemic insecticides are available for use on beef cattle. Timing of application, however, is important: It should be applied as soon as the active heel fly season ends. Once the grubs are in the back, the damage is done and, because of their size, destroying them then with insecticides may lead to serious tissue reaction. Be sure to follow directions carefully when using systemic insecticides. Unfortunately these systemic insecticides may not be used on lactating dairy cattle. At present, only rotenone is approved for application to the animal's back where presumably it comes in contact with the grubs through the breathing hole they have made. With only a few animals it's about equally effective to manually express the mature grubs and then step on them.

Sheep Nose Bot

The sheep nose bot *Oestrus ovis* spends part of its life cycle resident in the nasal passages and sinuses of sheep and goats. The adult flies terrify sheep as they zoom in and deposit larvae at the nostrils. When the flies are active it's not unusual to see sheep running or standing with their noses tucked tightly in each other's flanks. Sometimes, they will stand in a circle with their heads together for mutual protection in a defense posture reminiscent of the wagon train.

Once deposited, the larvae migrate into the nasal passages and develop slowly over a period of months. As the larvae get larger and more active the sheep sneeze and shake their heads in an attempt to dislodge them. Sufficient irritation may be produced to cause a blood-tinged mucopurulent discharge. At maturity the larvae find their way out to the ground, pupate, and emerge as flies to repeat the cycle.

Ruelene given as a drench is reported useful as a control procedure. If you have never drenched sheep before, get someone to show you how. It's about as easy to put the medication in the lungs and drown the sheep as it is to get it in the stomach where it belongs. Other drugs such as ivermectin and trichlorfon may be used in injectable form.

Until recent years not much consideration was given to reducing the ravages of parasitism through immunization. Emphasis was on reducing infection by breaking the life cycle by use of chemicals or changes in management where appropriate. Accelerating interest on the part of immunologists, parasitologists, and epidemiologists is now bringing us closer to the reality of immunizing agents for control of at least some of the internal parasites and external parasites that plague humans and animals.

Metabolic Diseases

METABOLIC DISEASES ARE INTRINSIC IN ORIGIN and represent a breakdown of normal body function. They are not contagious or infectious. However, the same external factors — nutrition, production, stress, and so on — that precipitate a disease such as ketosis in one cow may trigger it in others, giving the illusion of a contagious disease.

The metabolic diseases of livestock are not many in number but collectively each year they cost the industry millions of dollars. Fortunately, if one understands the basis for them most are preventable through management.

BOVINE KETOSIS (ACETONEMIA, HYPOGLYCEMIA)

This is an important problem of high-producing dairy cattle that is really not a discrete disease entity but is a symptom of a sequence of events leading to an excess of ketones in the blood.

Primary ketosis occurs when the cow mobilizes body fat for energy at a rate faster than ketones can be eliminated. This is most common during the peak of milk production when the cow is either not offered enough or cannot consume enough nutrients, particularly energy, to meet her needs for milk production as well as maintenance. **Secondary ketosis** may occur anytime appetite is depressed as a result of diseases such as mastitis, metritis, displaced abomasum, or as a result of malnutrition. It may be aggravated by feeding poor-quality grass silage that has a high butyric acid content.

The presence of a modest level of ketone bodies, acetoacetic acid, B-hydroxybutyric acid, and acetone in body tissues is normal. These are byproducts of the breakdown of stored fat into fatty acids and up to a point can be used by the cow as an energy source. However, when energy requirements exceed energy intake, the rate of body fat catabolism accelerates, with production of these ketones in excess of the cow's ability to utilize them. When this happens abnormal levels of ketones appear in blood, milk and urine where they are readily detectable by chemical means. Unfortunately, high ketone levels have a depressant effect on appetite, so that the cow who needs more energy intake to counteract the ketosis usually has no interest in high-energy feeds.

While the foregoing is a simple rational explanation, it leaves some questions unanswered. For example, why is ketosis more prevalent in a given herd some years than it is in others and why is it more common in some cow families than others? Why do some cows of equal body weight producing equal amounts of milk have ketosis year after year while others never do? These are questions for which we don't have the answers as yet although considerable research has been and is being done on these problems.

Several factors have been suggested that may lead to primary ketosis:

- **Glucose drain to meet lactation requirements.** Milk is high in lactose, which comes from glucose. It has been established that high-producing cows need as much as 1 kilogram of glucose daily from dietary carbohydrates to meet the need for lactose. If nutrient intake is inadequate the cow will make up the deficit from body fat. This may be the most important factor, since ketosis almost invariably coincides with peak lactation.

- **Endocrine disorders.** There is some evidence that exhaustion of the adrenal and pituitary glands during peak lactation accounts for gluconeogenesis failures. Substitution therapy, using ACTH or glucocorticoids, produces a favorable response in some ketotic cows, lending some credence to this hypothesis.

- **Liver dysfunction.** The liver is an important organ in the conversion of free fatty acids to glucose and plays a role in the detoxification of ketones. A consistent finding in ketosis cases of long duration is a degenerative change — fatty infiltration of the liver. A similar change is seen in cows that are obese, lending support to the theory that fat cows are more prone to develop ketosis.

- **Protein excess.** It has been reported that ketosis has been produced experimentally by feeding excess protein. Protein may add extra ketogenic amino acids to the diet. In herds with a major ketosis problem where protein was being fed in excess of requirements, reduction of protein intake has been beneficial.

- **Vitamin or mineral deficiencies.** Over the years ketosis has been ascribed to deficiency of a variety of minerals and vitamins. However, with the exception of cobalt, which is essential to the enzyme systems involved in gluconeogenesis, it is doubtful that deficiencies are a factor.

- **High intake of ketogenic materials.** It is reasonably well established that intake of ketogenic materials such as butyric acid found in poor-quality silage will contribute to a herd ketosis problem.

Clinical Signs

Almost invariably primary ketosis occurs in the range of one to six weeks after calving. Perhaps the earliest sign the alert herd managers will notice is a lack of eye lustre. This is followed by a decline in milk production and a selective loss of appetite. Typically, the cow will refuse first grain, then silage and finally hay. Concurrently there will be rapid loss of body weight and the manure will become dry and hard. Herd managers with a good sense of smell report that ketotic cows have a characteristic sweetish acetone odor in their milk and on their breath. Onset of the disease signs may be quite sudden or they may be insidious, stretching over several weeks.

A few (about 1 percent) cows with ketosis will exhibit signs of neurological disturbances such as pushing against walls, bellowing, and incoordination. Being a metabolic disorder rather than infectious in nature, ketosis rarely causes any elevation of body temperature.

A simple rapid chemical test is available for the detection of acetoacetic acid and acetone in the milk or urine. The test is more sensitive when used with urine because ketone levels are higher in urine than in milk. Discretion must be used in interpretation of test results. Many normal cows will show a positive reaction so test results must be correlated with clinical signs to reach a positive diagnosis. Also the test will not detect B-hydroxybutyic acid. In a few ketotic cows this compound will predominate and test results will be negative although all clinical signs indicate ketosis.

Treatment

Because of the complexity of the disease and the poor response to treatment of some cases, literally hundreds of compounds and concoctions have been tried over the years. Most are worthless, but a few have real value.

Ketotic cows are always low in blood glucose. The standard therapy that produces good results is glucose solution given intravenously. Unfortunately, while it is very effective, its effect is transitory, lasting only about two hours, after which blood glucose levels begin to fall again. However, for many cows the brief respite it affords is often sufficient to allow their metabolic equilibrium to return to normal and they proceed to recover. It may be given as often as necessary to promote recovery. A more dilute solution given by slow I.V. drip over a period of twenty-four to forty-eight hours is more effective, but the apparatus and restraint required are cumbersome.

Orally both propylene glycol and sodium propionate have been effective, and 6 to 8 ounces of either given three times daily to supplement I.V. glucose is helpful in refractory cases.

Use of steroid hormones such as dexamethasone provides good stimulus to gluconeogenesis and it is often used in conjunction with glucose. However, steroids have a depressant effect on antibody production that can lead to complications such as infection. For that reason, they should be used cautiously, keeping in mind that serious complications may result. The hormone ACTH to stimulate the adrenals is safer but somewhat less effective.

The diagnosis in unresponsive cases should be carefully reevaluated for the presence of other concurrent disease problems. Displaced abomasum typically presents a clinical picture not unlike ketosis even to the usual time of occurrence shortly after parturition.

Prevention

As with all diseases, prevention is far more valuable than treatment and some recommendations can be made that will reduce the prevalence of ketosis.

- Pay close attention to dry cows. Reduce energy intake during the early weeks to keep them from getting too fat.

- Begin to feed some grain, 2 to 4 pounds daily, during the last two weeks of the dry period to condition rumen bacteria to utilization of grain.

- Increase grain intake immediately after calving at the rate of 1½ to 2 pounds daily until milk production peaks. This will provide maximum energy intake when the cow needs it most. Increasing grain at a faster rate may induce indigestion with acidosis and precipitate ketosis.

- Use good quality hay and silage. Avoid using silage that has a spoiled or rancid odor.

OVINE KETOSIS
(PREGNANCY DISEASE, KETOSIS, PREGNANCY TOXEMIA)

Physiologically, this disease of sheep bears some resemblance to ketosis of cows in that the clinical signs are brought on by a metabolic failure resulting in an excess of ketones in the blood. The similarity ends there, although there are some common denominators.

Like bovine ketosis, ketosis in sheep is the result of a disparity in energy utilization compared with energy intake. In cows, the energy drain is from lactation; in sheep the loss is brought about by the needs of a developing single large lamb or, more often, twin lambs. Characteristically, pregnancy disease occurs late in gestation, often during the last week or two, in ewes that have been on a gradually declining plane of nutrition. To the inexperienced observer this may not appear to be the case when the body weight lost by the ewe is replaced by the bulk of the fetus. The disease can be precipitated in fat ewes by withholding feed twenty-four to forty-eight hours, abrupt change in diet, or the stress of inclement weather. Sometimes these factors combine to cause so many cases in a short period of time that it seems an infectious agent must be to blame.

Symptoms

Neurological signs characterize the disease in ewes. They will stand aloof from the flock, blunder into objects if they move, and sometimes stand with their heads pressing against a wall or fence for hours on end. Apparent blindness is common. As the disease progresses, muscle twitching, circling, and spasmodic jerking of the head may occur. Eventually convulsions occur with intervals of rest between. This pattern continues for three or four days followed by a period of prostration and death.

Treatment

While a dairy cow with ketosis will lose weight rapidly and milk production declines to a point where energy needs balance with energy intake, the cow recovers. Not so with sheep. Mortality from pregnancy toxemia with or without treatment is high. Once the clinical signs are fully developed, response to treatment is poor. Intravenous glucose repeated frequently will help and an occasional ewe can be saved by a prompt Caesarean if it can be done with minimal stress. Corticosteroids have not given consistently good results in sheep. Sodium propionate and propylene glycol given to other pregnant ewes in the flock may prevent additional cases from occurring if at the same time energy content of the ration is increased.

Management is the best prevention. Keep the ewe flock on a diet adequate for maintenance and raise the energy content gradually during gestation. Be sure ewes get adequate exercise and protect them from the stress of inclement weather during late pregnancy.

POSTPARTURIENT PARESIS (MILK FEVER, HYPOCALCEMIA)

Milk fever, sometimes called **parturient paresis,** is a metabolic disease seen primarily in dairy cattle manifested by onset at or near parturition, loss of appetite, stasis of the digestive tract, stilted gait, paresis, prostration, and death. This sequence of symptoms may occur over a period of two to twenty-four hours. There is usually some premonitory indication of the disease before the cow goes down. A similar condition is seen with less frequency in sheep and goats.

Calcium Loss

High-producing cows are most susceptible to milk fever and it is seen more commonly in the Jersey breed. However, high milk production is not essential to the onset of the disease because it is occasionally seen in beef cows and mediocre dairy cattle. The precipitating factor is the sudden loss of calcium (up to 20 grams/day) in colostrum in excess of the rate of calcium replacement from the digestive tract and stored reserves in bone. The result is a hypocalcemia which, if uncorrected, leads to progressive development of the symptoms listed above.

Serum calcium levels are controlled by an interrelationship between calcium (Ca) and phosphorus (P) intake, serum P levels, vitamin D, Ca and P reserves, the parathyroid and thyroid glands, and the age of the animal. The normal serum calcium level ranges from 9–12 mg/100 ml. With the onset of lactation, it may drop to 7 mg/100 ml and if it continues to fall below 5 mg/100 ml milk fever generally occurs. This physiologically normal decline to 7 mg is directly related to calcium loss in colostrum. It does not occur in mastectomized cows (cows with the mammary gland surgically removed).

Calcium Mobilization

Normally the lost calcium is replaced within a few hours through mobilization of stored calcium reserves in bone under the influence of parathyroid hormone and vitamin D. This happens only if the parathyroid is physiologically active. In cows that develop milk fever, the parathyroid is frequently inactive, resulting in failure of calcium mobilization. The rate of calcium intake has an important bearing on parathyroid activity. If the rate of intake is very high, as for example, on a high legume diet, absorption from the gut alone will be adequate to maintain serum calcium levels during the dry period. There will be little exchange of calcium in bone and the gland becomes more or less dormant. Second, Ca and P in serum are normally in equilibrium. A deficiency of one will simulate an excess of the other as far as the parathyroid is concerned. Therefore, to maintain parathyroid activity, Ca and P intakes should be approximately in balance and the total intake of each should be in line with established recommendations.

Vitamin D

Vitamin D has an important influence on calcium metabolism. It has some effect on the absorption of Ca from the intestine but has a profound influence on calcium in bone. Excessive doses will cause a rapid increase in serum calcium at the expense of bone reserve. The serum calcium level may increase beyond the animal's capacity to eliminate it, resulting in precipitation of calcium in soft tissues, especially heart muscle. At the same time there will be a loss of bone strength due to depletion of mineral content. Therefore, although many workers have established that the prevalence of milk fever can be reduced by administration of 20 million units of vitamin D daily for five days prior to calving, the procedure is not without risk.

The effect of vitamin D raises the question of deficiency. Under normal conditions in mature cattle, vitamin D deficiency probably does not occur. It is synthesized in the skin through the action of sunlight. However, in total confinement housing where the cattle are rarely, if ever, outside, our thinking may have to be revised and we may find it advantageous to supplement the diet with small amounts of vitamin D.

Age plays a part in Ca metabolism, too. As cows get older, the rate of absorption from the gut decreases. More important, calcium in bone tends to become more tightly bound with increasing age and therefore is not as readily mobilized on demand. This is a possible explanation of the observation that milk fever rarely occurs in first-calf heifers but increases in prevalence among older cows.

Treatment

It has been established that the thyroid gland has an indirect influence on calcium mobilization. Excessively high levels of serum calcium stimulate release of thyrocalcitonin from the thyroid, inhibiting the parathyroid. This mechanism can be triggered by intravenous administration of calcium. Standard treatment of milk fever is I.V. administration of 500 cc of 25 to 25 percent calcium gluconate. This will cause a transitory rise in serum calcium to about 20 mg/100 ml. The excess is dissipated rapidly so that within a few hours the serum calcium level is back down to normal or below normal again if some mobilization has not occurred. It is postulated that this sudden high increase in calcium may precipitate the thyrocalcitonin response, leading to the relapses that sometimes occur. Until a quantitative field test for serum calcium becomes available, this is probably one of the hazards of milk fever therapy that will continue to be accepted.

The alternative in treatment is to revert to the standard procedure of fifty years ago, namely insufflation of (inflating with air) the udder to suppress the flow of milk. This is effective although not as dramatic in response as I.V. therapy. Mastitis is a hazard, of course, but the relatively slow response (two to six hours) is a more important disadvantage.

Prevention

As with every disease, prevention is infinitely more valuable than treatment. Total intake of Ca and P must be adequate according to the body weight of the cow. The N.R.C. recommendations are a good guide. Second, the intake of each should be balanced so that there is not a substantial excess of either. The Ca:P ratio in the diet should not exceed 2:1 and should be close to 1:1. In problem herds, this need will usually necessitate a forage analysis and alteration of the ration and/or addition of additives such as dicalcium phosphate or other phosphorus supplement. Injection of large (10 million) units of vitamin D a week prior to calving seems to prevent some cases of milk fever.

The "Downer" Cow

One question that always arises in connection with milk fever is the problem of the alert "downer" cow. These cases usually begin as milk fever and respond to therapy to the extent that they are alert, eat reasonably well, and attempt to rise but cannot do so. At one time it was thought that this might be a manifestation of potassium deficiency. However, results of potassium replacement therapy were disappointing.

It now seems apparent from numerous necropsies that many of these cases are the result of muscular, ligamentous, or skeletal injuries sustained during the initial hypocalcemic paresis. Cows down with milk fever in a cramped position for as little as an hour have been shown to develop degenerative muscle changes that make them physically unable to rise. Ruptured ligaments and tendons and, occasionally, fractures have been found. These lesions are probably due to the weight of the animal and the exertion of trying to get up during the hypocalcemic period when coordination is poor. The problem is compounded when the cow is confined in a stanchion or is lying on a hard slippery surface with no bedding. Good nursing care is essential for "downer" cows and the longer they are down, the poorer the prognosis. Rotating them from one side to the other every hour helps prevent decubital sores and, if cows will tolerate it, use of a sling to help them to their feet frequently is worthwhile.

Most milk fever can be prevented by paying attention to Ca and P intake during the dry period. By forage analysis and arithmetical calculation you can keep intake of both within recommended limits and in proper ratio. For the few that don't respond to dietary management, don't delay treatment until the cow goes down. Milk fever almost always occurs within twenty-four hours of calving, and affected cows always have a glassy eye, absence of rumen activity and a stilted gait before they go down. Treatment before they go down brings about uneventful recovery although it may need repeating. Waiting until the cows are down carries with it a risk of injury from which they may never recover.

AZOTURIA (BLACK WATER, MONDAY MORNING DISEASE)

This once-common disease of horses has declined in frequency along with the passing of the draft horse. Nevertheless, it is still seen occasionally in horses that are worked hard and may bear some relationship to the more frequently reported "tying-up syndrome."

Typically, azoturia appears in a horse that has been routinely working hard and is maintained on full feed. Symptoms develop a few hours after work begins following a couple days or more of complete rest. The sobriquet, "Monday morning disease," came about because it was seen most often on Monday following a weekend of rest.

Clinical Signs

Clinical signs begin soon after strenuous exercise starts. These include profuse sweating, stiff gait, and reluctance to move. If the horse is forced to continue working signs get progressively more severe until the horse goes down in severe pain, unable to rise. If the horse is given complete rest as soon as signs begin, they may disappear in a few hours.

Theoretically the disease comes about because excess glycogen is stored in muscle tissue at rest. When exercise begins it is rapidly metabolized, with one of the metabolic products being lactic acid. If this acid accumulates faster than it can be carried away by the blood stream, coagulation necrosis of muscle tissue occurs. Whether the theory is correct or not, there is no doubt that muscle tissue necrosis occurs, involving especially the heavy muscles of the hip and loin. Breakdown of muscle cells releases myoglobin, which gives the urine a dark coffee-colored appearance — hence the name, "blackwater." The tying-up syndrome produces similar although less severe clinical signs under similar conditions.

The clinical signs of azoturia are sufficiently clear cut that diagnosis is generally not difficult. If there is doubt, several chemical tests on the blood serum will clarify the issue and indicate the extent of the muscle damage. Your veterinarian should be called without delay but what you do in the interim may determine whether the horse recovers, becomes permanently lame, or dies. The most important thing is to **stop working the horse immediately** and keep him at rest but on his feet. Even walking him to the barn should be avoided until the situation can be evaluated. Application of moist hot packs to loin and rump may ease the pain and improve circulation to lessen lactic acid concentration.

Prevention

To prevent azoturia, feed your horse like your car. Just as the car needs more gas when pulling a load, so the horse needs more feed to produce energy. But when it's idling the car doesn't need as much gas and neither does the horse. When the horse isn't working, cut his grain ration in half. He won't love you for it but he will be much healthier.

HYPOMAGNESEMIA (GRASS TETANY, GRASS STAGGERS)

This disease affecting lactating cattle, sheep, and occasionally goats is the result of a decreased serum magnesium level. It occurs most often when animals are grazing lush pasture early in the spring. Relatively low levels of magnesium in lush grass compared to potassium and nitrogen apparently are responsible for decreased magnesium absorption and the onset of clinical signs. Grass pastures top-dressed with either potassium or nitrogen or both have been shown to produce hypomagnesemia more often than those without such practices. Nitrogen and potassium apparently reduce the soil availability of magnesium so that grasses growing rapidly on such soils are themselves low in magnesium. The same circumstances prevail in some latitudes when fall rains again stimulate rapid pasture growth and on cereal crop pasture. In fact, in some areas the disease is called "wheat pasture poisoning."

The precise mechanism by which hypomagnesemia comes about is not well known. Magnesium is excreted primarily in urine, and to a lesser extent in milk. The ruminant lacks a good homeostatic mechanism for magnesium balance and is therefore more susceptible to rapid loss or lack of intake. In most cases of the tetanic form of the disease there is hypocalcemia as well and it is standard practice to treat grass tetany with I.V. solutions containing calcium and magnesium.

It appears there may be two phases to hypomagnesemia, one being a chronic low level of serum magnesium that causes the disease we know as "grass tetany" only when triggered by some other factor — hypocalcemia, brief starvation, shipping, or weather stress.

Symptoms

Clinically the symptoms range from chronic to acute. A few animals in a herd with low serum magnesium levels may show vague signs such as unthriftiness, poor appetite, and dullness. After a few days of this they may develop more definitive signs such as a wild attitude, throwing the head about, or unsteady gait with exaggerated leg movements. Loud noises or sudden movements may precipitate a convulsion lasting several minutes with paddling motions of the legs. Similar signs are occasionally seen in calves on an exclusive milk diet as they approach two to three months of age.

The acute form of the disease in cattle and sheep may appear without warning with the animal going from a normal grazing attitude to almost maniacal behavior. Tossing the head, bellowing, and galloping are common until the animal staggers and falls in a convulsion. During the convulsion the eyes twitch, and the legs paddle or are stiffly extended. Frothing and champing of the jaws are common. Pulse and respiration are rapid and temperature is elevated due to exertion. When the convulsion subsides, the animal lies quietly, but a noise or touch may precipitate a recurrence. Symptomatically, acute hypomagnesemia strongly resembles acute urea poisoning. Although response to treatment is good, mortality is high because it's generally only about an hour from onset of signs to death. Acute hypomagnesemia is one of the few diseases in livestock medicine that can be considered an emergency. Others become that way through neglect.

Control

Despite our lack of complete understanding of the pathogenesis of hypomagnesemia, control procedures have been worked out that are quite helpful. Feeding magnesium oxide as a feed additive during the period of greatest vulnerability, top-dressing pastures with dolomitic limestone or magnesium oxide, or placing one or more magnesium "bullets" in the animal's stomach with a balling gun have all given satisfactory results. A switch from all-grass to grass-legume pastures is helpful in climates where this is possible. Feeding some dry hay in addition to pasture will also help prevent the disease. Protection from cold, inclement weather also helps especially to prevent the winter tetany seen in cattle maintained on marginal diets.

BRISKET DISEASE

This is of concern only to the owners of cattle pastured for long periods in the high mountain areas, generally over 7,000 feet. The disease generally affects less than 2 percent of the herd and is the direct result of constant exposure to the low oxygen tension prevalent at that altitude and higher. In an attempt to meet the tissue demand for oxygenated blood the heart works harder at those altitudes. In some animals this causes enlargement of the right side of the heart, a self-defeating attempt at compensation. Unless the valves increase in size proportionately to the body of the heart, leakage occurs, resulting in liver congestion and a call for even more oxygen.

The end result is brisket disease, leaving an animal with an enlarged heart, subcutaneous edema especially around the brisket, lack of stamina and appetite, loss of weight, rapid pulse, and labored breathing or collapse after exercise.

Treatment of these individuals is usually not practical although obviously oxygen would help. The next best thing is to move them carefully and without excitement to a lower altitude where spontaneous clinical recovery sometimes results. Pneumonia is a common sequel and may be prevented with antibiotics. Recovered animals should not be returned to high altitudes, nor should they be used for breeding on the chance theirs may be a hereditary weakness.

Deficiency Diseases

STRANGE AS IT MAY SEEM, the most commonly reported deficiency disease is inadequate protein and energy intake, a polite term for starvation. Whether through ignorance or indifference on the part of their owners, thousands of animals are maintained in a state of malnutrition, particularly during the winter months when feed must be brought to them.

The business of raising livestock is certainly governed by economics and feed costs are generally the largest single item of expense. It's logical, then, that cutting back on feed costs by reducing consumption is the most likely place to save money. But is it? Cutting back on feed consumption will save money in the long run only if you are presently overfeeding and your animals are too fat. It's common practice to "rough" the young stock through giving them only enough to stay alive on the premise that since they aren't producing meat or milk, only growing, they don't need much to eat. That's a false assumption, resulting in retarded growth, delayed sexual maturity, and decreased disease resistance.

If breeding must be delayed several months because the animal didn't grow large enough fast enough on a marginal diet, it means that many more months must elapse before the animal starts producing income. Where is the economy in that? Similarly, if you can get a hog to market in six months, why hold back on feed and wait eight months? Restricting feed intake below the needs of the animal is false economy.

When animals are fed adequate quantities of a variety of feedstuffs such as hay or pasture, grains, and silage, deficiency diseases are generally not a problem. Occasionally, however, specific mineral, trace element, or vitamin deficiencies will occur as a result of such things as deficiency in the soil where the crop was grown, feed spoilage or weather damage, oxidation in storage, overabundance of one element tying up another to make it unavailable, and other such factors. The following deficiency diseases of livestock are of sufficient importance to warrant some discussion.

RICKETS

This is a disease of young animals caused by vitamin D or phosphorus deficiency resulting in a failure of normal bone mineralization. Lesions are most pronounced as enlargements at the ends of the long bones (epiphyses) where the longitudinal growth of bone occurs. Lameness and fractures are common, but by themselves they are not sufficient basis for an accurate diagnosis. Other diseases such as hyperparathyroidism can cause similar signs. Rickets is not common but is more likely to be found in young ani-

Crooked legs due to improper bone development such as rickets.

mals raised in total confinement in an area of the barn where there is little or no sunlight. Specialized cells in the skin produce vitamin D under stimulation of ultraviolet rays from the sun. Although vitamin D can be added to feed stuffs such as milk replacer or grain, it does not occur naturally in sufficient quantity to prevent deficiency signs from developing if the animal is deprived of sunlight.

Prevention of rickets is contingent upon adequate phosphorus intake and regular exposure to sunshine or vitamin D supplementation. It's important before embarking on treatment of suspected rickets with vitamin D to be sure of the diagnosis. If the condition is actually due to calcium deficiency, injection of vitamin D would only make matters worse. Examination of the animal, the diet, the serum calcium and phosphorus levels, and X-rays histopathological examination of bone sections are often all necessary for an accurate diagnosis. It's a job for your veterinarian.

NUTRITIONAL HYPERPARATHYROIDISM (OSTEODYSTROPHIA FIBROSA)

This is perhaps the most common disease of young growing animals. The underlying cause is a deficiency of calcium in the diet, but the clinical signs are attributable to overactivity of the parathyroid gland. You may recall in our earlier discussion of milk fever that, as serum calcium levels drop, the parathyroid

"Big-head."

gland mobilizes stored calcium reserves in bone. Although with this disease the problem is with dietary calcium deficiency rather than calcium metabolism, the parathyroid activity is triggered the same way.

When calcium is deficient in the diet over a period of weeks or months, parathyroid hormone pulls compensating amounts out of the bones. Eventually the bones become sufficiently demineralized that they become deformed or fracture. The disease is most common in pigs and horses, perhaps because calcium deficiency is more likely to occur in animals maintained on all-grain diets. In the horse the disease is occasionally referred to as "bran disease" or "big-head," the latter because of the characteristic changes that occur in the bones of the head.

Treatment

Once the diagnosis is made, treatment consists primarily of rest and addition of calcium to the diet in the form of calcium carbonate or limestone. Restoration of normal calcium levels will not make any significant change in bone deformities but will restore normal strength to the bone reducing the possibility of future fractures.

This disease is readily and economically preventable by keeping calcium and phosphorus intake adequate and in balance. Refer to the chapter on nutrition for specific recommendations.

PARAKERATOSIS

This skin disease occurs in pigs and occasionally calves raised in confinement and fed exclusively on commercial diets. It does not occur in animals with access to pasture. The cause is an actual zinc deficiency in the diet or a relative deficiency induced by an overabundance of calcium. It responds well to addition of zinc to the ration.

Symptoms

In pigs, the principal effect of the disease is reduced rate of gain due to depressed appetite and less efficient feed conversion. The skin lesions appear first as reddened areas. These areas become papules, which develop crusts that may coalesce. There is symmetrical involvement of limbs, ears, and head. The crusts become quite thick and crack easily. Secondary bacterial infection of the affected skin is not unusual.

The skin lesions in cattle may be more extensive with loss of hair (alopecia) and wrinkling of the skin over the joints, scrotum, and neck. The disease has been diagnosed in sheep grazed on zinc-deficient soils. Loss of wool, wrinkling of the skin, and ram infertility are the prominent signs in sheep.

Prevention

Zinc in the form of carbonate or sulfate added to the diet relieves the symptoms rather rapidly. The disease can be prevented by being certain, through analysis, that the diet contains adequate amounts of zinc and by supplementation if necessary. If the calcium level is excessive, adjusting the ration composition to bring it down to normal will have a sparing effect on zinc so that a marginal level will be adequate.

VITAMIN A DEFICIENCY (AVITAMINOSIS A)

Vitamin A is one of the most important vitamins for livestock and is required in comparatively large amounts. Green feeds pasture grasses, hay, and corn contain ample amounts of carotene and carotenoids that animals readily convert to vitamin A, and deficiency is unlikely to occur in animals with access to these feedstuffs. Very young animals depend on colostrum and milk for their vitamin A needs. If the dam's reserves are low, deficiency may occur in the offspring.

Carotene is absorbed as vitamin A in the intestine and converted back to carotene for storage in the liver. A high proportion of carotene may be destroyed in the intestine and the rate of absorption conversion is influenced by availability, presence of phosphorus, calcium-phosphorus ratio, vitamin E, and levels of serum vitamin A. Required intake is higher during any disease due to lowered efficiency of conversion. If carotene intake is marginal, the liver reserve will be depleted in two to three months and deficiency signs will begin to appear.

Carotene (vitamin A) is rather unstable, tending to oxidize quite rapidly. Hay that has been weather damaged or in storage more than six months will have a low carotene content and supplementation is recommended for animals maintained on this type of diet. Grains, especially corn, have a high carotene content, but most commercial grain ratios have vitamin A added as a precautionary measure. Vitamin A deficiency is most likely to occur in animals maintained on diets that do not include forage crops and during the late winter months when the carotene stored in the liver is depleted.

Symptoms

Vitamin A exerts its principal effect on epithelial tissue. Epithelial tissues include the skin and the lining of the gastrointestinal, respiratory, and reproductive tracts. Signs of deficiency relate to problems of these areas, particularly lowered resistance to such things as ringworm, respiratory disease, and reproductive disorders such as infertility and retained placenta. Classical descriptions of vitamin A deficiency include reference to such things as night blindness, swollen joints, convulsions, and diarrhea. These are extremes and long before these severe signs are seen other less definitive aberrations occur. The cumulative losses from lowered resistance, stillbirths, weak offspring, and so on, are much more significant and difficult to diagnose.

Prevention

Vitamin A deficiency can be prevented by including good quality hay in the diet or by addition of vitamin A to the grain ration. Where this is not feasible, intramuscular injection will provide a reserve lasting several months.

WATER DEPRIVATION

It seems so obvious that most texts don't even mention it, but water is the single most important dietary component for all species. Adult animals can go a week or two without feed but one day without water and they are pretty uncomfortable, two days and they are obviously sick and in three days many will be dead. Hot weather hastens the onset of clinical signs. These include restlessness, bellowing, depression of milk flow and appetite, dehydration, and constipation. Convulsions and coma may occur prior to death. Similar signs occur when there is overconsumption of salt with restricted water intake (salt poisoning).

It's important that animals have adequate fresh water available at all times. Check you watering equipment daily because equipment failures account for the vast majority of water deprivation problems.

GOITER

Goiter is enlargement of the thyroid gland due to deficiency of iodine. Soils in some areas notably the Upper Midwest and Far West, are deficient in iodine, and animals, as well as people, raised in these areas may have goiter. The condition is most prevalent in the newborn, and pigs and lambs are most susceptible although it can occur in any species. Severely deficient animals will be weak at birth or stillborn. Those that survive, if untreated, fail to grow and develop normally due to thyroid hormone deficiency. The disease is readily recognizable by the obvious enlargement of the gland located in the neck. Frequently the skin is thick, edematous, and flabby.

Those that are born alive respond reasonably well to supplementation of the diet with iodine. The disease is readily preventable by feeding iodized salt and this practice is now so general that the disease is rarely seen.

ANEMIA

Anemia has many causes — hemorrhage, parasitism, and diseases of red blood cells to name a few. Nutritional deficiencies can also result in depressed hemoglobin formation. **Iron deficiency anemia** of baby pigs is perhaps the most common and universal. Piglets are born with virtually no iron reserve and the iron content of sow's milk is usually inadequate to sustain them. Signs of iron deficiency anemia begin to appear at about one week of age, gradually increasing until the piglets are a month old. Affected piglets do not grow well, are prone to develop enteric infections, and usually show signs of respiratory distress. This takes the form of a rapid and forced respiration, giving rise to the common name of the disease, "thumps."

Although piglets are most susceptible, iron deficiency anemia can occur in any species raised on an exclusive milk diet. It is not uncommon in veal calves raised in total confinement on milk or milk replacer. In some parts of the country there is a premium market for fancy veal that requires a very pale meat. To achieve this, growers must maintain calves on an iron-deficient diet. Such calves are anemic and the stress of rough handling when they are being loaded may cause some to collapse.

Deficiency Correction

Iron deficiency anemia is most common in piglets raised in total confinement on impervious floors. If they are outside on the ground it rarely occurs, and one of the early and still effective control procedures is to place a shovelful of sod in the pen for them to root around in. But this doesn't fit into modern management schemes and is contraindicated for parasite control, therefore other means of supplementing iron have been devised. One is to add ferric citrate to the sow's diet for a couple weeks prior to farrowing in hopes of raising the iron content of her milk. This is not very effective, since the composition of milk remains quite stable regardless of diet. Swabbing the sow's udder daily with ferrous sulfate so the piglets get some when they nurse or dosing the piglets daily with a 1 percent solution is effective but laborious. The method adopted by most swine growers is to give each piglet an injectable iron preparation such as iron dextran at one week of age. For early weaned pigs, a single dose may be sufficient. If weaning is delayed to five or six weeks, a second dose may be necessary. The same preparation is suitable for the young of other species suffering from iron deficiency anemia.

Other Deficiencies

Deficiencies other than iron can also cause anemia in animals but are not as clear cut nor so easily diagnosed. **Deficiency of copper** is responsible for unthriftiness, depressed milk production, and anemia in many parts of the world. It may be **primary,** in which there simply isn't enough copper in the soil or forage, or **secondary,** in which case copper is there but made unavailable by an excess of molybdenum. The latter is most common on mucktype soils such as are found in many areas of the United States. **Cobalt deficiency** also causes anemia in ruminant animals and has been identified as one factor leading to reproductive inefficiency. Anemic animals do not come into heat regularly, nor do they readily conceive if they do.

Symptoms of copper or cobalt deficiency are often obscure and diagnosis is not easy and is often retrospective. If the animal improves when the specific element is added to the diet then the assumption is that deficiency is the cause. The best procedure is to prevent deficiency by adding trace mineralized salt to the ration or giving animals free choice access to it.

WHITE MUSCLE DISEASE
(WMD NUTRITIONAL MYOPATHY, STIFF LAMB DISEASE)

White muscle disease is a nutritional disease seen occasionally in young calves and lambs. In some areas it reaches serious proportions, causing losses of 50 percent or more of the calf or lamb crop. It is caused by a deficiency of the element selenium. The effect of selenium deficiency is more pronounced when levels of vitamin E are also low.

Selenium is a part of the enzyme glutatione peroxidase, which plays a part in detoxification of naturally occurring peroxide at the cellular level. Peroxides are toxic to cell membranes and unless detoxified cause muscle cell necrosis. This hyaline generation of muscle tissue gives the affected areas a white, cooked appearance, hence the name, "white muscle disease."

Vitamin E, also an antioxidant, has a sparing effect on selenium so that if selenium intake is low but vitamin E is adequate, clinical signs of WMD will not appear. However, if selenium is absent, vitamin E alone will not prevent symptoms from occurring.

Selenium is an essential trace element with a rather narrow margin of safety. A daily intake of as little as 0.1 ppm is adequate for health. Higher levels may be toxic, and the element in high doses has been shown to be carcinogenic for laboratory rodents.

Selenium content of soils varies widely. It is deficient in many parts of the Northeast but overabundant in some of the Western range areas. Some seleniferous plants growing in that area may contain in excess of 10 ppm, a level toxic to animals that eat those plants.

Although seen more commonly in the young, the effect of selenium deficiency is not limited to that age group. Adult animals can be affected as well. There is increasing evidence that retained placenta as a herd problem in dairy cattle may be due in part to inadequate selenium in the diet. Also, careful necropsy of so-called "downer cows" will sometimes reveal the lesions typical of WMD in the heavy muscles and particularly the heart.

Symptoms

The condition may be seen any time but it is most common in the age range of three weeks to three months. Clinical signs vary from stiffness of the hind limbs and reluctance to move, to sudden death with no premonitory signs. Exercise aggravates the condition, and a typical history is that the calves seemed healthy but when they were turned out on pasture the first time and started to run and play, several dropped dead.

Occasionally the condition may be manifested by a pneumonia-like syndrome with fever and labored breathing which is unresponsive to antibiotics.

Diagnosis

The disease can usually be readily diagnosed on the basis of clinical signs but the stiffness and stilted gait must be differentiated from injury, blackleg, and conditions such as foot rot. The age range at which it occurs usually precludes the latter.

At necropsy, characteristic white areas of degenerated muscle tissue will be seen in the heavy muscles of the hind leg, the loin area, the intercostal muscles and occasionally in the diaphragm and heart. In advanced cases, some calcification of the necrotic tissue occurs and it may have a gritty feel when cut with a knife. However, most cases terminate fatally before this occurs.

Treatment

If detected early, many cases respond well to injection of sodium selenite, vitamin E, or a proprietary combination of the two. However, sodium selenite is quite toxic and treatment should be administered only under direction of your veterinarian. Unfortunately, many cases are not detected until it is too late. The muscle damage that occurs is not reversible. The animal that survives may compensate to some degree but it is frequently unthrifty and therefore uneconomical. Like most diseases, prevention of WMD is easier and more effective than treatment.

Prevention

The disease is most prevalent in calves that are basically on a milk diet. The easiest and most logical preventative, therefore, is to be sure there is adequate selenium and vitamin E in the dam's milk.

One method is to buy hay and grain from a variety of sources on the assumption that at least some of it will be grown on soils adequate in selenium. A more practical method for most people is to inject the dam with a vitamin E/selenium preparation during the last month or two of gestation. A single injection usually is sufficient.

Alternatively, a smaller dose of the same material can be given to each calf when it is born. However, this won't help the occasional calf that is born with WMD or the few that are stillborn for the same reason. Creep feeding grain will help to prevent the disease in older calves.

Perhaps the most convenient way to assure adequate selenium intake is to incorporate small amounts of it in the grain. Because the amount required and legally permitted is so small, this should not be attempted with home mixing equipment. It can be done on a prescription basis by your feed dealer.

Miscellaneous Diseases

THERE ARE A NUMBER OF COMMONLY ENCOUNTERED disease conditions of livestock that cannot be readily grouped by cause. Nevertheless, they occur with sufficient frequency that the owner should have some knowledge of them. A few are uncontrollable, but the majority, if you know what to look for and plan ahead, can be prevented. These conditions are described briefly on the following pages.

ABSCESSES

These are accumulations of dead and living bacteria, cellular debris and body fluids, otherwise known as pus, walled off in a connective tissue capsule. They can occur anywhere and vary in size from microscopic to the size of a basketball. Microabscesses occur in liver, kidney, and occasionally the brain secondary to generalized bacterial infection. The larger abscesses are generally located subcutaneously or intramuscularly and are the result of wound infection. Subcutaneous abscesses due to *C. pyognes* are common in goats and the same organism commonly causes abscesses on the lateral side of the hocks and on the knees of cattle confined to stalls with inadequate bedding. The constant bruising they undergo each time the cow lies down injures and devitalizes tissue and infection results. This is a serious problem in some herds that can best be controlled by steam-cleaning the stall beds to reduce the bacterial population and then using more bedding and/or rubber mats. Poor sanitation aggravates the problem. Lung abscesses may be secondary to pneumonia. Umbilical abscess is not uncommon in animals about a week old due to infection occurring at or soon after birth. Dipping the navel in tincture of iodine usually prevents the problem.

When first detected, abscesses are usually hot and painful to the touch. They may or may not cause fever and lack of appetite. Without treatment, they commonly terminate in one of two ways: The abscess may continue to enlarge, with the capsule thinning out at the surface until it ruptures to discharge pus. Or active infection may subside, with inflammation disappearing and pus remaining inside the capsule. These so-called "sterile" abscesses may persist for months, with the pus gradually being replaced by scar tissue.

Treatment

Treatment of abscesses is determined by the location. Long-term antibiotic therapy is the only way to handle abscesses in the internal organs such as the lung and it isn't always successful. Fair success has been obtained in controlling liver abscesses of cattle and hogs by constant low-level antibiotic feeding.

Surgical drainage of abscesses that are accessible is the treatment of choice followed by daily irrigation with antiseptics and concurrent systemic administration of antibiotics. If you decide to open an abscess yourself, be sure you know what you are doing. Abscesses can easily be confused with hematomas, joint capsule distention such as bog spavin, and umbilical hernia.

On more than one occasion, I have been called upon to rescue a calf that supposedly had an umbilical abscess that the herdsman incised, only to find himself holding a handful of intestines rather than pus. When in doubt, call your veterinarian!

ALLERGY

Like people, some animals suffer from allergies, most notably horses and cattle and occasionally goats. The mechanism of allergy is complex and beyond the scope of this text. Suffice to say it is a generalized adverse reaction to prior sensitization by an allergen. In animals the allergenic substance is usually certain weeds or grasses, mold spores, or drugs. The reaction may take the form of urticaria or hives, characterized by edema of the eyelids and hairless skin area such as the vulva and by raised areas (wheals) on the neck and back. **Pulmonary edema** is a complication of hives in which the lungs fill with fluid, causing respiratory distress and hypersalivation. It can be rapidly fatal if untreated. **Allergic dermatitis** occurs as a result of insect bites and contact with chemicals or harness.

Photosensitization is a form of allergy that occurs when animals ingest certain plants such as St. John's Wort, rape, white clover, and sometimes alfalfa. Substances in the plant render the animal more susceptible to sunlight and the lesions resemble sunburn. The lower leg and muscle are the main areas affected.

Although allergy is usually an individual problem, it occasionally affects a high proportion of the herd. A good example is the acute respiratory disease seen in cattle grazing on aftermath or improved pastures. This disease is more common in climates noted for wet weather and frequent fogs, hence the name "fog fever." It is rarely reported in the United States as a herd problem, although we do see a similar condition in individuals, sometimes called "summer snuffles."

An unusual type of allergy occurs in a small percentage of dairy cattle allergic to their own milk. Signs of urticaria develop when the udder is distended and subside when the cow is milked out.

Generally speaking, allergy is a self-limiting individual problem that disappears spontaneously in most cases. An exception is the complication of pulmonary edema that can be very rapidly fatal. It requires prompt treatment with epinephrine, antihistamines, or corticosteroids and sometimes all three. In such cases, until your veterinarian arrives the best you can do is keep the animal as quiet as possible to reduce the demand for oxygen. Urticaria that doesn't disappear promptly when the diet is changed can be successfully treated with antihistamines.

ANAPHYLAXIS

This can best be described as a peracute, rapidly fatal allergic response to a foreign protein. In livestock the triggering factor is usually injection of a vaccine, bacterin, or antiserum. The reaction can occur following the initial dose but is more likely following a second or subsequent dose, with the first acting as a sensitizing dose. Products containing serum from another animal species (heterologous serum) cause anaphylactic shock more than any other. The older leptospirosis bacterins containing small amounts of rabbit serum frequently caused anaphylactic reactions.

Symptoms

Signs of anaphylaxis occur usually within an hour of the time of injection and often within minutes. These may include hypersalivation; rapid, labored breathing; shivering; and rapid temperature rise. Pulmonary edema or emphysema in the less acute case is common. Bloat in ruminants and diarrhea are occasionally seen. Release of large amounts of histamine from muscle tissue occurs, which in turn contributes to rumen atony (failure of normal rumen contractions) and vasodilation (dilation of blood vessels) with a fall in blood pressure and eventual collapse of the animal.

The biological products in use today are highly purified to reduce the risk of anaphylaxis but it still occurs occasionally. It's a good idea therefore to keep animals under close observation for an hour after vaccination. Immediate treatment is important if the affected animal is to survive, using drugs such as epinephrine and antihistamines. Laminitis is a common sequel in the horse.

BLOAT

Bloat is a condition unique to ruminant animals and is generally more of a problem in cattle than sheep or goats. It is distention of the rumen with trapped gas that can become severe enough to cause death in an hour or less. That bloat is more than a simple mechanical problem of accumulated gas has been demonstrated by experimental inflation of the rumen with air with no adverse effect on the animal. They just burp the air out as fast as it is pumped in. With bloat, however, rumen contractions are sluggish or totally absent and eructation (burping) does not occur so the distention continues as long as gas evolves from the rumen contents.

Bloat is more likely to occur when animals are grazed for the first time on lush legume pasture, which is especially dangerous when it is wet with early morning dew or rain. Bloat is also a problem in the feedlots when cattle or lambs are placed on full feed. Some of them become chronic bloaters and fail to gain as they should. Early marketing is the best answer for them. Chronic bloat is occasionally seen in cattle whose rumen function is impaired by irritation of the vagus nerve, either from traumatic gastritis (hardware disease) or tumors.

Legume bloat is not a simple matter of free gas trapped in the rumen but is often called "frothy bloat" because the gas is trapped in bubbles. This greatly complicates solution of the problem.

Diagnosis

Diagnosis of bloat is a simple matter. Affected animals usually stop eating and stand apart from the herd. When viewed from the rear, the animal shows a pronounced swelling on the upper left side back of the last rib and below the lateral processes of the lumbar vertebrae. When palpated, this area feels as tight as a drumhead. Depending on severity the animal may breathe in rapid, short breaths with the mouth open. The least exertion aggravates the shortness of breath and the animal may fall to the ground and expire from anoxia (lack of oxygen). Death due to bloat may be acute, with animals found dead in the pasture. For that reason, it's a good idea to check them periodically for the first few days they are put into a legume pasture. If no clinical signs are seen prior to death and a dead bloated animal is all you see, a distinction must be made between death due to bloat and other diseases such as anthrax, blackleg, and urea poisoning.

Prevention

Bloat can be largely prevented through management. Feeding some dry hay to cattle or sheep prior to putting them in legume pasture and waiting until the grass is dry before turning them out are very helpful procedures. Leaving them in the pasture for only half an hour or so until they are accustomed to it also helps. Feedlot bloat is not so easy to manage, but various techniques have been used with fair success. Addition of surface tension reducing agents such as poloxalene or vegetable oils to the feed are helpful. Incorporating antibiotics such as penicillin in the feed to alter the rumen flora is also helpful in reducing losses, but it is not approved by the Federal Drug Administration.

Treatment

Severe bloat requires prompt emergency treatment. Call your veterinarian, but while you wait there are some things you can do to help. Get all the animals out of the pasture immediately. A couple tablespoons of household detergent given orally helps reduce surface tension of bubbles in the rumen, releasing trapped gas. A pint of vegetable or mineral oil will do the same thing but the volume of fluid makes it more risky to give orally. Tying a one-inch diameter piece of wood in the mouth like a bit in a horse will stimulate salivation and eructation. This procedure has saved many animals. If veterinary help is not available, a makeshift cow stomach tube can be made using a ten-foot length of smooth garden hose. Lubricate it with mineral oil and pass it gently down the throat into the rumen to relieve the pressure. This procedure takes practice but if you can't get professional help in a hurry, it's worth a try. As a last resort, use a **trocar and cannula,** if available. This instrument, available from most livestock supply houses, is especially made to relieve bloat by inserting a short pipe directly into the rumen. Medication such as poloxalene, detergent, or oil can be put directly into the rumen via stomach tube or through the cannula. Use of the cannula is quick in an emergency to save the animal's life but infection frequently follows so routine use is not recommended.

CALCULI

Urinary calculi are sometimes a problem in feedlot steers or wethers and less often in intact males as well. These are hard aggregations of mineral salts and epithelial cells that form either in the renal pelvis or the bladder where they may produce a mechanical irritation and a chronic cystitis. A more serious complication results when they become lodged in the urethra to block partially or completely the flow of urine.

Symptoms

Affected animals evidence colicky pain such as kicking at the belly, treading with the hind feet, and switching the tail. Attempts to urinate are frequent with straining and grating the teeth. Urine passage is scanty, often blood-tinged, and sometimes totally absent. When the obstruction is complete, the urethra or bladder ruptures. Rupture of the urethra results in diffusion of urine into the subcutaneous tissues of the belly extending toward the chest, causing obvious fluid swelling. This is often accompanied by infection and occasionally by sloughing of a section of skin, which permits urine to escape. Rupture of the bladder brings immediate relief from pain but urine accumulating in the abdomen causes a toxemia and death in about forty-eight hours. The characteristic appearance of animals with abdomen distended by urine gives the disease the common name of "water belly."

Treatment

Surgical intervention is the only effective treatment once the clinical signs appear but dietary management helps to reduce prevalence of the condition. Adequate and balanced amounts of calcium and phosphorus are important, as is adequate vitamin A. Addition of sodium chloride to the diet up to 5 percent of daily dry matter intake will prevent the problem almost entirely — provided adequate amounts of fresh water are available. Feeding ammonium chloride to alter urine pH has also been found to reduce the formation of calculi.

COLIC

This is really not a disease but a group of symptoms in response to abdominal pain. The underlying cause is almost always a gastrointestinal disturbance and it occurs in the horse far more often than any other species. It may range from simple indigestion with gas formation to mechanical blockages such as a twist in the bowel (volvulus) or telescoping of the bowel (intussusception). A not-infrequent occurrence in the horse is thrombus (clot of blood) formation in the mesenteric arteries due to strongyle larvae. When a thrombus forms in an artery, the blood supply to tissue served by it is cut off and that section of the bowel dies. Large masses of bots may cause sufficient inflammation of the stomach wall in the horse and even partially obstruct the pyloric end to cause gastric distress. Engorgement and impaction often occur when a horse gets accidental access to the feed bin or is fed finely chopped indigestible hay. Some horses get chronic indigestion because their teeth are bad and they can't chew properly.

Symptoms

Regardless of the cause, clinical signs of colic in the horse are essentially the same varying only in severity. Restlessness, kicking at the belly, getting up and down frequently, and rolling are common. Standing in a stretched out "sawhorse" attitude is characteristic. More severe pain causes sweating, rapid pulse, and onset of a shocklike syndrome. Movements may be quite violent with self-inflicted injury common. With volvulus or cecal torsion, onset is sudden; with impaction, engorgement, or simple indigestion, it is more gradual.

Early accurate diagnosis is important in the management of colic. Volvulus, torsion, and sometimes impaction require surgery to save the animal's life and the longer it is delayed, the poorer the prognosis. Aside from calling a veterinarian immediately, the most useful thing an owner can do is to keep the horse from injuring himself. The best way to do this is to keep the horse on his feet and walking. Walking also helps to stimulate peristalsis (rhythmic contraction of the gut) and passage of gas and manure.

Prevention

As with everything else, prevention is far better than treatment and several things should be done as a matter of routine good husbandry. Control internal parasites and have the horse's teeth checked and floated at least once a year. Make any feed change gradually, and above all be sure the horse doesn't have an opportunity to overeat grain. Feed coarsely ground rather than finely ground grain, and avoid hay composed primarily of young tender legumes. Some horses develop a habit of bolting their grain as soon as it is put out and regularly get indigestion as a result. Putting a couple of stones the size of soft-balls in their feed bucket will slow down consumption because they have to work around the stones to get at the grain. Some horses regularly get indiges-tion from eating straw used as bedding. The logical thing to do in this case is switch to shavings or sawdust for bedding.

DISPLACED ABOMASUM

This is a problem of the dairy cow close to the time of parturition, seen almost exclusively in cows on high concentrate, high silage, or complete feed diets. The condition is one of torsion of the fourth stomach (abomasum) either to the left or the right, resulting in depressed appetite and reduced milk pro-duction. The majority of displacements are to the left, with the abomasum sliding under the anterior part of the rumen and upward where it becomes dis-tended with gas. The clinical signs are almost identical to ketosis, with the cow showing preference for hay and silage over grain, intermittent constipation, and occasionally diarrhea and gradual weight loss. The test for ketones in urine and milk is positive.

Many theories have been advanced as to the cause, including abomasal and rumen atony due to hypocalcemia, vitamin E or selenium deficiency, and lifting of the rumen by the gravid uterus to allow the abomasum to slip under-neath. Diet, however, appears to play the most important role, since the condition can be prevented almost entirely by feeding four to five pounds or more of long hay daily.

Treatment

Conservative treatment consists of rolling the cow on her back and rock-ing her back and forth to get the abomasum back in position. This sometimes produces dramatic recovery but relapses are frequent. A heavy suture placed through the abomasum from the outside will hold it in place but this approach carries a risk of infection. Many veterinarians have found the rate of relapse declines if the animal is given calcium gluconate and a laxative. When these methods fail, surgery is the only resort and is quite successful.

FOUNDER (LAMINITIS)

This painful condition of the foot occurs in all hooved animals but is more commonly thought of in connection with horses and ponies. The predispos-ing factors in the horse are well defined, but the mechanism by which they cause founder is less well understood. These factors include overeating grain, consumption of large amounts of cold water when the animal is hot, serious illness such as pneumonia or metritis, and concussion during fast road work, especially by an unconditioned horse. Overeating grain or pasture is the most common cause. Acute allergic reactions may also produce founder.

Normally only a small portion of the animal's weight is borne on the sole of the foot. Most of the weight is borne on the walls through soft laminae which attach the op pedis or coffin bone to the wall. With acute founder, swelling of the laminae occurs and since the walls of the hoof can't expand to accommodate the swelling, excruciating pain results. The swelling is probably the result of excess histamine combined with impairment of circulation in the foot. In more advanced cases, separation of the laminae occurs with rotation of the coffin bone down-

Laminitis and founder from inexcusable neglect.

ward at the tip — even to the point in extreme cases where it protrudes through the sole. This rotation results in deformity of the foot and chronic lameness.

Symptoms

Acute laminitis in the horse has a sudden onset with acute pain, sweating, fever, and extreme reluctance to move. The horse will stand with the feet tucked up or stretched out to relieve pain and after considerable effort may lie down and refuse to get up. Prompt treatment is required if the animal is to recover without permanent lameness. Antihistamines, analgesics, a laxative, and packing the feet in ice are the usual therapy.

The horse may recover in a few days or the disease may become chronic with the coffin bone rotating downward, the forward part of the hoof wall becoming concave and the entire wall assuming a corrugated appearance. The effects of chronic laminitis can be relieved somewhat by corrective shoeing but the foundered horse is usually unable to do hard work without again becoming lame.

Laminitis in the other livestock species is more insidious and occurs over a period of time. It is rarely acute, as in the horse. Almost invariably it is the result of high grain feeding and is a particular problem for exhibitors of beef cattle who want their animals fat at show time. The high concentrate feeding necessary to get adequate fat covering contributes to laminitis. Because their feet hurt, cattle with laminitis don't gain weight or produce milk as they should, and in some herds the resulting economic loss is substantial. Alleviation

Laminitis. Note deformity of the bottom claw compared with the normal at on top.

of the problem, once it occurs, is difficult. Frequent trimming of the feet to be sure they bear weight evenly is about the best that can be done. Prevention through dietary management is the most important thing.

FRACTURES

Fortunately, fractures don't occur very often in livestock, although the frequency increases in the presence of other conditions such as rickets and phosphorus deficiency. From a theoretical medical standpoint, fractures in livestock should heal as well as they do in smaller animals and people. And they do, depending on location. Broken ribs due to kicks, crowding through gates, or fighting are not unusual and they heal uneventfully. But leg fractures are a different matter in mature animals and the problem is mechanical rather than medical. It's extremely difficult to immobilize a long bone fracture in an animal weighing 1000 pounds or more, particularly when the animal doesn't understand what you are trying to do and does its best to get the splint or cast off. With calves, foals, sheep, and goats the problem is not as great, but even then it taxes the ingenuity of the orthopedic surgeon. Fractures of the small tarsal and carpal bones occurring most frequently in the horse are amenable to surgical repair using internal fixation such as screws, nails and/or external casts.

But given the guarded prognosis for long bone fractures and the finite value of commercial livestock, most owners elect euthanasia. The expense and tribulations of fracture repair generally can be justified only for valuable purebred animals.

Prevention

Fractures are accidents, and most accidents are preventable if one uses a little forethought. In this case the owner has to do the thinking for his animals. Try to foresee the hazards and take steps to remove them. Simple things — such as putting sand on slippery floors to prevent falls and keeping animal confined when it's icy outside — will help. Keeping machinery and junk out of the pastures will reduce accidents of all kinds. Cattle frequently fracture the end of the tuber coxae (hip) when crowding through narrow doors especially when some impatient soul is chasing them from behind. Padding the sides of the door frame and moving them slowly will keep this type of injury from occurring. All it takes is a little forethought, a little more intelligence than the animals possess and the realization that "whatever can go wrong will."

HEAT STROKE

This is a seasonal problem encountered primarily in swine, but any animal can be affected. High temperatures, high humidity, and inadequate ventilation are the predisposing factors and fat animals are more susceptible. Panting, collapse, and very high body temperature are the principal signs.

The condition requires prompt treatment and the most effective procedure is to reduce body temperature with cold showers. As soon as the animal can stand, move it to a shady or cooler area.

Prevention measures are obvious. In hot weather provide shade for pastured animals and cool the barn with fans and/or evaporative coolers. Avoid the stress of trucking animals during the hot period of the day and don't overcrowd them in the pens.

HEMATOMA

This is an accumulation of blood, generally subcutaneously, resulting from rupture of a blood vessel. Injury is the usual cause and the location can be anywhere. Swelling is the obvious clinical sign and bleeding may continue for several hours, with the hematoma becoming quite large. Hematomata must be distinguished from abscesses and depending on location, hernias. Compared with an abscess they develop rapidly, are not hot to the touch, and generally are not acutely painful.

In most cases, no special treatment is necessary and the blood will eventually be reabsorbed, although some scar tissue may remain. Surgical drainage may be necessary if the hematoma is located in a position to cause interference with breathing or eating. Occasionally secondary infection will occur, and what started as hematoma becomes an abscess. In dairy cattle, hematomata of the tests due to injury are difficult to handle. The teat becomes swollen, hard, and difficult to milk. Soaking the teat frequently in a warm water and epsom salt solution (1 tbsp/pt) will help reduce the swelling but a cannula may have to be used for several days to remove the milk without further injury. When using a teat cannula use careful aseptic procedures to avoid causing mastitis.

HERNIA

Hernias occur in all species and are usually umbilical, scrotal or inguinal in location. Hernias at other sites are ruptures — the result of injury. A hernia is an interruption of the continuity of the abdominal wall with an outpouching of the peritoneum. The condition is serious if a loop of intestine passes through the opening. It may become strangulated, causing severe pain with necrosis of that part of the bowel due to interruption of the circulation, and death of the

Calf with umbilical hernia.

animal. If the intestine has been there long enough for adhesions to form, surgery is the only solution to the problem.

Umbilical hernias are obvious at or soon after birth, but must be distinguished from an umbilical abscess or hematoma. They are most common in calves and there is good evidence the condition is hereditary; therefore calves with umbilical hernia should not be used for breeding purposes. Small hernias of an inch or so in diameter will usually close spontaneously. Closure can be hastened by maintaining reduction of the hernia with a band of wide adhesive tape around the abdomen. Larger hernias require surgical repair.

Scrotal hernias are found most commonly in baby pigs usually at the time of castration. Anyone who castrates very many pigs soon learns to keep suture and needle handy to make on-the-spot repairs. This lesson is brought home rather forcefully the first time one sees a just-castrated piglet run to the far side of the pen dragging a loop of intestine behind him. Closure of the external inguinal ring with a few sutures is a simple matter if you have the materials at hand. Scrotal hernia is really an extended inguinal hernia.

Strangulated inguinal hernias occur in stallions and occasionally bulls and are extensions of bowel through the internal inguinal ring. Such a hernia is often manifested as colicky pain immediately after breeding and the diagnosis can be made by rectal examination. If the hernia cannot be reduced per rectum, surgery is necessary.

Hernias result from omission of nature or accident and, except in the case of hereditary umbilical hernia of calves, little can be done to prevent them. Although a definite hereditary link has not been established, it would be prudent not to use littermates of pigs with scrotal hernia as breeding stock.

ISOIMMUNE HEMOLYTIC ANEMIA

This disease is unique in that it is rarely reported in species other than the horse and is most common in the Thoroughbred breed. It occurs when, through placental injury, some of the foal's blood enters the mare's circulation. This acts as an antigen and the mare produces antibody in response. When the newborn foal then nurses colostrum he also gets a dose of antibody against his own red blood cells. This results in hemolysis and agglutination of red cells, causing the foal to show signs of anemia in twelve to ninety-six hours. The severity of signs is governed by concentration of antibody in the colostrum and how much colostrum the foal consumed.

Affected foals are lethargic, weak, and have accelerated heart and respiratory rates without fever. Jaundice and hemoglobinuria appear as the disease progresses. These signs, coupled with age at onset and the breed, are presumptive evidence of isoimmune hemolytic anemia. Diagnosis can be confirmed by hemagglutination of the foal's red cells with serum or colostrum from the dam. The disease is more likely to occur in second or subsequent foals born of the same mating.

Treatment

Treatment depends on severity of clinical signs, but in any case the foal should not receive additional colostrum from the mare. Mild cases recover with good nursing care. Blood transfusion is indicated for those more severely affected and in extreme cases a complete blood exchange may be necessary.

Prevalence of the disease can be reduced by test matching serum from the mare with red cells from the stallion prior to breeding. If agglutination occurs, use another stallion. Alternatively, follow the same procedure with red cells from the foal before it nurses. If agglutination occurs, don't let the foal nurse. Instead, use colostrum from a different mare, if available, or a milk substitute. Milk the mare out for forty-eight hours and then let the foal nurse. By that time most of the antibody will be gone but bear in mind that foals deprived of colostrum will be more susceptible to infection and will require special care.

EQUINE LAMENESS

Lameness in horses has many causes, but perhaps the single most important factor is the stress of training to race as two-year-olds. This has nothing to do with the horse but is a reflection of human greed, to get horses on the track and earning money as soon as possible. The skeletal development of horses until they are about three is not sufficiently progressed to withstand the concussion and the stresses of hard work. An analogous situation is the disproportionately high prevalence of injuries on the football field sustained by high school athletes.

Because sound feet and legs are so important to the horse, diagnosis and management of lameness should be left to the experienced veterinarian. Over the years a bewildering variety of terms has evolved to name the various lamenesses, many of which make no sense at all. The following definitions may help the reader to understand the various lamenesses, making it possible to converse intelligently with the veterinarian when the diagnosis is made.

Bog Spavin: Accumulation of fluid causing distention of the joint capsules of the hock.

Bowed Tendon: Severe strain on the flexor tendons of the foreleg. Swelling gives a "bowed" appearance from the knee to the ankle.

Bucked Shins: Seen in overworked young horses. Swelling and heat appear on the front of the foreleg from the knee to the ankle.

Canker: Inflammation or infection of the frog, resulting in an overgrowth of imperfect frog tissue.

Capped Elbow (shoe boils): Swelling at the point of the elbow. Caused by bruising due to inadequate bedding, or self-inflicted in high-stepping horses.

Capped Hock: More or less chronic swelling at the point of the hock as a result of injury.

Coffin Joint: The joint formed by the second and third phalanges and the navicular bone. It lies within the wall of the hoof.

Contracted Tendon: Shortening of the flexor tendons of the leg. Seen primarily in young horses.

Corns: A bruise resulting from pressure from the heel of the shoe. Occurs at the angle of the sole between the bar and the wall.

Curb: A swelling starting about four inches below the point of the hock. Results from ligament rupture due to strain from jumping, running, or slipping.

Founder (laminitis): An inflammation of the sensitive laminae inside the wall of the hoof. It is seen most commonly in overweight horses and ponies and in mares as a complication of foaling. Congestion within the hoof weakens the attachment of the sensitive laminae, and the sole drops so that it appears convex instead of concave. The condition is acutely painful in the early stages.

Knee Spavin: Injury to the inside of the knee produced when turning at high speeds. May result in a chronic arthritis.

Navicular Disease: A chronic inflammation of the navicular bone which with the coffin bone and the second phalanx forms the coffin joint. Usually starts as a bursitis and continues with erosion and exostosis. Most common in Quarterhorses.

Osselet: Hot, painful, and relatively soft swelling at onset along the front margin of the fetlock. Due to bone disease in the area of the joint capsule attachment. The affected area later becomes calcified.

Quittor: A draining sinus at the coronet, usually from infection or necrosis of the lateral cartilage.

Ringbone: A term generally applied to erosion of bone at the joint surfaces from the fetlock down. May be called high or low depending on which joint is affected. With "false ringbone" there is excess bone (exostosis) formed at the edges of the joint surface, but the joint surface is unaffected. In true ringbone it is affected.

Sandcrack: A crack starting at the wearing surface and extending part way up the wall of the hoof. Quarter cracks may start at the hairline and extend downward.

Seedy Toes: A separation of the toe between the wall and the sensitive lamina of the foot. The space is filled with a crumbly type of horn tissue, hence the name "seedy toe." May be evidence of past foundering.

Sidebone: Bone formed as a result of ossification of the lateral cartilage of the foot.

Spavin: True or "jack" spavin is an inflammation of the covering (periosteum) of the bones on the inside of the hock, resulting in bone enlargement at this point. Blind spavin is an inflammation of the joint surfaces of the bones at the hock, with no visible bony enlargement.

Splints: Excess bone growth (exostoses) occurring usually on the inside of the foreleg just below the knee. They may also occur on the outside of the foreleg below the knee and rarely appear on the rear leg. They are found principally in young horses and though they may be present in older horses, they usually are not a cause of lameness in this group.

Stringhalt: A condition in which the hock is overflexed and forcefully extended when the horse moves, causing a jerky motion. The true cause is unknown.

Thoroughpin: Soft swelling due to distention of the tendon sheath of the hollow area forward of the point of the hock.

LIGHTNING STROKE

In pastured animals, death due to lightning stroke can be confused with other diseases causing sudden death such as anthrax, blackleg, and bloat. Lightning stroke is usually fatal, so one might wonder what difference a diagnosis makes. There are two good reasons why diagnosis is important. First, if death was due to lightning, insurance may cover the loss. Second, if it was due to an infectious disease or bloat, steps can be taken to protect the balance of the herd.

Symptoms

Obviously, lightning stroke occurs only in conjunction with electrical storms. On several occasions I have had farmers try to convince me that a cow found dead on a bright day was killed by lightning. These were blatant attempts at insurance fraud. Death due to lightning strike is sudden, with no evidence of struggle such as trampled ground. Sometimes the animals even have the last bite of grass in their mouths. Occasionally singed hair will be found around the muzzle or lower leg where sparks have jumped. Necropsies are frequently entirely negative so that circumstantial evidence is all there is to go on. Often the animals are found lying near a fence or gathered around an isolated tree that shows evidence of having been hit by lightning.

Surprisingly, lightning strike is not always fatal. It may render the animal unconscious for a time with no other injury. It may also cause partial or complete paralysis, from which the animal may or may not recover. The most unusual case I ever saw was a cow with a clean cut all the way through the skin and subcutaneous tissue extending from the backbone in a straight line to a point below the hock, a distance of almost three feet! A sharp knife couldn't have done better and after the wound was sutured she made an uneventful recovery. Three others in the pasture with her were killed instantly.

Little can be done to protect against lightning strike. The safest place for animals during an electrical storm is in a barn equipped with lightning rods. But if these are nonexistent or not functioning properly, cattle confined in steel stanchions may all be electrocuted if lightning hits the barn or they may suffocate if the barn burns. Most people philosophically accept lightning strike as one of the risks of raising livestock.

MYOCLONIA CONGENITA

This is a disease of piglets, the cause of which is obscure. It begins as fine tremors at or shortly after birth. The trembling increases to a point where the piglets have difficulty nursing and they die of starvation. Those less severely affected gradually improve over a period of several days.

At one time, vaccination of pregnant sows for hog cholera was thought to be a factor, but since vaccination is no longer permitted and the disease has been eradicated this is not a factor. However, other unidentified viruses infecting the sow and thus the piglets during gestation may be a factor. Nutritional deficiencies have been suggested but not proven. Heredity may be a factor and it is suggested that boars that have sired litters in which the disease appeared not be used for further breeding. For the same reason, recovered pigs should not be used for breeding stock. Assuming a virus is responsible for some cases, it may be useful to expose open sows and gilts to affected piglets so they become infected and develop immunity prior to breeding.

OBTURATOR PARALYSIS

This partial paralysis of the rear legs is the result of trauma to the dam's obturator nerves during a difficult birth. It is seen in cattle more than any other species. For part of their length the right and left obturator nerves run along the inside forward edge of the pelvis inlet against the bone where there is no protective fat covering. Prolonged pressure from an oversized or malpresented calf injures the nerve, causing paralysis of the adductor muscles that the cow uses to hold her hind legs together. The cow with obturator paralysis is either unable to stand or, if she does, may lose control of the legs so they spread outward. When this happens, dislocation of the hip or splitting of the pubic symphysis frequently occurs.

Treatment

Affected animals may or may not recover depending on the extent of the nerve injury and the quality of the nursing care. Use of lots of bedding to prevent decubital sores and turning the paralyzed cow from one side to the other every hour or so are important parts of the nursing care. Tying the hocks together with soft rope will help prevent "splitting" of the hind legs. If the cow will tolerate it, supporting her for a few minutes several times a day with a hip sling is very helpful. When using a sling, raise the animal just high enough so the feet touch the floor in the normal extended position. The idea is to encourage her to support her own weight with the sling in place to keep her from falling. The longer the paralysis persists the poorer the prognosis and those that don't recover within a week usually don't recover at all.

The moral of the story is to be sure the fetus is in a normal position for delivery and then use gentle traction rather than brute force. Refer to Chapter 4 for more detail on normal and abnormal delivery.

PROLAPSE

This can be simply defined as an eversion through a normal body opening of the rectum, vagina, uterus, or prepuce.

Prolapse of the Rectum

This is the result of prolonged straining due to enteritis or constipation. It is most common in young animals, particularly pigs. The rectum everts through the anus and appears as a red inflamed cylindrical mass. This soon becomes black and necrotic due to interruption of circulation. The condition is fatal if not promptly corrected. If detected early, the mass can be replaced and retained with a purse string suture in the anus. Longstanding cases require amputation and resection. In either case, it's a job for the veterinarian. The condition is most likely to occur when the straining is induced by chronic diarrhea or constipation. Prevention, therefore, depends either on control of diarrhea or modification of the diet to produce a normal soft stool. High-fiber diets for young pigs should be avoided.

Prolapsed rectum and vagina.

Prolapse of the Vagina

This condition occurs during advanced pregnancy and is first noticeable when the animal is lying down, especially if her hindquarters are lower than the front. It is most common in fat cows that have unusually relaxed pelvic ligaments. The increased intraabdominal pressure when the cow lies down cause the vagina to balloon outward through the vulva. In most cases it slides back into place when the animal gets up. However, exposure of the vaginal mucosa to the elements causes irritation and swelling and the swelling may become so great that the vagina does not go back into place. The protruding vagina stimulates a straining reflex which further aggravates the problem. There are several ways to alleviate the problem. It is helpful to confine the animal in a straight stall with the floor built up higher under the rear legs to throw the abdominal weight forward. For cattle a truss is commercially available that has been used with some success. It is simply a heavy aluminum rod shaped in the form of a Y. Placed so that the arms of the Y pass on each side of the vulva and tied tightly to the neck with rope, it provides enough external pressure to keep the vagina in place. If these methods fail, surgical repair is the only recourse. Once parturition takes place the problem is solved. Vaginal prolapse is much less common in animals that have ample exercise and are not too fat.

Uterine Prolapse

This is a serious complication that is often a sequel to vaginal prolapse because the same conditions that foster the one lead to the other. Uterine prolapse is a complete eversion of the uterus following parturition. It can occur in any species but is more frequent in cattle, and in most cases muscular atony induced by hypocalcemia is a contributing factor. To the uninitiated, a prolapsed uterus is a terrifying sight. The only thing good to be said about it is that it makes it easy to remove the placenta because you can see what you are doing. The sooner it can be replaced the better for the life of the animal and her future productivity, but replacement is a job for the veterinarian. It is physically difficult due to the bulk and weight of the organ if nothing else so be prepared to help your veterinarian do the work. Until then, the best you can do is to protect the uterus from injury. Confine the animal so she can't bang the pendulous uterus around when walking. Wrap it in a clean cloth (a bedsheet is ideal) to protect it from dirt and manure and keep it moist with warm water. Cows that continue to strain after the calf is born are more likely to prolapse their uterus (cast their withers). If you have one in that category, have your veterinarian give her an epidural anesthetic to block the straining reflex.

Prolapse of the Prepuce

This occurs in some bulls, particularly those with Brahma breeding. The preputial tissue protrudes from the sheath where it is subject to injury, infection, and scarring, which may be sufficiently severe to prevent coitus. Surgical removal of the excess tissue is the only alternative to salvage by slaughter.

PULMONARY EMPHYSEMA (HEAVES)

This is a chronic, irreversible, noninfectious disease seen primarily in the horse. Pathologically the condition is one of rupture of the walls of the lung alveoli with some escape of air into the surrounding tissue. The result is loss of lung elasticity so that they fail to collapse during expiration. Since they don't collapse completely neither do they fill completely during inspiration and the seriously affected animal has difficulty inhaling sufficient air to meet its oxygen needs.

Pulmonary emphysema occurs secondary to pneumonia in all species, but in the horse the condition appears to be more of an allergic response with dusty surroundings and mold spores from spoiled hay being triggering factors. A few horses develop signs of heaves in the spring when put out to pasture, but most cases originate when animals are stabled. The symptoms may be more pronounced in hot weather.

Symptoms

The disease is progressive, with dry hacking cough, especially after exercise, gradual weight loss, flaring of the nostrils during inspiration, and contraction of the abdominal muscles during expiration. The latter is noticeable at the margin of the ribs (heave line) and by a pumping action of the anus as the horse tries to expel the residual air. There is no specific treatment for heaves, although antihistamines, corticosteroids, and aminophylline may relieve the symptoms in some cases. Keeping the barn free of dust and well ventilated, using shavings instead of hay or straw for bedding, and substitution of feeds such as beet pulp for hay in the ration are all helpful.

Prevention by keeping horses in dust-free surroundings and avoiding the use of moldy hay is most important.

QUITTOR

This is a nondescript term that means different things to different people. To the horse owner it means chronic inflammation of the lateral cartilage in the foot with pus formation, necrosis, and sinus tracts extending from the cartilage to the outside at the coronary band. It is the result of penetrating wounds either down from the coronet or up through the sole and surgery to remove the diseased tissue is the only recourse.

Quittor.

To the cattle owner quittor means protrusion of a pad of fat and connective tissue down into the interdigital space, which in time may extend halfway to the tip of the toe. This pad, or quittor, keeps the toes splayed apart when the animal walks and chafes to cause chronic lameness. It is most common in fat cattle and surgical removal is the only lasting cure.

SILO GAS POISONING

This is not a common problem, fortunately, but it occurs often enough to deserve mention, particularly since it is also a hazard to people. Early in the fermentation of ensiled corn, oxides of nitrogen form that are very irritating to lung tissue and may even involve an allergic response. Most texts describe the first three weeks after the silo is filled as being the most dangerous period but I have seen acute respiratory distress in cattle caused by silo gas toxicity as long as three months after the silo was filled. This is probably the exception rather than the rule.

The condition is more likely to occur when cattle are fed corn silage in a tightly closed barn. The first signs noted are coughing when the silage is placed in front of them. Continued exposure leads to copious salivation, labored breathing, elevated temperature, and depressed milk flow. In severe cases, abnormal lung sounds can be heard even without the aid of a stethoscope. Continued exposure without treatment may cause death due to anoxia.

In most cases, removal of the offending silage from the diet brings about spontaneous recovery, although the cough may persist for several months. More severely affected animals require treatment with atropine, antihistamines, and corticosteroids as well as antibiotics to prevent secondary bacterial pneumonia.

It's best to wait several weeks before feeding out of a newly filled silo and to observe cattle carefully the first day or two when feeding begins. If they seem to cough excessively stop feeding the silage or aerate it outside for a few hours prior to feeding and keep the barn well ventilated during the feeding period. If these measures don't control the problem it may be necessary to wait several months before the silage can be safely fed.

SPASTIC SYNDROME (STRETCHES)

This is a hereditary disease of dairy cattle that unfortunately doesn't make its appearance until they reach maturity. Signs are most evident when the cow gets to her feet. Crampiness is apparent and the animal treads from one hind leg to the other intermittently extending one leg rapidly backward and then the other. Concurrent muscular tremors of the leg and back may occur. The condition gets progressively worse and eventually affected animals stand in an abnormal posture with the rear legs extended backward. They are in constant discomfort and have difficulty walking. As a result milk flow drops to a point where they are uneconomical to keep.

Metallic debris adhering to rumen magnets.

Treatment is of no value and prevention through selective breeding is the only recourse. Unfortunately, because of the long delay in onset this is easier said than done but certainly offspring of cattle known to have the disease should not be used for breeding purposes.

TRAUMATIC GASTRITIS
(HARDWARE DISEASE, TRAUMATIC RETICULITIS)

This is a disease almost exclusively of cattle and occurs because of the eating habits of the cow coupled with the anatomical arrangement of the stomach compartments. Cattle swallow forage with minimal chewing and regurgitate it later for more complete mastication. Because they don't chew initially and only wad the forage sufficiently to swallow it, they occasionally swallow nails and pieces of wire that are mixed in with it. Being heavier than grass or silage these gravitate to the lowest part of the stomach, the reticulum. Since the outlet from the reticulum to the omasum is not located at the bottom of the reticulum, accumulated hardware remains there sometimes until it rusts out.

When field choppers and pick-up balers first came into use as a method of harvesting the hay crop, "hardware disease" was almost an epidemic on some farms because all the stray wire lying in the fields was chopped into pieces about two inches long and harvested along with the hay. Now that most of this debris has been gleaned from the fields, the condition is much less common.

Symptoms

The vast majority of cows have some metal lying loose in the reticulum and it normally does no harm. Occasionally, though, a piece will become lodged in such a way that during the normal reticulum contractions it perforates through the wall. This causes immediate pain, cessation of stomach contractions, loss of appetite, and typically a low-grade fever of 103°–104°F. Affected cows are reluctant to move and may stand with a "humped up" appearance. When forced to move they do so very gingerly because every movement causes pain. Local abscessation or peritonitis or even sudden death due to penetration of the heart by the foreign object may occur.

Treatment

In an attempt to prevent damage to the heart, it is standard practice in cases of traumatic gastritis to confine the cow in a stall with her front legs raised on a platform about four inches high. The objective of this procedure is to direct the center of gravity back away from the forward wall of the reticulum. In early cases, if the wire or whatever has not passed all the way through the wall, this technique alone may bring about recovery. Special cylindrical magnets given to the cow orally with a balling gun are a further aid to retrieval of the metal from the rumen or reticulum wall. These magnets last as long as the cow, and given prophylactically to every cow in the herd they will prevent "hardware disease" almost entirely.

If these conservative methods fail, the only recourse for the affected cow is a surgical operation known as a **rumenotomy.** Through an opening in the rumen, the surgeon, preferably one with a long arm, reaches in and removes the offending object. If undertaken before too much damage is done, the surgery is highly successful. Vigorous antibiotic therapy is necessary, of course, to combat the peritonitis that invariably accompanies the condition.

Keeping nails, wire, and so on separated from the feed and putting a magnet in each cow will almost completely prevent "hardware disease." As an interesting sidelight, it is sometimes a question whether a cow has had a magnet put in her or not. It's easy to find out by holding a magnetic compass near her left elbow. If she has a magnet, north will always be toward the cow no matter which way she is headed.

TUMORS (NEOPLASMS, CANCER)

With the exception of bovine lymphosarcoma and papillomatosi, the cause of cancer in animals as well as man is unknown. Although many substances have been proven carcinogenic in massive doses it is doubtful that normal limited exposure to any of these is responsible for cancer in animals. The cause therefore remains unknown.

Tumors can occur in any tissue or organ and where there is organ involvement the symptoms are usually those of malfunction of that organ. For example, tumors in the brain result in abnormal behavior or problems with locomotion. Tumors may be benign or malignant, in which case they metastasize to other parts of the body. Surgical removal is the only practical cure in livestock. While some tumors are responsive to radiation therapy or chemotherapy, the cost — except perhaps for valuable race horses — cannot be justified.

One of the most frequently encountered and therefore costly tumors of livestock is adenocarcinoma of the third eyelid (cancer eye), seen almost exclusively in Hereford cattle. Other breeds are rarely affected. In some herds a rather high percentage of cattle develops this tumor each year, leading to the possibility that a transmissible agent may be involved, although none has yet been demonstrated. Lack of pigment in the eye and constant exposure to bright sunlight seem to increase the frequency of these tumors. Treatment is surgical removal. When the tumor is small with no evidence of spread to adjacent structures, removal of the tumor alone is adequate. With more extensive involvement the entire eyeball and adjacent structures must be removed.

Urea Poisoning

The economic advantage of adding urea to cattle feeds as a substitute for part of the protein has made this one of the more common poisonings of dairy and beef cattle.

Urea is highly toxic to livestock not conditioned to it. However, through repeated daily exposure to small amounts, rumen microorganisms adapt to it and covert the nitrogen in urea to amino acids that are absorbed and utilized by the animal. Without this bacterial intervention, urea hydrolyzes to ammonia, which is rapidly absorbed from the rumen and highly fatal. It takes about six weeks to build a rumen flora that can safely handle sizeable amounts of urea. However, if urea feeding is interrupted for as little as forty-eight hours this urea-adapted population dies off. If urea feeding is then resumed at the previous level, toxicity may result. Most cases of urea poisoning occur following interruption of urea feeding, following inadequate mixing of urea in the grain or silage, following accidental addition of too much, or when cattle accidentally get access to a bag of urea.

Symptoms

Regardless of the cause, acute urea poisoning is a dramatic disease. Onset usually occurs within half an hour of consumption and the first sign is hyperesthesia with the animal appearing unusually alert and responsive to external stimuli. They move quickly in the pen or pasture finally breaking into a full run, bawling as they go. This progresses to more aggressive mindless behavior, and they run into walls or fences and occasionally charge other animals or people in the pasture. This progresses to staggering and they crawl before finally collapsing. Hypersalivation, bloat, panting, and fever are constant findings. The symptoms closely parallel those of acute grass tetany. The entire episode from onset of signs to death usually takes less than an hour.

Treatment

Treatment of animals that have consumed a fatal dose is, in my experience, of little value. Theoretically neutralization of the ammonia with weak acids such as vinegar given orally or pumped directly into the rumen should help. But it takes a couple of gallons to do any good, and it's rare occasion when that much vinegar is available in time.

Most commercial dairy rations contain some urea and it is a perfectly safe protein substitute when properly used. The important thing is to be sure that cattle are conditioned to it and that it is thoroughly mixed. It's also important that cattle being fed urea get sufficient high energy feed to maintain a rumen flora adequate to handle it.

Wounds

These come in a variety of shapes, sizes and locations and about the same variations in severity. Management of them is determined by all these factors. If there is hemorrhage the most urgent thing is to stop the bleeding, either with a tourniquet or pressure applied to the wound. Once the bleeding is arrested, then a decision can be made whether sutures are required or whether it should merely be treated with antiseptics and left to heal as an open wound. As a general rule, lacerations extending through the skin will heal faster if they are sutured. However, a ragged, heavily contaminated gash may be better if left to heal in from the bottom.

Dairy Cattle

A fairly common accident in dairy cattle is a puncture wound through the mammary vein, usually acquired going through a barbed wire fence. These bleed profusely and, in fact, the hemorrhage can be fatal. The area does not lend itself well to application of a pressure pack or tourniquet. A trick that often works as an emergency measure is to apply a spring-type clothespin directly on the puncture wound. This shuts off the hole through which bleeding occurs and will suffice until the veterinarian arrives to suture it.

Horses

The horse is perhaps more susceptible to lacerations than other species because of a comparatively thin skin and less protective hair covering. By nature horses are also more prone to accidents because of their normally quick movements and excitability. Cuts on the lower legs, where there is only a little connective tissue between skin and bone, and over the joints, where there is constant movement, frequently develop a complication known as **granulation tissue** or **proud flesh.** Granulation is a normal part of the healing process for open wounds and granulation tissue is basically unorganized, highly vascular connective tissue. In the horse it tends to grow exuberantly, filling the entire wound cavity and bulbing cauliflower-like beyond the margins of the skin. At that point it actually impedes healing, since the skin won't cover it and it bleeds and becomes infected easily. Proud flesh can be retarded by keeping a pressure bandage over wounds on the lower leg. If it does overgrow, it must be cut back surgically or with chemicals until the skin heals.

Management of wounds is largely a matter of good judgment and nursing care. Sheep and horses with lacerations should routinely be given a prophylactic dose of tetanus antitoxin, and during the fly season wounds in all species should be covered with bandage, ointment, or repellents to protect against myiasis. This is particularly important in screwworm areas.

Foreign Animal Diseases

THE CASUAL READER SEEING THE HEADING ON THIS CHAPTER may wonder why a discussion of foreign animal diseases is included. If we don't have a disease here why worry about it? It's precisely because we don't have some of these catastrophic foreign animal diseases that we should worry about them. Our livestock have no prior experience with these diseases and therefore no immunity, making them highly susceptible. A rapidly spreading disease such as foot-and-mouth could decimate our cattle, sheep, and swine industries in a matter of weeks, causing an economic disaster the magnitude of which cannot be appreciated until it happens. The word "until" in the preceding sentence was used intentionally. It is not a question of **if** one of these major diseases enters this country; it's only a question of **when.**

The foot-and-mouth virus can readily be transported via animals, meat and dairy products, frozen semen, and even on clothing of people who have recently visited infected farms. The magnitude of traffic in people and goods from foreign countries makes it inevitable that disease will be imported someday.

Although a major outbreak of a foreign animal disease is sure to be costly, the speed with which it can be contained will determine how costly. Early diagnosis is most essential, and the first person to see a cow with foot-and-mouth disease or a pig with African swine fever in all probability will be the owner. If that owner or herd manager recognizes that the animal may have a foreign animal disease and calls the veterinarian immediately, the disease may be contained before it can spread very far.

That's the reason for the brief description of the major foreign animal diseases that follows. If you learn the clinical signs, you may some day be instrumental in preventing a catastrophic disease outbreak.

FOOT-AND-MOUTH DISEASE (FMD)

This viral disease is prevalent in most parts of the world except North and Central America, Australia, and New Zealand. It is widespread in Europe, Africa, the Middle East, and South America. It is one of the most contagious of all animal diseases and affects all cloven-hooved animals such as cattle, sheep, goats, swine, and deer.

Symptoms

Symptoms include fever, vesicles (blisters) in the mouth, on the tongue, at the bulb of the heel, and between the toes and on the teats. Copious salivation accompanies the mouth lesions. The vesicles rupture and slough leaving raw, denuded areas. Lameness is common with the foot lesions; affected animals are reluctant to move and they stand with the feet tucked up under them to relieve pain. Lacrimation and nasal discharge are common. Affected animals refuse feed during the acute phase and lose weight rapidly. Milk production may stop entirely. The disease is usually not fatal but lasts about a month in the individual animal. It takes several months longer for weight to be regained and milk production to resume. The economic loss is severe.

In some countries where the decision has been made to live with the disease rather than attempt eradication, annual vaccination is the only control program. It is a major continuing expense and occasional outbreaks still occur. In the United States, for example, with about 200 million susceptible animals, the cost of a vaccination program would approach a billion dollars annually. Furthermore, there are seven distinct serotypes of FMD virus and sixty-two subtypes. No single vaccine will protect against all these different strains of virus.

Prevention

The most important thing is to keep out foot-and-mouth disease. The second most important is to identify it immediately when it does get here.

SWINE VESICULAR DISEASE (SVD)

The lesions of this virus disease of swine closely resemble those of foot-and-mouth disease, vesicular exanthema, and vesicular stomatitis. In swine these four vesicular diseases are indistinguishable except by serological means. It has been reported in Europe and the Far East. The virus is an enterovirus of the picornavirus group and is closely related to human Coxsackie B-5 virus. In fact, there is some speculation that it is Coxsackie virus that has become adapted to pigs. Infection with it has occurred among laboratory workers, so it must be considered a public health hazard.

Symptoms

SVD starts with high fever quickly followed by numerous vesicles on the snout, in the mouth and on the feet. Affected pigs refuse feed and are very lame. The vesicles rupture in a day or two, leaving raw denuded areas that, in the mouth, heal rather quickly. Although the lesions are similar, the disease is not generally as severe as FMD; fewer pigs are affected and recovery is more rapid. Encephalitis is an occasional complication, with shivering and an unsteady gait. Experimentally the virus has been shown to be lethal for baby pigs, but the principal economic effect is due to weight loss and a protracted recovery period. Additional loss occurs due to the embargo placed on pork products from countries where the disease exists by those that are free of the disease.

SVD virus, like FMD, is very hardy and has been shown, for example, to survive in salami for over 200 days. Feeding contaminated garbage to swine is the route by which most outbreaks have occurred.

VESICULAR EXANTHEMA (VE)

This swine disease, identical in appearance to FMD and SVD, is no longer important. It was first reported in California and during the 1950s became widespread in the United States. Restrictions on the movement of swine and the feeding of garbage coupled with slaughter of infected herds resulted in eradication of the disease and it has not been reported elsewhere in the world.

However, a virus isolated recently from sea lions off the coast of California and designated "San Miguel sea lion virus" has been shown to be physically and chemically identical to VE virus. Moreover, when injected into swine it produces disease very similar to VE. Serologically there is some difference but, at the moment, there is debate about whether the sea lion virus is a new virus or a different antigenic strain of VE. The major concern is that it will come ashore one way or another and start a new wave of infection in swine.

AFRICAN SWINE FEVER (ASF)

As the name implies, this swine disease was first found in Africa and is endemic there. In Africa, wart hogs appear to be the natural reservoir of the virus and most outbreaks in African domestic swine have occurred when wart hogs were seen in the vicinity. Aside from Africa, the disease is now endemic in Spain and Portugal. Outbreaks have occurred in France, Italy, Haiti, and Cuba but the disease has apparently been eradicated from those countries. In the latter two countries the disease was eradicated by slaughtering the swine population.

Symptoms

The African strain of SF virus is particularly lethal for domestic swine. Persistent high fever ranging up to 105°F is the earliest clinical sign noted but characteristically pigs continue to eat and act normally during the early febrile period. After about four days more definite signs develop including lack of appetite, huddling together, reluctance to move, and rear leg weakness. Very rapid pulse, cough, labored breathing, discharge from eyes and nose, and occasionally vomiting and diarrhea follow the high fever. Reddish blotches on the ears and legs are common. Death due to the African strain usually occurs about seven days from the onset of fever. Serial passage of virus through domestic swine such as occurred in Spain and Portugal renders it less virulent, and in those countries more swine survive.

African swine fever closely resembles hog cholera, a serious swine disease present in the United States until the mid-1970s. While vaccination played an important role in hog cholera control and eradication, as yet there is no vaccine for ASF. Preventing its introduction therefore is of utmost importance.

AFRICAN HORSE SICKNESS

This equine disease is transmitted by biting flies and mosquitoes. It is endemic in most of Africa and since the late 1950s outbreaks have occurred in Turkey and the nearby island of Cyprus. Several outbreaks have been reported in Spain, the latest in 1989. Clinically the disease can be confused with equine piroplasmosis, equine infectious anemia, and viral arteritis. However, the mortality is much higher ranging up to 90 percent.

Symptoms

High fever lasting four to five days and obvious discomfort are consistent findings. Edema of the eyelids, conjunctiva, and along the jugular veins extending to the brisket are the most obvious external signs. In the later stages there may be copious frothy exudate from the nostrils. Oddly, most horses continue to eat until they die, leading to speculation that there may be some central nervous system involvement as well.

At least seven types of African horse sickness virus have been identified and a polyvalent vaccine that apparently protects against all types has been used effectively to control outbreaks. Should the disease appear in the United States, whether via imported horses or via accidentally imported vectors, it is virtually certain that many thousands of horses would die before adequate numbers could be vaccinated.

CONTAGIOUS BOVINE PLEUROPNEUMONIA

This disease, caused by *Mycoplasma mycoides* var. *mycoides,* at one time was one of the major cattle epizootics in the world. It has been eradicated from Europe, North American, South Africa, and Australia but still persists in other areas of southern Africa and parts of Asia, China, and Mongolia. A related organism, *Mycoplasma mycoides* var. *capri,* has been isolated from goats in the United States but does not cause disease in cattle.

The disease has an incubation period lasting up to three months or more. It is spread primarily through inhalation of aerosol droplets exhaled or coughed by infected cattle. High concentrations of cattle therefore encourage spread of the disease.

Symptoms

The principal clinical sign is pneumonia which may be very severe prior to death. Fever, lack of appetite, depression, and evidence of acute chest pain are characteristic. Respiration is shallow and rapid with frequent coughing. Mortality is about 50 percent and many of those that recover become chronic carriers. Carrier animals are the source of greatest risk for new infections.

In terms of what we are familiar with, contagious bovine pleuropneumonia perhaps resembles severe shipping fever pneumonia more closely than anything else. Areas of necrosis occur in the lungs and adhesions occur between the lungs and chest wall. Large amounts of fluid accumulate in the chest cavity further increasing respiratory difficulty. In calves the organism invades the joints to cause arthritis more often than pneumonia. Serological testing to detect carrier animals and vaccination have been useful in controlling spread of the disease.

SHEEP POX

At present this pox disease is limited to southeastern Europe, North Africa, and Asia. It is the most severe of the pox diseases of domestic animals. Pox eruptions occur on the cheeks, nostrils, lips, and wool-free skin. Unlike most pox diseases, systemic reactions occur frequently with lesions occurring in the trachea, lungs, and digestive tract. The pox vesicles frequently become hemorrhagic with development of pustules.

Goat pox virus is closely related to sheep pox but the lesions in the goat are less extensive. Mortality from sheep pox may be as high as 50 percent. Sheep or goat pox can easily be confused with sore mouth.

In areas where these diseases occur, vaccines are used to control the outbreaks.

RINDERPEST

This viral disease of cattle is one of the oldest recognized cattle diseases. Since the fourth century it has occurred in many parts of the world. Its distribution at present is limited to parts of Africa, India, and southeast Asia. Although cattle are the only species to be seriously affected, the virus is capable of infecting sheep, goats, and swine, some of which may become unaffected carriers.

Symptoms

The clinical signs in cattle vary with the pathogenicity of the particular virus strain and with the natural resistance of the animal. Infection occurs via the respiratory or digestive tracts resulting in fever, depression, lack of appetite, and decreased milk production. The mucus membrane of the mouth, eye, and vulva become reddened and congested and the muzzle is dry. This is followed by lacrimation and a clear nasal discharge which becomes mucopurulent.

After four or five days of fever, small necrotic areas form on the lips, gums, tongue, and on the inside of the cheek. These coalesce to form larger areas of ulceration. Excessive salivation coincides with the appearance of mouth lesions. Weight loss is quite rapid, with dehydration due to diarrhea prior to coma and death. In highly susceptible herds, mortality may be as high as 90 percent. On the basis of clinical signs alone, rinderpest is virtually indistinguishable from virus diarrhea and malignant catarrhal fever, making laboratory confirmation essential.

Bovine Spongiform Encephalopathy (BSE)

This apparently new disease of cattle was first reported in Great Britain in 1986. It has not yet been reported in the United States. The disease closely resembles scrapie in sheep and goats in that it is primarily neurological, has a long incubation period, and is slowly progressive terminating in death.

Clinical signs which appear over a period of several weeks or months include apprehension, reduced milk yield, loss of weight, hyperesthesia, aggression, frenzy, incoordination, ataxia, and paresis. The intense itching characteristic of scrapie is not seen with BSE. The clinical signs could be confused with rabies, urea poisoning, or hypomagnesemia but these are of much shorter duration.

The assumption in Great Britain is that the source of the virus was scrapie-contaminated processed protein and bone meal in cattle feed. Feeding ruminant origin animal protein in ruminant rations is now prohibited.

Summary

We must constantly be on guard against introduction of any of these diseases because our livestock, having no immunity through prior exposure or vaccination, are completely susceptible. Inspectors of the Animal and Plant Health Inspection Service (APHIS) do an excellent job at our ports of entry, but the task they face in our mobile society is awesome. For example, during 1975, 77 million pieces of baggage were inspected at customs stations. From that baggage over 200 tons of animal products possibly contaminated with animal disease virus were confiscated.

Scientists working under tight security precautions at the Plum Island Animal Disease Center, USDA/APHIS, are constantly seeking additional knowledge about foreign animal diseases and working on development of vaccines to prevent them. Much of what they have learned is being applied in those areas of the world where these diseases are rampant.

But they can't do it all. The ultimate responsibility lies with you and me and everyone else who either works with livestock or is tempted to bring back from abroad animals or animal products that could harbor disease agents.

APPENDIX

Recommended References

For those seeking more information there are many excellent references in the field of veterinary medicine. Following is a partial list of the texts available.

Current Therapy in Equine Medicine. N.E. Robinson, W.B. Saunders Co., Philadelphia, PA. 1983.

Diseases of Feedlot Cattle. Jensen and Mackey. Lea and Febiger Co., Philadelphia, PA. Second edition, 1971.

Diseases of Sheep. Rue Jensen. Lea and Febiger Co., Philadelphia, PA. First edition, 1974.

Diseases of Swine. Dunne and Leman. The Iowa State University Press, Ames, IA. Fourth edition, 1975.

Equine Medicine & Surgery. R.A. Mansman and E.S. McAllister. American Veterinary Publications, Santa Barbara, CA. Third edition, 1982.

Feeding and Care of the Horse. L.D. Lewis, Lea & Febiger, Philadelphia, PA. 1982.

Management and Diseases of the Dairy Goat. S.B. Guss. Dairy Goat Journal, Scottsdale, AZ.

Merck Veterinary Manual. Merck and Company, Rahway, NJ. Seventh edition, 1991.

Parasitology for Veterinarians. J.R. Georgi. W.B. Saunders Co., Philadelphia, PA. Fourth edition, 1985.

Veterinary Medicine. Blood. Radostits and Henderson. W.B. Saunders Co., Philadelphia, PA. Sixth edition, 1983.

Veterinary Obstetrics and Genital Diseases. S.J. Roberts. Edward Brothers, Inc., Ann Arbor, MI. Third edition, 1984.

Veterinary Pharmaceuticals and Biologicals 1982/83. Veterinary Medicine Publishing Co., Edwardsville, KS.

Veterinary Toxicology. R.D. Radeleff. Lea and Febiger, Philadelphia, PA. Second edition, 1970.

Viral Diseases of Cattle. Robert F. Kahrs, Iowa State University Press, Ames, IA. 1981.

Glossary

Abomasum. The fourth or true digestive stomach of a ruminant.

Acidosis. A disturbance in the acid-base balance of the body in which there is an accumulation of acids.

Adjuvants. Chemicals added to a prescription to enhance therapeutic action.

Ad libitum. At pleasure, or as much as is wanted.

Aerosol dispersion. Spraying through the air.

Agalactia. Absence of milk secretion after delivering young.

Aneurysm. Localized abnormal enlargement of a blood vessel.

Anoxia. Deficiency of oxygen.

Anthelmintics. An agent useful in treating parasitic intestinal worms.

Arthritis. Inflammation of a joint.

Ataxia. A disorder of irregularity; affected by muscular incoordination.

Atony. Lack of normal tone.

Attenuation. Lessening of pathogenicity of an organism.

Bacterins. Suspensions of killed bacteria used to immunize against a specific disease.

Ballotting (or **ballottement**). A technique of feeling for a floating object in the body, such as an organ or fetus.

Biuret. A crystalline substance formed from urea.

Brucellae. Organisms in animals causing a disease called "Brucellosis." Plural of Brucella.

Carcinogenicity. The property of being able to induce cancer.

Carotene. A yellow crystalline pigment present in various plant and animal tissues. It is stored in the liver where it is converted to vitamin A.

Cerebellar hypoplasia. Incomplete development of the cerebellum.

Circling disease. Common name for listeriosis.

Collagen. A fibrous protein found in the connective tissue.

Comatose. In condition of a coma; a deep, abnormal sleep.

Conjunctivitis. Inflammation of eyelid lining.

Coronary Band. Junction of skin and hoof wall.

Corticosteroid. Adrenal gland hormone. Natural or synthetic.

Cyanosis. Slightly bluish or grayish discoloration of skin because of reduced hemoglobin in blood.

Cyclopean. Malformed, having one eye.

Demyelination. Process of removing sheath (called myelin) of nerve tissue.

Dystocia. Difficult labor.

Edematous. Swollen.

Electrolyte. A chemical salt that ionizes in solution. Ions increase the electrical conductivity of solutions, hence the name.

Encephalomyelitis. Acute inflammation of the brain.

Endometrium. The mucous membrane lining the inner surface of the uterus.

Enteric. Pertaining to the intestinal tract.

Enterotoxemia. Disease caused by toxins in the intestinal tract.

Epididymis. Small oblong body resting upon and beside the posterior surface of the testes. A part of the vas deferens or spermatic duct.

Epileptiform. Having the form of epilepsy.

Epithelium. Layer of cells forming the outer layer of skin and the surface layer of mucous membranes.

Eructation. Belching.

Estrum. The phase of the heat cycle during which the female is receptive to the male.

Etiology. Cause of disease.

Exudate. Accumulation of fluid containing tissue cells, bacteria, and other debris of infection.

FA test. Fluorescent antibody test.

Febrile. Feverish.

Fistulous tracts. A group of abnormal tubelike passages from one part of the body to another, usually resulting from infection.

Founder. Lameness caused by separation of the sensitive laminae from the wall of the hoof.

Gilt. A young pig that has yet to produce a litter.

Goitrogenic. Tending to cause goiters.

Granulomatous mastitis. Inflammation of the udder due to granular tumors.

Hemoglobinuria. The presence of hemoglobin in the urine.

Hemolytic. Pertaining to breaking down of red blood cells.

Hernia. Bulging of an organ through the wall of the cavity which normally holds it.

Herpes. A class of virus.

Host-specific. An organism that matures in only one species of host.

Humoral. Pertaining to circulating body fluids such as blood.

Hypocalcemia. Abnormally low blood calcium.

Ingesta. Food and drink received into the body through the mouth.

Inguinal. Pertaining to the region of the groin.

Insufflation. Blowing air into udder to increase intramammary pressure and suppress milk flow. An old treatment for milk fever.

Intradermal. Within the substance of the skin.

Intranasal instillation. Dropping or spraying a liquid into nasal cavity.

I.V. Intravenous.

Ketones. Substances of an acid nature in the body that are the end products of fat metabolism.

Ketosis. Incomplete metabolism of fatty acids, usually from carbohydrate deficiency or inadequate utilization. Commonly seen in starvation, high fat diet, following anesthesia, and in diabetes. A metabolic disease of cattle and sheep.

Lacrimation. Secretion and discharge of tears.

Lactate. To form or secrete milk.

Laminitis. Inflammation of the sensitive lamina of the hoof. Commonly called *founder*.

Leukopenia. Abnormal decrease of white blood cells.

Lymphosarcoma. A malignant disease of lymphatic tissue.

Mastectomized. Having had the udder removed.

Metritis. Inflammation of the uterus.

Mucopurulent. Consisting of mucus and pus.

Multiparous. Having borne more than one offspring.

Mycotoxins. Substances produced by mold growing in animal feed, causing illness or death.

Myiasis. Condition arising from infestation with larvae of flies or maggots.

Myositis. Inflammation of muscle tissue.

Necropsy. Examination of dead body to determine cause of death.

Necrotic hematoma. A swelling or mass of blood signifying death of a portion of tissue.

Neurotoxin. A toxin or poison that attacks the nervous system.

"Obligate" parasite. Parasite completely dependent on its host.

Oocyst. A reproductive cell inside a cyst.

Opisthotonos. An arched-back position of the head, caused by spasm induced by such things as strychnine poisoning or by brain disease.

Osmotic. Having to do with the passage of solvents, such as water, through semipermeable membranes.

Palpable crepitation. Crackling feeling due to gas accumulation in the subcutaneous tissue.

Parasite. Organism that lives within or upon another one, which is known as the host.

Parenteral. Pertains to route of administration of drugs. Intravenous, subcutaneous and intradermal are parenteral routes.

Paresis. Partial paralysis.

Parturition. Act of giving birth.

Pathogens. Organisms capable of producing disease.

Peracute. Very acute or violent.

Perineal. Relating to the perineum, the area at the outlet of the pelvic region.

Peripheral. Pertaining to the outer part or surface of the body.

Peristalsis. Involuntary wavelike movement in the alimentary canal.

Peritonitis. Inflammation of the lining of the abdominal cavity.

Petechial. Small, hemorrhagic spots.

Placenta. The structure in the uterus through which the fetus derives its nourishment. It is an organ of the fetus and is expelled from the uterus at or soon after birth.

Ppm. Parts per million.

Propionate. A salt or ester or propionic acid.

Protozoan. A one-celled organism. The lowest division of the animal kingdom.

Pyometra. Pus accumulation in the uterine cavity.

Pyruvate. A salt or ester of pyruvic acid that plays an important role in the metabolism of carbohydrates, fats, and amino acids.

Rarefaction. Making bone more porous because of loss of mineral substances, or osteolysis.

Rumen. Large first stomach compartment of a cud-chewing animal.

Rumen atony. Lack of normal tone of the rumen.

Rumenitis. Inflammation of the rumen.

Ruminants. Cud-chewing animals, including cattle, sheep, and goats.

Salmonella. A genus of bacteria causing intestinal disorders, sometimes fatal.

Saprophytes. Organisms living on decaying or dead organic matter. Nonpathogenic.

Schizonts. A stage appearing in the life cycle of coccidia.

Scours. Severe diarrhea in farm animals.

Septicemic. Relating to infection, when an animal's bloodstream has been invaded by disease-producing organisms.

Septicemic infections. Those in which disease organisms invade the bloodstream.

Serologic testing. Lab examination of blood or blood serum.

Sloughing. Dead matter separated from living tissue.

Somatic. Pertaining to the body.

Sporulation. Production of spores (one-celled reproductive organisms).

Staphylococci. A genus of bacteria.

Stasis. Stagnation of normal flow of fluids, as of blood, urine, or intestinal products.

Subepithelial. Beneath the epithelium (layer of cells forming the outer layer of the skin).

Symmetrical. Equally distributed throughout.

Systemic. Pertaining to a whole body.

Systemically. Pertaining to the whole body.

Taxonomists. Specialists in the study of scientific classification.

Teratogenic. Contributing to the development of an abnormal embryo or fetus.

Titer. Standard of strength per volume.

Turbinates. That portion of the upper respiratory tract between the nostrils and the pharynx through which air passes.

Uniparous. Producing or having produced a single offspring.

Urolithiasis. Formation of urinary stones and the illness associated with that condition.

Vasodilation. Dilation of blood vessels.

Vector. An insect acting as a carrier of disease from an infected animal to an uninfected one.

Vegetative. Growing or having the ability to grow.

Viscosity. State of being sticky or gummy.

W.B.C. White blood cells, or, commonly, white blood cell count.

Index

Page references in *italics* indicate illustrations; page references in **bold** indicate tables.

335